THE EXPERTS SPEAK 1996

The Role of Nutrition In Medicine

THE EXPERTS SPEAK 1996

The Role of Nutrition
In Medicine

Edited By

Kristine Simpson
Jan Ekdahl
Karen Rae Hamilton
Janine Bellissimo
Courtney Sauer

Kirk Hamilton PA-C

I.T.Services
Health Associates Medical Group
Sacramento, California USA

This book is for educational purposes only and is directed towards health professionals and those with focused interests in the fields of nutrition and preventive medicine. It is **not** a recommendation for the specific therapies and concepts reviewed. The information enclosed is **not** a treatment or recommendation for the lay public. Those with medical problems should consult with their personal physician for their specific health problem.

Great effort has been made to relate the facts as the interviewees have shared them. This author takes no responsibility for errors, inaccuracies, omissions or inconsistencies in these interviews. This author encourages retrieval of the original articles for complete details of the specific research or correspondence with the original authors. Authors' and publisher addresses are enclosed for requesting reprints, correspondence or professional networking purposes.

Published by

I.T.Services
3301 Alta Arden #2
Sacramento, CA 95825 USA
(916) 483-1085
(916) 483-1431 (FAX)

ISBN 0-9628840-9-X
Second Printing June, 1996

Printed in the United States of America
On Recycled Paper

TABLE OF CONTENTS

INTERVIEWS - TOPICS AND AUTHORS
EXPERTS SPEAK 1996

ii

iii

We would like to Acknowledge the Generous Contributions of the following Companies...

BIO-TECH PHARMACAL, INC.
P.O. Box 1992
Fayetteville, AR 72707 U.S.A.
(800) 345-1199 / (501) 443-9148 / (501) 443-5643 (FAX)

BIO-TECH Pharmacal manufactures an extensive line of pharmaceutical grade nutritional products - **Rx** and non-**Rx** maintaining standards of excellence in manufacturing and customer service. AZEC, BIO-STATIN, BROMASE, PROS-TECH, QUENCH, THYROID.

METAMETRIX, INC.
MEDICAL RESEARCH LABORATORY
5000 Peachtree Ind. Blvd.
Norcross, GA 30071 U.S.A.
(770) 446-5483 / (770) 441-2237 (FAX)

MetaMetrix specializes in nutritional-metabolic testing including: Vitamins, minerals, toxic metals, antioxidants, amino acids, fatty acids, organic acids, food allergy testing and bone loss markers.

DOCTOR'S DATA, INC.
P.O. Box 111
West Chicago, IL 60186 U.S.A.
(800) 323-2784 / (708) 231-3649 / (708) 231-9190 (FAX)

Doctors Data, Inc. performs elemental testing of blood, hair and urine and amino acids assays from plasma and urine. These tests are used by health professionals to determine nutritional adequacy and heavy metal burden.

SPECTRACELL LABORATORIES, INC.
515 Post Oak Blvd., Suite 830
Houston, TX 77027 U.S.A.
(800) 227-5227 / (713) 621-3101 / (713) 621-3234 (FAX)

SpectraCell Laboratories' EMA™ blood tests measure the intracellular function of vitamins, minerals, antioxidants and other essential nutrients. DNA synthesis measured in peripheral lymphocytes identifies deficiencies limiting mitogenic responses or cell-mediated immune function.

EUROPEAN LABORATORY OF NUTRIENTS/VITAMIN DIAGNOSTICS
Industrial Drive and Route 35
Cliffwood Beach, NJ 07735 U.S.A.
(908) 583-7773 / (908) 583-7774 (FAX)
Netherlands 31 30287 1492 / 31 30280 2688 (FAX)

ELN/Vitamin Diagnostics specializes in testing concerning the status of nutrients in the body such as (trace) elements, vitamins, essential fatty acids, amino acids in the blood, urine, hair and food allergy testing.

NATIONAL BIOTECH LABORATORY
3212 N.E. 125th Street, Suite D
Seattle, WA 98125 U.S.A.
(800) 846-6285 / (206) 363-6606 / (206) 363-2025 (FAX)

A federally licensed diagnostic laboratory for Nutritional Medicine: Allergy Testing (ELISA IgE/IgG4), Salivary Hormones (Adrenal, Female, Male), Cardiovascular Risk (Homocysteine), Liver Detoxification (Phase I/II), Stool Analysis, Amino Acids, Vitamins, Minerals. Accepts Insurance/Medicare.

SUPPLEMENTS PLUS
317 Adelaide Street West, Suite 503
Toronto, Ontario M5V 1P9 Canada
(800) 387-4761 / (416) 977-3088 / (416) 977-3099 (FAX)

Supplements Plus sells quality vitamins, herbs and homeopathic preparations through their stores and delivers worldwide. Supplements Plus is committed to providing information and quality products to practitioners, patients and the public.

NATURAL OVENS OF MANITOWOC
430 Country Road
P.O. Box 730
Manitowoc, WI 54221-0730 U.S.A.
(800) 558-3535 / (414) 758-2594 (FAX)

Natural Ovens makes scientifically designed food fortified with 15 vitamins and minerals and omega-3 fatty acids (flax). These products do not contain preservatives or dairy products. Some products are certified organic.

We would like to Acknowledge the Generous Contributions of the following Companies...

We would like to Acknowledge the Generous Contributions of the following Companies...

We would like to Acknowledge the Generous Contributions of the following Companies...

ACKNOWLEDGEMENTS

I have so many people to thank...

To the authors who took the time to share their work with us. Who have worked so hard on their particular topic of interest to research, test and write about it.

To Karen Rae, Courtney, Karen Young, Roni, Traci, Jennifer, Jan, and Kris for doing your jobs so well that I could continue to create freely.

To Stacia for really understanding my journey like few people do.

To Janine for the hope and that wonderful laughter. You are a great teacher and friend. Also, thanks for the last minute help.

To Dharmaja for your patience, skill and creativity with the cover of the book.

To Jan, for your "11th" hour effort with such a great attitude. It was and is appreciated more than you will ever know. Thank you so very much. That "enjoyed" intensity sets the tone for success at ITServices in 1996.

To the Health Associates Staff for your love and support.

To my patients for your constant teaching which helps steer me through the maze of information to find what is clinically important.

To the companies who contributed financially so this book could be printed.

To Michael Kwiker for your constant love, friendship and support in allowing me the space to create my path and contribute without totally understanding where I was going.

To my daughter, Mya. You are truly my spirit and support. Always there to encourage and understand. You are beyond your years. You don't know how many times I have looked at the phone recorder that says "never give up" and thanked God that he has blessed me with you... I love you.

To Sai Baba for continually bringing the full meaning of service into my life.

"Love All, Serve All"
Sai Baba

FOREWORD

Recent decades have seen remarkable progress in the control of many diseases, resulting in present expected human longevities of 70 to 80 years. It is now becoming increasingly clear that further improvements will require a focus on health maintenance and disease prevention, rather than control of acute, catastrophic events such as a heart attack or widespread cancer. Nutrition is all that we put into our bodies. Intuitively, one would expect nutrition to play a crucial role in health maintenance. A vast amount of data now corroborates this seemingly obvious notion. As illustrated in the collection of interviews by Kirk Hamilton, many experts consider nutritional agents to be important in diverse situations ranging from behavior disorders to heart disease to cancer. Equally diverse is the group of agents which play a role, ranging from simple minerals to antioxidant vitamins to fatty acids and fish oil.

As expected from the complexity of the human diet, this is a difficult area in which to conduct clarifying research that would enlighten us on the role of one individual substance or another. In nature, these compounds are found widely distributed in varying quantities and in different food stuffs. Similarly, easy availability and lack of toxicity of many of these compounds makes it difficult to do the simple and often conclusive clinical trials that are possible when testing a drug against a disease. Such trials are further made impossible because the endpoint -- prevention of disease -- is such that it would require large numbers of participants involved for long periods of time to do the usual type of study. Thus, information on the potential health benefits of one nutrient or another often derives from a perusal of varying lines of evidence, from epidemiologic surveys to laboratory studies to investigations in animal models or particularly high-risk human groups, rather than a single clinical study. It is in this context that Mr. Hamilton's collection of interviews constitute a fascinating, well-written and readable group of articles that provide useful information to readers from all backgrounds, ranging from the lay person to the health professional. Mr. Hamilton has taken care to ensure that each of the interviewees has the necessary credentials and background to provide an educated opinion based on the scientific evidence available in a particular area. I would hope that readers would use these interviews as a stepping stone from which to embark on a more comprehensive study of the areas of interest to them.

The 20th Century leaves us with little doubt that nutritional agents are of tremendous significance in health maintenance. Research goals for the remaining years and into the next century will target individual nutritional agents and access their interactions with one another as well as the significance of each one's contribution. Anyone interested in this subject, or the subject of health maintenance in general, will benefit from these series of articles. The breadth and range of topics is, indeed, remarkable. There is something for everyone in this collection.

Harinder S. Garewal, M.D., Ph.D.
Arizona Cancer Center, College of Medicine
Assistant Director of the Cancer Prevention and Control Program
Tucson, Arizona, U.S.A.

FOREWORD

Nutrition, including minerals and herbs, is the essence of medical science. Many of the earliest medical breakthroughs have been related to a rediscovery of ancient cures. William Withering reported on an account of foxglove more than 200 years ago, taking a page from traditional therapy's use of digoxin. This type of connection continues today. Many disorders in medicine are related to abnormalities in nutrition. It is a recognition of these types of problems that will allow medicine to advance and science to become more helpful to the common man.

Because the amount of written information about nutrition and its role in medicine is overwhelming, many individuals may believe yet another book about it is unnecessary. There are, however, many exceptional reasons to consider this work. Of the many books on nutrition with special references to physiology and medicine, few have been authored by as many leading experts in the field as this one. Kirk Hamilton has done an exceptional job in finding individuals who not only know their field, but also are practicing and researching their subject. Each of the interviews were conducted around the time of an important publication, most of which are on the cutting edge of their respective fields.

This compilation is also important because the issues addressed in each interview are important. The information is not focused strictly on a research level, but is presented in a very readable fashion. This work can be read by and instructed to medical doctors, lay people and all other disciplines. This is, therefore, a valuable collection of information for a variety of individuals seeking information on nutrition and medicine. This work is particularly helpful and valuable, and adds to the available armamentarium of information about nutrition and medicine.

Michael Brodsky, M.D.
University of California, Irvine, Medical Center
Director of the Cardiac Arrhythmia Service
Division of Cardiology
Orange, California, U.S.A.

INTRODUCTION

This book excites me! It excites me because of the cutting-edge information it contains and the wonderful authors who have contributed to it from around the world. It further excites me because this collection of 110 interviews begins to bring to fruition a picture of a new kind of medical approach that is low risk, clinically effective and is more cost efficient than our present disease care/drug treatment model. On more than one occasion, I have had my heart race with excitement as I reviewed an interview that I know provides information that will help busy clinicians deliver -- and patients receive -- better health care.

Another reason this book excites me is that it took on a life of its own. It "wanted" to come into existence. Initially, I was looking for one to two interviews a month as a new feature for our health letter, *Clinical Pearls News*. I received too many responses to the interview requests. The information was so significant and the authors were so excited about sharing their work, that a compilation of their efforts was the only possible option. Thus, the *Experts Speak 1996* was born. My only regret is that I did not have the resources to have 200 to 300 interviews. The information and "Experts" are there...Next year!

Nutritional supplementation and diet can work along side traditional therapy or it can work by itself. What makes nutritional biochemistry/pharmacology so unique as a specialty is that it is the only specialty, aside from psycho-somatic and "energy" medicines, that intimately permeates *every* discipline. There is no specialty where nutrition (biochemistry) does not play a *significant* role. Just look at the wide variety of specialties and topics represented in this year's *The Experts Speak* -- from cancer and cardiology to oncology and psychiatry. Nutrients are nothing more than molecular substances that, when used at the right time and in the right metabolic pathway, create optimal functioning for an individual. Drugs manipulate these same pathways and are usually made after observing how these molecular substances work. Why not use the exact substance, which is usually less expensive and has a lower risk of adverse effects?

Many people are beginning to accept the fact that nutrition is a powerful force in preventing disease and in reducing our reliance on crisis-care medicine. If we do not alter our present reliance on disease-care, we will continue on our spiralling course towards financial insolvency.

Nothing would do more for the health of this country than adherence to the government's recommendation of 5 daily servings of fruits and vegetables by 80% to 90% of the population, as opposed to the reality -- 9% to 20%. That important point aside, I will go one statement and philosophy further about nutrition's role in medicine. Nutrition, the use of molecular substances innate to the human body, will provide some of the most powerful treatments for acute disease. The use of nutrition will rival drug medicine within the next decade, provided economic and political "turf wars" do not completely control its destiny. Read through the interviews about nutrition's role in acute problems such as heart attacks, liver failure, cardiac surgery and pancreatitis, among others. It is quite impressive. I believe the data shows the results are real.

Looking through a thousand medical journals a month, summarizing 150 to 200 articles pertaining to nutrition in medicine, and talking to hundreds of researchers, gives me the awareness that the information is there to create a much better health care delivery system. It is all about better delivery of this information, the tempering of egos, and where the money goes.

Personally, I would like to get rid of the terms "conventional medicine" and "alternative medicine." Therapies that work and have scientific backing are "real medicine" whether they are labeled traditional or alternative. Labeling does nothing more than build walls and reduce communication. It is my sincere hope that the way this collection of interviews is packaged will help network people from different specialties and from different health-care philosophies. I further hope it will encourage improved communication and open-mindedness. I say this as emphatically for those in the alternative community, where I have practiced for the last 12 years, as I do for those in the conventional medicine community.

For those of you who were trained in conventional medicine, I ask you to put aside your beliefs of nutrition as some ancillary diet therapy or something that is promoted by fringe individuals. Look at it from a biochemical perspective. Drugs manipulate biochemical pathways. They were made by mimicking the structure of molecular substances. It is not a far reach to expect some type of positive response by using the same substances that the drugs you use were modeled after. Also, look at where the information in this book comes from -- your own peer-reviewed medical journals and some of the most esteemed academic medical centers in the world.

For those in the alternative medicine arena, be ready to be scrutinized. You want nutrition and yourselves to be looked at as credible. You want to say there is scientific data to support what you do. The data is accumulating and showing that nutrition is very powerful. But with that new data and evidence, some of your old paradigms and reasonings why things worked will change. We are going to find that many treatments worked, but for different reasons than were stated. You are also going to find that some things do not work. And you are going to find out that some of these nutrients are very powerful and treat acute disease which may be beyond the expertise of some "alternative" practitioners. Even though I strongly believe the use of molecular substances (nutrition) is considerably safer and less expensive than drug medicine, more side effects of nutrients will be discovered as their use becomes prevalent. You only have to follow the emerging story of vitamin A dosage and birth defects to understand some of the possibilities of the things to come.

I urge all of us to have less ego and to think more of the common good that we all have talents to contribute to. It is an exciting time and I am very thankful for those who have contributed to this book and to those who have the interest to read it. I am sure you will find something that will be helpful to you in delivering good health care, or will help you participate in your own health-care journey.

Kirk Hamilton PA-C
I.T.Services
Health Associates Medical Group
Sacramento, California, U.S.A.

HOW TO USE THIS RESOURCE

This resource can be helpful to the health professional, policy maker and progressive lay person.

The topics are arranged in alphabetical order with the appropriate disease listed first in the heading. The author, along with their address, fax, phone numbers and full reference are included at the top of each interview. From this information, it should be easy to obtain a reprint of the author's work and dialogue via correspondence, fax or phone. The goal is to make it as easy as possible to exchange information and ideas so we can progress forward in evolving a better health care system.

Generally, the table of contents will be the quickest way to find a general topic of interest. For a more in-depth view of the subject matter, please turn to page 209 which offers a very extensive cross-referenced subject index.

For the health professional I hope this is a networking tool so you can exchange ideas of similar interest with these researchers. It may also open up new ideas regarding treatment approaches for you. These interviews can be used to communicate better with your colleagues who may be just becoming open to the role of nutrition in medicine. Some of these interviews will be applicable for patient education.

For health educators and policy makers, there is enough information enclosed to really help the development of a better health care model that is more sustainable. This book can be a statement of introduction for public officials that nutrition, implemented to its fullest, does not only have a solid scientific base, but can be applied immediately to dramatically change the health, and costs of health, in this country.

For the lay person who picks up this book, don't be put off initially by the medical sounding terminology. A majority of these interviews have very practical information in them that can be applied directly to your health. Also, this is an excellent tool to share with your health care provider if you would like to have nutrition and lifestyle play a bigger part in your health care management.

Feel free to use the format of the postcard on the next page to design your own postcard for article reprint requests. Simply fill out the postcard with the information provided in each interview (address and reference), and you will receive a free article reprint within 1-4 weeks. Take advantage of this simple, cost-effective way of obtaining important health information.

SAMPLE POSTCARD - REPRINT REQUEST

_____

_____   **STAMP**

_____

Author's Address: _____

                        _____

                        _____

                        _____

"Reprint Request"

REPRINT REQUEST INFORMATION
(Please fill out completely)

Please send a reprint of your article - Title	
Author:	
Journal:	
Vol/No.: Page(s):	Date:

Dear Sender: Please place self-addressed label here. Press firmly.	Dear Author: Please use return label and press firmly on envelope.
	THANK YOU

The Experts Speak 1996
Order Form

I.T.Services
3301 Alta Arden #2
Sacramento, CA 95825 U.S.A.

(916) 483-1085
(916) 483-1431 (FAX)

_____ Copies of *Experts Speak 1996* (**U.S.A.**) @ $35.00 $ _____

_____ Copies of *Experts Speak 1996* (**California Resident**) @ $37.71 $ _____

_____ Copies of *Experts Speak 1996* (**Canada & Mexico**) @ $40.00 $ _____

_____ Copies of *Experts Speak 1996* (**Foreign**) @ $45.00 $ _____

Subtotal Enclosed $ _____

Volume Discount If Applicable
(multiply total by appropriate discount)   X _____

Total Enclosed $ _____

VOLUME DISCOUNTS

5-10	25% Discount (multiply total x .75)
11-20	30% Discount (multiply total x .70)
21-30	35% Discount (multiply total x .65)
31 or more	40% Discount (multiply total x .60)

PAYMENT: BY **VISA** OR **MASTERCARD**; ALL CHECKS IN U.S DOLLARS ONLY

Bankcard #: _____ - _____ - _____ - _____   Ex. Date _____

Phone: _____ FAX: _____

Company: _____

Name: _____

Address: _____

City: _____ Country: _____

I.T.Services Order Form

PRINT

Clinical Pearls 1989
(6000 Citations, Keywords & Phrases Without Summaries)
- $53.82 ☐ **California** Residents (Includes 7¾% Sales Tax)
- $49.95 ☐ U.S.A.
- $59.95 ☐ Canada, Mexico
- $74.95 ☐ Foreign **Air Mail**

Clinical Pearls 1990
(1000 Summarized Articles)
- $32.27 ☐ **California** Residents (Includes 7¾% Sales Tax)
- $29.95 ☐ U.S.A.
- $34.95 ☐ Canada, Mexico
- $42.95 ☐ Foreign **Air Mail**

Clinical Pearls 1991
(2000 Summarized Articles)
- $64.60 ☐ **California** Residents (Includes 7¾% Sales Tax)
- $59.95 ☐ U.S.A.
- $69.95 ☐ Canada, Mexico
- $85.95 ☐ Foreign **Air Mail**

Clinical Pearls 1992
(2000 Summarized Articles)
- $64.60 ☐ **California** Residents (Includes 7¾% Sales Tax)
- $59.95 ☐ U.S.A.
- $69.95 ☐ Canada, Mexico
- $85.95 ☐ Foreign **Air Mail**

Clinical Pearls 1993
(1800 Summarized Articles)
- $64.60 ☐ **California** Residents (Includes 7¾% Sales Tax)
- $59.95 ☐ U.S.A.
- $69.95 ☐ Canada, Mexico
- $85.95 ☐ Foreign **Air Mail**

Clinical Pearls 1994
(2000 Summarized Articles)
- $64.60 ☐ **California** Residents (Includes 7¾% Sales Tax)
- $59.95 ☐ U.S.A.
- $69.95 ☐ Canada, Mexico
- $85.95 ☐ Foreign **Air Mail**

Clinical Pearls 1995
(1500 Summarized Articles)
- $53.82 ☐ **California** Residents (Includes 7¾% Sales Tax)
- $49.95 ☐ U.S.A.
- $59.95 ☐ Canada, Mexico
- $74.95 ☐ Foreign **Air Mail**

Clinical Pearls News Health Letter
(11 Issues Yearly - 50-65 Summaries & Encapsulations Per Issue)
- $79.00 ☐ U.S.A.
- $84.00 ☐ Canada & Mexico
- $90.00 ☐ Foreign **Air Mail**

Clinical Pearls News Health Letter 1991-92 Bound Volume
(430 Summarized Articles With Commentary)
- $32.33 ☐ **California** Residents (Includes 7¾% Sales Tax)
- $30.00 ☐ U.S.A.
- $35.00 ☐ Canada, Mexico
- $40.00 ☐ Foreign **Air Mail**

Clinical Pearls News Health Letter - 1993 Bound Volume
(400 Summarized Articles With Commentary)
- $32.33 ☐ **California** Residents (Includes 7¾% Sales Tax)
- $30.00 ☐ U.S.A.
- $35.00 ☐ Canada, Mexico
- $40.00 ☐ Foreign **Air Mail**

Clinical Pearls News Health Letter - 1994 Bound Volume
(500 Summarized Articles With Commentary)
- $32.33 ☐ **California** Residents (Includes 7¾% Sales Tax)
- $30.00 ☐ U.S.A.
- $35.00 ☐ Canada, Mexico
- $40.00 ☐ Foreign **Air Mail**

Clinical Pearls News Health Letter - 1995 Bound Volume
(500 Summarized Articles With Commentary)
- $32.33 ☐ **California** Residents (Includes 7¾% Sales Tax)
- $30.00 ☐ U.S.A.
- $35.00 ☐ Canada, Mexico
- $40.00 ☐ Foreign **Air Mail**

_____ = Total Column 1

COMPUTER DISKETTE
CPdsk - 1989-95

Clinical Pearls 1989, 90, 91, 92, 93, 94 & 95 Books On Computer Diskette
(10,500 Summarized Articles Plus 6000 Citations Plus Keywords and Short Phrases In ASCII/DOS Format)
- $646.50 ☐ - **California** Residents (Includes 7¾% Sales Tax) (I.B.M. Compatible)
- $600.00 ☐ - U.S.A. & Foreign (I.B.M. Compatible)
- $610.00 ☐ - Noncompressed DOS/ASCII Diskettes for *Macintosh Users* - Need DOS conversion program.

Clinical Pearls 1989 On Computer Diskette
(6000 Citations, Author's Address, Keywords, Short Phrases)
- $107.75 ☐ - **California** Residents (Includes 7¾ % Sales Tax) (I.B.M. Compatible)
- $100.00 ☐ - U.S.A. & Foreign (I.B.M. Compatible)
- $110.00 ☐ - Noncompressed DOS/ASCII Diskettes for *Macintosh Users* - Need DOS conversion program.

Clinical Pearls 1994 on Computer Diskette
(2000 Summarized Articles In ASCII/DOS Format)
- $134.69 ☐ - **California** Residents (Includes 7¾ % Sales Tax) (I.B.M. Compatible)
- $125.00 ☐ - U.S.A. & Foreign (I.B.M. Compatible)
- $135.00 ☐ - Noncompressed DOS/ASCII Diskettes for *Macintosh Users* - Need DOS conversion program.

Clinical Pearls 1995 On Computer Diskette
(1500 Summarized Articles In ASCII/DOS Format)
- $107.75 ☐ - **California** Residents (Includes 7¾ % Sales Tax) (I.B.M. Compatible)
- $100.00 ☐ - U.S.A. & Foreign (I.B.M. Compatible)
- $110.00 ☐ - Noncompressed DOS/ASCII Diskettes for *Macintosh Users* - Need DOS conversion program.

Clinical Pearls News 1991-95 On Computer Diskette
(200 Summaries With Commentary In ASCII/DOS Format)
- $200.00 ☐ - U.S.A. & Foreign
- $215.50 ☐ - California Residents
- $210.00 ☐ - Noncompressed DOS/ASCII Diskettes for *Macintosh Users* - Need DOS conversion program.

Clinical Pearls News 1995 on Computer Diskette
(500 Summarized Articles With Commentary and Interviews In ASCII/DOS Format)
- $75.43 ☐ - **California** Residents (Includes 7¾ % Sales Tax) (I.B.M. Compatible)
- $70.00 ☐ - U.S.A. & Foreign (I.B.M. Compatible)
- $80.00 ☐ - Noncompressed DOS/ASCII Diskettes for *Macintosh Users* - Need DOS conversion program.

ISYS Indexing Program

ISYS For: Windows_____ DOS_____
(Not Available In Macintosh Format)
- $435.00 ☐ U.S.A.
- $468.71 ☐ **California** Resident (7.75% Sales Tax)
- $455.00 ☐ Outside North America - Includes shipping

_____ + _____ = _____
Total Column 1   Total Column 2   Total 1 & 2

Phone:_____ FAX:_____

Bankcard # _____ Ex. Date_____
(VISA or MASTERCARD only)

Name:_____

Company:_____

Address:_____

_____

Country:_____

(Please Print Clearly)
Send Payment To: *I.T.Services*
3301 Alta Arden #2, Sacramento, CA 95825, U.S.A.
(916)483-1085/FAX(916)483-1431
Check Or Money Order Payable In U.S. Funds Only

The Nutrition Information Family
Clinical Pearls and Clinical Pearls News
~PRINT~

Clinical Pearls - 1989: The "original" **Clinical Pearls** contains over 6000 references with author's addresses, keywords, short phrases, monthly and cumulative indexes. *It does not contain summaries*. Spiral bound printed on a full 8½ x 11 page. **$49.95**

Clinical Pearls - 1990: The top "1,000" articles from 1990 in nutrition and preventive medicine. Summaries are between 100-500 words, complete with references and author addresses. An in-depth, fully cross-referenced, subject index is provided. Summaries are organized under the disease category in alphabetical order. Spiral bound, half page, clinical manual size with more than 450 *information packed* pages. **$29.95**

Clinical Pearls 1991, 1992, 1993, 1994 & 1995: These volumes of **Clinical Pearls** maintain the same user friendly style as 1990 edition, yet are double in content and are printed on a full 8½ x 11 page. **$59.95, ($49.95 *Clinical Pearls 1995* only)**

Clinical Pearls News (CP News): A monthly health letter for the public and professionals, summarizing and encapsulating the "best" 50-65 articles in nutrition and preventive medicine from that month's research. Practical commentary follows approximately 20-30 summaries called a "**Pearl**". Each summary is fully referenced, including the author's address for reprint requests. Each issue has 1-2 interviews with key researchers in the fields of nutrition and preventive medicine. Published 11 times yearly. **$69.00**

Clinical Pearls News 1991-92, 1993, 1994 & 1995/Bound Volumes: The 1991-92 bound volume is a compilation of 14 back issues from September 1991 through December 1992. More than 430 of the most exciting articles from that time period are summarized with an in-depth, cross-referenced subject index and table of contents. The newsletters are bound for easy retrievability and durability. The 1993 issue contains more than 400 summaries of articles while the 1994 & 1995 bound volumes contain 500 articles each with interviews from key researchers in the fields of nutrition and preventive medicine. **$30.00 each**

~COMPUTER DISKETTE~

Clinical Pearls *Dsk* - 1989-95: **CP*dsk*** allows for the access to over 6000 citations with author's addresses, keywords and short phrases in **Clinical Pearls 1989** and over 10,500 summarized articles from **Clinical Pearls 1990, 1991, 1992, 1993, 1994** and **1995** on computer diskette in an ***ASCII/DOS*** format. This is approximately 20 megabytes of information compressed onto 5 - 3 ½ inch diskettes. **$600.00**

Clinical Pearls *Dsk* - 1989: The original **"Clinical Pearls"** has never before been available on diskette. It provides over 6000 references with author's addresses, keywords and short phrases. *It does not contain summaries*. It has approximately 2 megabytes of data. **$100.00**

Clinical Pearls *Dsk* - 1995: This volume allows access to 1500 summarized articles from **Clinical Pearls 1995** on computer diskette in an ***ASCII/DOS*** format. Approximately 2.5 megabytes of information compressed onto 1 - 3 ½ inch diskette. **$100.00**

Clinical Pearls News *Dsk* - 1991-95: 2000 summarized articles with full references and author's addresses are available with clinical commentary, a "**Pearl**", in the majority of summaries. Clinician and researcher interviews, and an important reference section are included. Over 4 megabytes of information are compressed in an ***ASCII/DOS*** format. **$200.00**

SPECIAL NOTE: For users of Clinical Pearls Products On Computer Diskette: This data comes in an ASCII/DOS format. The data does not include a search or indexing program on the diskettes. This information can be retrieved into a basic word processor, in general, word processors have slow and simplistic searching capabilities and can search only a word or an exact group of words. With fast computers (486 DX2s or Pentium processors) this *may* be adequate. We recommend indexing programs or "search engines" to allow for multiple word searches with specific conditions. These programs allow for much greater speed in searching. ISYS is an excellent and simple indexing program which we recommend for **IBM** compatible computers. They have excellent customer support. Some MacIntosh users can use noncompressed ASCII/DOS files but you will need a *DOS conversion program* and the "know how" to retrieve *ASCII/DOS* files.

THE INFORMATION SOURCE - Kirk Hamilton, PA-C is a practicing physician assistant, specializing in nutrition and preventive medicine since 1983. Mr. Hamilton is also founder of I.T.Services, a company focused on information transfer to the public and health professionals. The services provided by I.T.Services come from an ever-accumulating database of more than 24,000 articles on nutrition and preventive medicine from 1,000-1,500 medical journals scanned on a monthly basis. The goal of I.T.Services is to present current, accessible, organized, clinically applicable and credible information to its readership in a timely fashion.

Aging, Immune Function and Zinc

Christina Fortes, MSc
Osservatorio Epidemiologico Regione Lazio
Via di Santa Costanza
53-00198 Roma, Italy
39 6 8610040 / 39 6 8603752 (FAX)

"Aging, Zinc and Cell-Mediated Immune Response",
Aging and Clinical and Experimental Research, 1995;7(2):75-76. #23041

Kirk Hamilton: *Could you please share with me your educational background and current position?*

Christina Fortes: I am a nutritionist with a Masters of Science (MSc) in human nutrition at London School of Hygiene and Tropical Medicine, University of London. At the moment, I am finishing my external part-time Ph.D. in epidemiology at the Royal Free Hospital, Department of Public Health, University of London. At the same time I am also working as a researcher in epidemiology at the Institute of Epidemiology Latium Health Authority, Rome.

KH: *How did you get interested in the role of zinc and aging?*

CF: My interest in the role of zinc in aging started in 1987. At that time, zinc deficiency was suggested as an important etiologic factor in the development of kwashiorkor. Golden had presented convincing evidence of an improvement in delayed immune response of children with protein-calorie nutrition (P.E.M.) to supplementary zinc. Golden had also demonstrated that thymic atrophy is reversed when malnourished children were given zinc supplements. Zinc deficient children had atrophy of the thymolymphatic system, depressed cell-mediated immunity and increased susceptibility to infection. Children with P.E.M. have similar immunological changes and also have decreased concentration of zinc in their liver, muscle and plasma. Elderly populations are also vulnerable to zinc deficiency with depressed cell-mediated immune response. As aging is also associated with thymus atrophy, and I thought that zinc could be a key element in improving immune function. Those observations and linkages were raised during my masters thesis, entitled "Nutrition, Immunity and Aging," in which I reviewed the theories of aging, the causes of morbidity and mortality, and nutrition surveys conducted in elderly from both developed and developing countries.

KH: *What are some of the major biological functions of zinc?*

CF: Zinc might be considered the most relevant trace element in the body for its great variety of biological functions. Zinc is required as a catalytic component for more than 70 different enzymes, and as a structural constituent of many proteins and hormone receptors. Besides, it has been implicated in cell division, differentiation, and programmed cell death and may be considered as a secondary antioxidant.

KH: *Why are elderly people at risk for zinc deficiency?*

CF: Elderly populations are at risk to zinc deficiency due to a complex combination of social, economic and physiologic factors which include impaired absorption, drug interactions, inadequate intake of zinc rich foods, specifically red meats.

KH: *Can zinc supplementation enhance immune response in the elderly?*

CF: Very few studies have been performed on the effect of zinc supplementation and immunocompetence in the elderly and the results are not very clear. It is probably due to the small sample sizes and lack of subjects randomization. Nonetheless, zinc supplementation has been shown to have a beneficial effect on the delayed hypersensitivity response, on circulating T lymphocytes and on IgG antibody response to the tetanus vaccine. A recent finding regarding zinc supplementation in the elderly is the improvement in plasma thymulin activity. Thymulin, a zinc containing thymic hormone, induces several T-cell markers and promotes T-cell function. This result suggests that zinc induces change in thymic function in elderly people. As I already mentioned, the thymus undergoes age-dependent atrophy with severe loss of thymocytes. Therefore, it might be possible that the decline in immune response which occurs with aging could be reversed by zinc supplementation.

KH: *What kind of preventive strategies with regards to diet and/or supplementation might we need to recommend for the elderly?*

CF: Elderly people present with low levels of plasma zinc and also have a low intake of zinc. Therefore, preventive measures could be to advise elderly people to increase the consumption of foods rich in zinc such as seafoods and lean red meats. Another preventive measure could be to fortify some foods normally consumed by the elderly. Regarding zinc supplementation, I would only recommend zinc tablets to elderly who are known to be zinc deficient, since little is known regarding zinc toxicity.

KH: *How significant was the zinc deficiency initially in the elderly when you looked at their overall health?*

CF: Zinc deficiency is known to be associated with depressive immune response and a higher risk of infections. Elderly people have low plasma levels of zinc, depressed immune response and also a high prevalence of infections. Therefore, zinc deficiency in the elderly might play an extremely important role in the overall health of the elderly. ◆

Aggressive Feelings and Tryptophan

Dr. A.J. Cleare

Clinical Lecturer in Psychiatry
Maudsley Hospital and Institute of Psychiatry
Denmark Hill
London SE5 8AZ, United Kingdom
44 171 703 5411 / 44 171 740 5129 (FAX)

"Effects of Alterations in Plasma Tryptophan Levels on Aggressive Feelings",
Archives of General Psychiatry, December 1994;51:1004-1005. #21426

Kirk Hamilton: *What is your educational background since your university studies?*

Anthony J. Cleare: I studied medicine at Guys Hospital Medical School, University of London, qualifying in 1990. After interning, I completed the residency training program in psychiatry at the Maudsley Hospital, London. Since then I have been carrying out research at the Institute of Psychiatry as a clinical lecturer. My main areas of interest have been in the psychopharmacology of aggression and affective disorders.

KH: *How did you get interested in the role of tryptophan and aggressive behavior?*

AC: I became interested in the role of serotonin in the control of aggressive impulses because there seemed to be a lot of work implicating lowered serotonin activity as important in producing this type of aggression. Most work was, however, looking at cross-sectional correlations between aggression and serotonin measures. We believed it was important to see if experimentally manipulating brain serotonin levels could produce changes in aggression. Tryptophan is, of course, the precursor amino acid for serotonin synthesis, and there is good evidence that changing blood levels of tryptophan subsequently alters brain levels of both tryptophan and serotonin. We, therefore, devised an experiment to alter acutely blood tryptophan levels and measure subsequent aggressive feelings and behaviors.

KH: *How does a sudden drop in tryptophan result in a change of mood?*

AC: In order to cause a rapid lowering of blood tryptophan, we gave a mixture of 50 amino acids without tryptophan. What happens is that the amino acid mixture stimulates protein synthesis and, because the mixture is tryptophan free, this uses up the body's stores of tryptophan, primarily in the blood. Thus, blood tryptophan is rapidly lowered, and this subsequently lowers the amount available for serotonin synthesis in the brain. It has been known for some time that depressed mood is associated with lowered measures of serotonin in the central nervous system. We confirmed the results of previous investigators that lowering serotonin acutely -- via this tryptophan depletion -- precipitates feelings of depression in healthy individuals. The exact location within the brain where the lowered serotonin is effecting this lowering of mood is not yet clear; however, there are dense collections of serotonergic neurons in the limbic areas, and it is probable that these are playing a large role in these effects.

KH: *What are the results of your study of 24 male subjects who had high levels of traits of aggression, based on the Buss-Dorkee Hostility Inventory, and their use of a tryptophan-free mixture of 15 amino acids or a tryptophan included amino acid mixture?*

AC: In this study, we wanted to see if aggressive feelings would be affected by changes in plasma tryptophan concentrations. We looked at both tryptophan depletion and tryptophan enhancement using the amino acid mixtures you described. They were balanced mixtures in the ratio of human breast milk, with or without 10.6 g of tryptophan. We thought if there were any changes, they would be largest in those with high levels of trait aggression. We, therefore, chose aggressive subjects from a volunteer pool of healthy males. We measured subjective feelings before and 5 hours after the drinks using a visual analog rating scale. We also confirmed using blood tests that depletion and enhancement of tryptophan from rest levels occurred. Subjects given the tryptophan depletion become significantly more angry, aggressive, hostile, quarrelsome, annoyed and more aggressive on the overall mean of 13 items. Subjects given the tryptophan enhancement responded in an equal, but opposite, direction on these variables, feeling substantially less aggressive overall. We also looked at mood changes after tryptophan drink in these subjects. Tryptophan depletion induced feelings of discontent on visual analog scales, while again, tryptophan enhancement had the opposite effect, producing feelings of increased well-being. We have since extended our studies to look at behavior measures of aggression in addition to these subjective feelings. We found that after tryptophan depletion, subjects behaved more aggressively on an experimental measure involving subjecting imaginary opponents to unpleasantly loud noises. Thus, not only does tryptophan depletion produce increased feelings of aggression, but subjects behave more aggressively, too. We also looked at subjects selected to have lower levels of trait aggression. In contrast to the high aggressive subjects, there were no consistent effects of tryptophan alterations in these subjects. This may have been either because they are less expensive to do tryptophan manipulations, or because the experimental methods are less sensitive to the smaller changes, which are nonetheless still occurring.

KH: *Is there a risk when giving an amino acid mixture that does not contain tryptophan in triggering a rebound depression?*

AC: These concerns have rightly been raised recently because not all amino acid mixtures now contain tryptophan. We use large amounts of tryptophan-free mixtures in our studies, 100 gm. However, it has been shown that as little as 30 gm of only 7 amino acids can cause the same degree of depletion as we found. Our subjects were also fasted from midnight on the day before, and received no breakfast or lunch on the test day. There is little doubt, though, that if people do take supplements in sufficiently large quantities without other food, that a significant proportion will suffer some degree of tryptophan depletion. This would put them at high risk of suffering depressive or aggressive symptoms as we have found in our subjects. Those at the highest risk would be aggressive people for the aggressive symptoms, and those with a history of depression for depressive symptoms. Particularly worrying would be people such as strength athletes, who frequently take large quantities of amino acid supplements, and who may also be using anabolic steroids, which also have pro-aggressive effects in some people.

KH: Do you believe tryptophan is a safe supplement with regards to the concern about tryptophan being a cause of eosinophilia-myalgia syndrome?

AC: The relationship between tryptophan and EMS is still controversial. While I think it is fairly clear that a number of fatal cases of EMS were associated with tryptophan use, it seems there was probably a contaminant in the manufacturing process that was responsible. However, no cases were associated with amino acid supplements, which often use different ingredients as the tryptophan source. There is, therefore, perhaps less compelling evidence for the continuing absence of tryptophan from some mixtures. I think the licensing authorities were correct to withdraw the drug at the time, and should now proceed cautiously reintroducing it for specific uses. This is now being done in Britain, where tryptophan can be prescribed for resistant cases of depression with close monitoring.

KH: Do your results suggest that tryptophan could be used as not only an antidepressive agent, but also a substance that may help normalize aggressive behavior in certain individuals?

AC: I think there is a suggestion from our work that raising tryptophan levels has an anti-aggressive effect. This is not quite the same as administering tryptophan because we also administered other substances, namely other amino acids. However, it is likely that administering tryptophan alone would raise blood tryptophan levels. There have been a number of small pilot studies looking at tryptophan in aggressive psychiatric patients, with promising results. There is clearly a need for larger, more controlled studies, using a wider range of individuals. Our work provides a theoretical rationale for this.

KH: Have you done any studies with behavioral and/or violent individuals and tryptophan supplementation?

AC: When we gave tryptophan enhancement to the subjects with high levels of trait aggression, they responded less aggressively in the experimental model previously described before involving noise administration to an opponent. This was in contrast to the tryptophan depleted individuals who responded more aggressively. We have not yet used this on a clinical population. ◆

Alzheimer's Disease, Dementia and Vitamin B1

Michael Gold, M.D.,
MDC 55, Assistant Professor
Departments of Neurology and Psychiatry
The University of South Florida
1209 Bruce B. Downs Blvd., Box 19
Tampa, FL 33612 U.S.A.
(813) 974-3100 / (813) 974-2580 (FAX)

"Plasma and Red Blood Cell Thiamin Deficiency in Patients With Dementia of the Alzheimer's Type," Archives of Neurology, November, 1995;52:1081-1085. #23739

Kirk Hamilton: Can you please share with me your educational background and current position?

Michael Gold: I am currently an assistant professor at the University of South Florida College of Medicine, with appointments in the Departments of Neurology and Psychiatry. I obtained my medical degree from the University of Miami School of Medicine. I proceeded to obtain my neurology training at Albert Einstein College of Medicine in New York and pursued a fellowship in behavioral neurology at the University of Florida College of Medicine.

KH: When did you get interested in the role of vitamin B1 in Alzheimer's Disease?

MG: I became interested in the role of thiamin (vitamin B1) in Alzheimer's Disease during my fellowship. I developed an interest in mitochondrial diseases during my residency and became interested in the role of faulty oxidative metabolism in neurodegenerative disorders. The specific interest in Alzheimer's Disease was related to the publication of several articles resulting deficits in thiamin-dependent enzymes in Alzheimer's Disease.

KH: What did you find in your study with regards to thiamin levels and Alzheimer's Disease compared to other types of dementia?

MG: We found that patients with Alzheimer's Disease had significantly lower levels of plasma thiamin than did patients with other forms of dementia. In addition, we found a disproportionally higher number of patients with Alzheimer's Disease that had deficiencies in plasma thiamin.

KH: Why did you not use a functional test of thiamin such as erythrocyte transketolase activity or the thiamin pyrophosphate?

MG: We did not use erythrocyte transketolase activity (ETKA) or thiamin pyrophosphate because those tests are dependent on RBC thiamin. Additional data also proved that the biological assay we used had a better correlation between known thiamin doses and plasma levels. Another factor is the working assumption that plasma thiamin is transported into the CNS, not RBC bound thiamin.

KH: What were the results of your study?

MG: In our study we found that plasma and RBC levels did not correlate. That is, we had a number of patients with deficient plasma thiamin who had normal RBC thiamin. The converse was not noted. In addition, RBC thiamin did not segregate out between the patient groups.

KH: What significance does this finding have?

MG: This finding, if substantiated, has serious implications for the assessment and treatment of Alzheimer's Disease. There may be a subset of patients with Alzheimer's Disease who are thiamin deficient. Our data suggests that this may be a large subset, but the actual extent of thiamin deficiency will need to be established using much larger numbers of patients. It is not known whether these patients have a unique cognitive profile or have a unique natural history. In terms of treatment, these patients have not been studied in a systematic fashion. So it is not known if these patients would respond to treatment with thiamin. Anecdotally, I have had reports of functional improvement from a few patients whom I have empirically treated with high doses of thiamin at 3-5 gm per day.

KH: Do Alzheimer's Disease patients have a dysmetabolism of thiamin or do they have a tendency towards deficiency?

MG: That is a tough question and the answer we do not know yet. There are conflicting data on the issue of the nutritional state of patients with Alzheimer's Disease. It is possible that there may be a degree of malabsorption, however, the normal RBC thiamin levels would argue against that. We believe that the metabolic derangement in the central nervous system may cause a more rapid shuttling of thiamin from the plasma into the central nervous system and that the thiamin is then rapidly cleared. The honest answer is that there are several potential mechanisms that have yet to be explored. The finding of plasma deficiency needs to be replicated before we begin to tease apart the mechanisms.

KH: Have there been any trials using thiamin in Alzheimer's Disease patients either orally or by injection?

MG: There have been 3 pilot studies of orally administered thiamin. Two of the three studies reported mild beneficial effects. One study did not find an effect. All these studies use very small patient samples, varied in the maximum dose of thiamin and in the duration of treatment. It is important to note that none of these pilot studies measured or selected their patients on the basis of thiamin deficiency, therefore the minimal beneficial effect reported in 2 of those studies may underestimate the effect of thiamin replacement. ◆

Angina Pectoris and Fish Oil

A. Salachas, M.D.
6 Diagora St.
116 36 Athens, Greece
30 1 748 6609 (FAX)

"Effects of a Low-Dose Fish Oil Concentrate on Angina, Exercise Tolerance Time, Serum Triglycerides and Platelet Function", <u>Angiology</u>, December 1994;45(12):1023-1031). #21511

Kirk Hamilton: *What is your educational background and present position?*

A. Salachas: I received my undergraduate medical school training at the University of Athens in Greece. I interned as a clinical assistant at a cardiothoracic unit of Northern General Hospital in Sheffield, United Kingdom. I did my training in cardiology at the same unit. I completed my residency in 1987. In October 1990, I joined the invasive cardiology medical staff at Evangelismos Hospital in Athens, Greece.

KH: *How did you get interested in fish oil's role in angina pectoris?*

AS: During my training in Sheffield, I had the opportunity to meet a well-known investigator in the field of fish oil, Dr. R. Saynor, and I became involved in a big project studying the effects of fish oils in patients with coronary disease. My interest for fish oils was triggered from the encouraging results of fish-oil studies in patients with angina, conducted by Dr. Saynor and his team.

KH: *What did you find from your study of fish oil?*

AS: A reduction in anginal attacks, glyceryl trinitrate consumption and triglycerides was expected. This has also been reported in previous studies. We were impressed by the increase of exercise tolerance time. As far as I am concerned, this parameter has not been studied in previous trials relating patients with coronary artery disease to taking fish oil. Although we did not expect a significant increase in exercise tolerance time, it seems that it is an encouraging finding for further trials.

KH: *From your study can fish oil be recommended for angina?*

AS: I believe further trials are needed before we can advocate fish oil as a therapy for angina patients. On the other hand, there is no doubt that fish oils constitute an effective therapy against hypertriglyceridemia.

KH: *Were there any problems with fish oil supplementation in your study?*

AS: The most frequent complaints by patients consuming large quantities of fish oil are related to the gastrointestinal tract. Mild dyspepsia, belching, increased flatulence, diarrhea or a fish after taste occur, and about 10% of patients will decline to continue the preparation. In our study, the gastrointestinal effects were lessened because of the relatively small dose and because the preparation was taken with food.

KH: *Is there any research showing fish oil consumption reducing atherosclerosis or cardiovascular mortality?*

AS: I believe there is a long-term effectiveness of fish oils on atherosclerosis. One large mortality trial recently has been published and showed a favorable effect of fish oil consumption on mortality in survivors of myocardial infarction, but additional studies are clearly needed. (Burr M., Fehily A., Gilbert, J.,et al., <u>Lancet</u>, 1991;2:757-761).

KH: *Is there variation in fish oil quality, and are there components of fish oil to be concerned about?*

AS: Most fish oil concentrates are low in vitamins A and D content, but preparations mainly derived from cod liver oil are not. Such preparations can contain 2 to 4 times the recommended daily requirement of these vitamins. Although considerably high doses of these vitamins are necessary to produce toxic effects, the effect of high dose fish oil over prolonged periods is unknown. Another potential detrimental effect is that some fatty fish and commercial fish oil supplements may contain concentrated quantities of mercury or polychlorinated dibenzodioxins and dibenzofurans as an unfortunate consequence of water pollution. These toxins can be removed during processing if appropriate steps are taken. Accordingly, it is advisable to obtain fish oils from a reputable source. Finally, many fatty fish contain cholesterol, some of the initial commercial concentrates also contain large quantities of cholesterol. Cholesterol is now removed from the majority of preparations available, so increasing cholesterol intake by fish oil is no longer a major concern. In our study, there were no harmful side effects of fish oil.

KH: *Should we be concerned about the oxidation of fish oil?*

AS:. Because consumption of large quantities of fish or fish oil concentrates increases the likelihood of lipid peroxidation and autooxidation, I believe that it is necessary to take vitamin E as an antioxidant. In fact, many commercial fish oil preparations contain vitamin E.

KH: *What actions of fish oil may affect angina pectoris?*

AS: I believe the vasodilatory and antiaggregatory effects of fish oil may help reduce or prevent angina pectoris (A. Leaf, <u>Circulation</u>, 1990;82(2):624-628/Dehmer, <u>Circulation</u>, 1990;82(2):739-742.).

KH: *Is there any evidence that fish oil can prevent atherosclerosis?*

AS: There is an increasing amount of experimental and clinical data to support the thought that fish oils could modify the occurrence and course of atherosclerosis. If well designed clinical trials confirm this effect, there may be a day where dietary supplementation with fish oil could become one of the simplest interventions against atherosclerosis and its complications. ◆

Antioxidants and Health

Jeffrey Blumberg, Ph.D., Associate Director,
USDA Human Nutrition Research Center on Aging
Tufts University/Chief of the Antioxidant Research Lab
711 Washington Street
Boston, MA 02111 U.S.A.
(617) 556-3330 / (617) 556-3295 (FAX)

"Considerations of the Scientific Substantiation For Antioxidant Vitamins and β-Carotene in Disease Prevention,", American Journal of Clinical Nutrition, 1995;62(Suppl.):1521S-6S. #23859

KH: How did your education prepare you for a career in human nutrition research?

JB: After undergraduate training in pharmacy and psychology at Washington State University, I received my doctorate in pharmacology from Vanderbilt University and then went on to a NIH post-doctoral fellowship in biochemistry at the University of Calgary. While on the faculty at Northeastern University I became interested in environmental toxicology and examined the mechanism of action, to many pollutants - the generation of free radicals. After moving to Tufts, I flipped the coin over again and began to study how the body protects itself against free radical pathology with antioxidant nutrients.

KH: What is your position at Tufts?

JB: I wear a few different hats: I am a professor in the School of Nutrition at the Jean-Mayer USDA Human Nutrition Research Center on Aging at Tufts University. I serve as the Associate Director of the Center and the Chief of Antioxidants Research Lab there.

KH: How would you say, over the last 12 years, has the view of public health officials on antioxidants changed?

JB: The enormous body of research, which is continuing to grow, has been compelling in its suggestion that antioxidant nutrients, particularly vitamins C, E and beta-carotene play an important role in promoting health and reducing the risk of many chronic diseases, including cancer and heart disease. Recently, some studies have also implicated antioxidants in reducing the risk of cataracts and age-related macular degeneration, certain neurologic diseases and infectious diseases. As a whole, the data are remarkably consistent across experimental, clinical, and epidemiologic investigations of antioxidants. Some of the more provocative results indicate a dose-response relationship continuing through supra-dietary intakes via supplements. However, despite the information available, a consensus about the health benefits of antioxidants has not been achieved as many people consider the potential of these nutrients as promising but not proven. Thus, there is a call for more research - particularly large scale clinical trials of long duration - until definitive, unequivocal results are obtained. Given the nature of the scientific enterprise, I am not sure that it will ever be possible to reach that objective.

KH: Two recent, well publicized antioxidant studies, one in Finnish smokers looking at lung cancer and one in American patients with colorectal adenomatous polyps - indicated no beneficial effect of the intervention. If these clinical trials had had positive results, do you think federal officials would have approved a health claim for antioxidants?

JB: It is impossible to know what would have happened. But I doubt the FDA would have found evidence from just two more studies sufficiently convincing that a significant scientific agreement was suddenly present to satisfy their regulatory requirements for making a health claim. Importantly, the fact that these studies were negative, especially with the increase in lung cancer incidents seen in the Finnish men taking beta-carotene, will undoubtedly prove to be a major setback in any official health claim being allowed for antioxidants. This is rather ironic as health claims on food and supplement labels are intended to promote primarily disease prevention in the general population while both these studies were attempts at secondary prevention in high risk populations with early signs of disease likely or definitely present.

KH: Did the results of these two studies change your opinion that there is a probable benefit in generous consumption of vitamin C, E and beta-carotene?

JB: Certainly not. I don't think that any one or two studies, no matter how large or well conducted, should or can undermine the totality of scientific information available. It is important to keep in mind the limitations of clinical trials - at best they can test only one or two antioxidants at one or two doses and the population selected must be at an elevated risk for the one or two principal disease end points selected for study as the intervention must be of very limited duration. However, the studies you are asking about are more pertinent to therapeutic efficacy than health promotion and disease prevention. Thus, it becomes apparent that every clinical trial will result in the need for further studies employing different combinations and/or doses of nutrients given to various populations for longer amounts of time. The development of public health policy today, such as recommending increased consumption of antioxidants, must be based on consistency, strength, and quality of all the knowledge we have now. Efforts to define vitamin requirements, dietary guidelines and health claims for nutrients must also weigh the potential benefits and the potential risks when establishing such a policy. While the conduct of clinical trials will always remain important, they should not be the only references when making decisions about these issues.

KH: Does the Finnish study suggest that there is a harmful effect from taking beta-carotene supplements?

JB: I don't believe so. The real message of the Finnish study is that smokers cannot expect from beta-carotene or any other nutrient a magic bullet to reverse the impact of a lifetime of heavy smoking. While there is some suggestion from *in vitro* studies that high doses of a single antioxidant in the absence of other antioxidants necessary to recycle them may become pro-oxidants, it is not clear that this occurs *in vivo*. The data which would help us better understand the nature of the increased incidence of lung cancer seen in the Finnish men randomized to the beta-carotene arm of this study have not yet been published. I would like to see answers to questions like: How many of those who got lung cancer actually took their supplements? How many were also consuming high amounts of alcohol (which interferes with beta-carotene metabolism) and low amounts of vitamin C and other dietary antioxidants? How many got lung cancer within the first few years of this 6 year study? It is important to note that the beneficial effects of smoking cessation on lung cancer mortality are not usually evident for 10 years. Following publication of the Finnish data, I understand that the NCI and all the U.S. investigators conducting clinical trials with beta-carotene reviewed their data from ongoing studies and found no suggestion of any adverse effect of beta-carotene. Thus, it would appear these results from the Finnish study represent a chance observation.

KH: Five servings of fruit and vegetable consumption obviously is one of the strongest dietary recommendations by the government. In your opinion are there any other phytochemicals that could have potent antioxidant capabilities aside from the classic ones we talk about - vitamins C, E, and beta-carotene?

JB: Absolutely. The biochemical and experimental data from studies of several phytochemicals, e.g., many of the bioflavonoid compounds, indicate that they are potent antioxidants - scavenging oxyradicals, sequestering metal ions via liganding, inhibiting cyclooxygenase, etc. The apparent dynamic interrelationships between the phytochemical antioxidants and vitamins C, E, and beta-carotene (and the other antioxidant carotenoids) may explain the failure of some clinical trials employing only the antioxidant vitamins to confirm the epidemiological observations. Nonetheless, it is important to recognize that the information about the antioxidant phytochemicals is still very limited. Few human studies have been conducted and there is a serious lack of values present for these compounds in the nutrient databases used in the analysis of diet records from epidemiologic surveys.

KH: You were quoted in a magazine once as stating that there was not enough information about vitamins to make public recommendations but there was enough information for an intelligent person to make an individual decision on their own to take supplements.

JB: It depends about which vitamins you are talking about. There is certainly enough information now for public recommendations for women of child bearing age to take a supplement containing 400 ug of folic acid to reduce the risk of neural tube and other birth defects. However, with regard to antioxidant nutrients, I am not unsympathetic with the dilemma the FDA, the CDC and the Surgeon General face when making health claim proclamations for vitamins because they have such wide ranging implications for food labeling and fortification policies and for all the federal nutrition programs including school lunches, WIC (Women Infant and Children) and Meals-On-Wheels. This is not a matter to be taken lightly.

On the other hand, we are facing a health crisis of dramatic proportions today which require the best solutions we can implement now. People are dying prematurely of heart disease and cancer and we must treat increasing numbers of older Americans for cataracts, osteoporosis, and other degenerative conditions. The financial costs as well as the personal costs in terms of dependence and suffering,

are enormous. This challenge should make us a little more courageous in making recommendations today in the presence of some uncertainty about efficacy but a great deal of confidence about safety of vitamins like antioxidants. We know we can begin to separate biology from chronology by changing nutritional status - frailty and chronic diseases are not inevitable consequences of aging. I do not mean to suggest that taking antioxidant supplements or improving one's dietary choices are the sole means for preventing all diseases or halting the ageing process - but they do represent one of the most effective and practical approaches we have today for health promotion.

KH: Do you take supplements yourself and at what doses? I realize these are not public recommendations.

JB: In responding to that question, I always have to make the disclaimer that what I do may be right for me but not necessarily relevant to someone much younger or older or women or someone at high risk for a particular disease. I take a multivitamin-multimineral supplement formulated around the RDA levels. With regards to antioxidants, I take total daily intakes of vitamin C between 250-1000 mg, vitamin E between 100-400 I.U. and beta-carotene between 6-30 mg would place most people among the groups found to be at the lowest risk for the diseases which appear effected by antioxidants. I don't feel we have sufficient data today to be more precise than offering these wide ranges. I also don't mean to imply that we can distinguish differences in efficacy between the low and the high end of these ranges. I take supplements of these antioxidants within these ranges.

KH: So you think that a tremendous health benefit can be gained by taking antioxidant supplements?

JB: It is important not to over-promise the potential of antioxidants. They represent one pro-active positive health behavior by which people can easily and inexpensively empower themselves to help achieve optimal health. But they may only reduce the risk of some chronic diseases by 10, 20 or 30% - and important benefit but not a guarantee of never getting ill. A rational approach to nutritional supplementation, particularly antioxidant supplements, is akin to wearing a seat belt - it provides a degree of protection against injury but it doesn't give you a license to drive recklessly. You cannot eat a diet high in fat, salt and sugar, never exercise, smoke cigarettes and practice unsafe sex and think that taking a nutritional supplement will provide you with optimal health. It is interesting to note that positive health behaviors clustered together - people who take supplements generally eat better, exercise more and smoke less than those who do not. ◆

Antioxidant and Coronary Heart Disease

Pauli V. Luoma, M.D.
Regional Institute of Occupational Health
Aapistie 1
FIN-90220 Oulu, Finland
358 81 5375661 / 358 81 5376000 (FAX)

"High Serum Alpha-Tocopherol, Albumin, Selenium and Cholesterol, and Low Mortality From Coronary Heart Disease in Northern Finland,"
Journal of Internal Medicine 1995;237:49-54. #21749

Kirk Hamilton: Could you please share with me your present position?

Pauli Luoma: I am currently doing research in the Department of Public Health Science at the University of Oulu, Finland. I am an assistant professor of internal medicine at the University of Oulu and an assistant professor of clinical pharmacology at the University of Tampe, Finland.

KH: How did you get interested in the role of antioxidants and coronary heart disease?

PL: The mortality from coronary heart disease (CHD) in Finland is one of the highest in the world. I got interested in antioxidants and coronary heart disease in the early 1980s when the association of low serum selenium and high risk of CHD in Finland was reported. I have been interested in lipid and apolipoprotein risk factors and liver microsomes, cytochrome P-450, lipids and proteins. Serum selenium is related to liver cytochrome P-450, and hepatic microsomal induction (increase in cytochrome P-450) is associated with a beneficial, antiatherogenic change in the serum lipoprotein profile. Antioxidants protect microsomes, low density lipoproteins and whole organs against oxidative damage, and may prevent atherogenesis and retard the manifestation of CHD.

KH: Were there any surprises to this study in particular, higher levels of cholesterol in the group that had the lower incidence of coronary heart disease?

PL: It is of particular interest to study reasons for a low CHD mortality in this country, well known for its high CHD mortality. The explanation for the association of high cholesterol and low CHD mortality might be found in some factor in genotype, diet, lifestyle or environment. The men of Sami origin (ethnic minority) living in northernmost Finland show a high frequency of apolipoprotein phenotype E4/4 and e4 allele which may in part explain the high concentration of serum cholesterol observed in the low mortality area. However, a major factor in the low CHD mortality in the north may be an adequate antioxidant status preventing the atherogenic modification of LDL also in people with a high serum cholesterol level.

KH: How would antioxidants protect against CHD?

PL: The antioxidants prevent the oxidative modification of LDL that has been suggested to have a major role in the development and progression of atherosclerosis and coronary heart disease.

KH: Why does reindeer meat have higher amounts of the antioxidants selenium and vitamin E? Are there other foods that are higher in these antioxidants that the Sami consume?

PL: Vitamin E and selenium in reindeer meat are derived from natural sources. Reindeer researchers report that particularly lichens and mushrooms are rich in selenium. The consumption of margarine, plus vegetable oils and cereals, which are important sources of vitamin E, is higher in the Sami area than the neighboring regions to the south. Serum selenium is related to the consumption of fish, which is an important constituent of the diet in the north.

KH: How about the effect of omega-3 fatty acids in not only the fish but also in the Northern Reindeer fat even though the total fat is less?

PL: There are some differences in the consumption of food items between the two areas which may have significance. The consumption of reindeer meat and margarine plus vegetable oils is higher and that of milk lower in the low mortality area than the reference area. The intake of fat and saturated fats is lower in the low mortality area than the reference area. Reindeer meat has relatively high contents of unsaturated oleic acid. It has one double bond and is much more resistant to oxidation than linoleic acid which contains two double bonds. An increase in the consumption of oleic acid may beneficially reduce the atherogenicity of the diet. There are differences in the consumption of saturated and unsaturated fats between the two areas but we do not have data on omega-3 fatty acids.

KH: Do you consume basic antioxidants in supplemental form (C,E or beta-carotene) as part of a preventive approach to CAD?

PL: Sometimes, but not regularly. A Mediterranean type of diet is a good goal. Further studies are needed for a general recommendation to use antioxidants in the prevention of cardiovascular diseases. ♦

Arrhythmias, Cardiac Surgery and Magnesium

Riyad Karmy-Jones, M.D., FRCSC, FRSCS (CT)
Henry Ford Hospital
Department of Surgery
2799 Grand Blvd.
Detroit, MI 48202-2689 U.S.A.
(313) 876-3053 / (313) 876-8007 (FAX)

"Magnesium Sulfate Prophylaxis After Cardiac Operations",
Annals of Thoracic Surgery, 1995;59:502-507. #23393

Kirk Hamilton: *Could you please share with me your educational background and current position?*

Riyad Karmy-Jones: I obtained my M.D. degree from the University of Alberta (Edmonton) in 1983. I completed my residency in general surgery at George Washington University (Washington, D.C.), critical care and trauma training at the Washington Hospital Center (Washington, D.C.) and cardiothoracic training at the University of Alberta (Edmonton). I am board-certified in critical care, cardiothoracic surgery and general surgery. Currently I am on staff at Henry Ford Hospital (Detroit) in the divisions of Trauma/Critical Care and Thoracic Surgery.

KH: *When did you start to get interested in the role of magnesium in cardiovascular surgery?*

RKJ: I became interested initially during my trauma/critical care residency when I saw that there was conflicting data regarding the significance of ventricular tachyarrhythmias (VTs) and supraventricular tachyarrhythmias (SVTs) both following myocardial infarction and following surgery. Much of the data used to justify treatment in the surgical population was based on data obtained in the post infarction patient, not post surgical patients. Further, the data regarding risk-benefit ratio of commonly used agents were becoming more murky. While a CVT fellow, I noticed that my patients were kept in monitored settings and treated for asymptomatic VTs. This represented a significant burden.

KH: *What were the major findings of your study?*

RKJ: The study demonstrated that magnesium supplementation reduced the incidence and severity of VTs following surgery. It suggested that many VTs need not be treated with drugs as they had little clinical importance, and tended to resolve with time. There was no impact on SVTs.

KH: *How does magnesium tend to work in reducing the incidence of ventricular tachyarrhythmias?*

RKJ: Magnesium has several cellular effects. Possibly the most important ones are by affecting sodium Na^+-K^+ ATPase to stabilize membranes and to maintain intracellular potassium levels.

KH: *Does this reduction in ventricular arrhythmias result in enhanced myocardial protection?*

RKJ: Because we gave the magnesium sulfate post pump, it is hard to prove better myocardial protection, but there was some

suggestion that this might be occurring to a degree as the patients with magnesium sulfate supplementation had reductions in CPK-MBs which also correlated with reduced VTs.

KH: *Why do you think there has been a discrepancy in the use of magnesium in myocardial infarction where some studies in which magnesium is given early on, before thrombolytic therapy, shows benefit while other studies show no benefit.*

RKJ: I don't know that anyone can absolutely answer this one. I suspect that part of the deal is with the timing (i.e.; before inducing reperfusion injury and how long before) as well as how the effects are measured. Perhaps using newer methods, such as Troponin I, will give clearer answers. Certainly, the surgical population is different because we create a situation where the myocardium is acutely cooled then rewarmed.

KH: *Do you think magnesium should be routinely used in cardiovascular surgical patients?*

RKJ: Absolutely. It should be added to the cardioplegia at the very least. Other possibilities include Allopurinol given by mouth preoperatively. ◆

Arrhythmias, Selenium and Magnesium

David Lehr, M.D., FACP, FACC
Professor Emeritus of Pharmacology
New York Medical College
125 West 96th Street
New York, NY 10025-6421 U.S.A.
(212) 866-6084 / (212) 666-1726 (FAX)

"A Possible Beneficial Effect of Selenium Administration in Antiarrhythmic Therapy,"
Journal of the American College of Nutrition, 1994;13(5):496-498. #21220

Kirk Hamilton: *What is your educational background from college and your current position now?*

David Lehr: I attended the Medical School of the University of Vienna and received my M.D. degree in 1935. I was appointed thereafter to the faculty as a member of the Pharmacological Institute of the medical school for a three year term. In July of 1938, I went to Sweden where I served as a research assistant at The Pharmacological Institute of the Royal University of Lund. I arrived in the United States in the fall of 1939, where after a year's stay at the Department of Pathology at Newark Beth Israel Hospital, as a research associate, I joined the faculty of New York Medical College as an instructor in medicine and pharmacology. I remained at New York Medical College for 41 years from 1940 until 1981. I rose through the ranks to a full professorship in pharmacology. In 1949 I established for the first time at this school a separate department of pharmacology and served as its first chairman for 25 years. At present I am still a member of New York Medical College as professor emeritus of pharmacology. Actually, I spent most of my professional life at this institution.

KH   And, what do you do at this moment?

DL: I have a license for the private practice of medicine, but I do only consultant work in the area of my specialty. I have never engaged in private practice because I was a full-time faculty member in the medical school.

KH: And what is your specialty in consulting?

DL: It is clinical pharmacology and therapeutics which encompasses the beneficial and toxic effects of chemical agents and their fate in the human body when used as drugs in the prevention and treatment of disease.

KH: How did you get involved with selenium and its effects on arrhythmias?

DL: This is an unusual story. Permit me first to digress for a moment. You were kind enough to send me an issue of *Clinical Pearls News* and I was fascinated by the interview you conducted with Dr. Michael Brodsky, regarding his study of "Magnesium Therapy in New Onset Atrial Fibrillation." My own interest in magnesium goes far back, actually to the beginning of my career. From 1935 to 1938, the late Dr. Eduard von Hueber and I carried out a major study on the therapeutic effect of magnesium in life-threatening, experimental ventricular arrhythmias. The beneficial effect of magnesium on arrhythmias was shown for the first time by Zwillinger in Czechoslovakia in 1935. He demonstrated the life-saving effect of intravenously injected magnesium sulfate in digitalis poisoning of human beings. Our experimental study confirmed the therapeutic effect of magnesium in severe, aconite-induced

arrhythmias in 3 species of animals. Our investigation was published in 1938. But at that time the transmission of scientific journals from Austria had been interrupted because of the Anschluss and the subsequent outbreak of World War II. Hence, our study is not well-known here. This early and intense preoccupation with the beneficial effect of magnesium upon the heart became my life-long interest. I later worked for more than 2 decades on the pharmacological and physiological effects of magnesium upon the myocardium. Now to return to your question about my interest in selenium, this is a rather different story. I would say it was pure serendipity. Fourteen years ago, I suddenly developed episodes of non-sustained and sustained ventricular tachycardia, a rather precarious situation. I was treated, for 4 years, with a battery of the most potent antiarrhythmic agents available at that time, unfortunately without much success. Ultimately, the noted Boston cardiologist, Dr. Bernard Lown, found that flecainide, then still an experimental drug, effectively eliminated my ventricular tachycardia (for a period of 9 years now), yet it did not completely remove my arrhythmias. I still had frequent episodes of ventricular bigeminy, less dangerous but rather disabling. Then one day, two years ago, I began taking a substantially larger dose of selenium.

KH: What was that dosage?

DL: Well that is an important point. The dosage of selenium in commercially available multivitamin/mineral preparations is usually 5 or 10 mcgs. This is a very small dose, actually a ridiculously small dose. The daily requirement for human beings is anywhere between 60 and 100 mcg. In order to take an effective dose of this well-known antioxidant, I raised my daily intake by 100 mcg, for a total of 110 mcg. I never thought about any effect upon my heart. I still had runs of ventricular bigeminy and many premature beats. Unexpectedly, one week after I started taking this larger dose of selenium, these arrhythmias completely vanished. I did not immediately think of selenium but I found that nothing in my life-style, in my habits, in my food intake had changed. The only thing I could think of as being different was that I was taking a 10 times larger dose of selenium. I then started looking into the medical literature and found that there is considerable recent information on selenium. I learned that there is a disease called Keshan's disease, a dilated cardiomyopathy which may be accompanied by severe arrhythmias and may lead to death. This disease has been reported to occur endemicly in the Keshan province of China, an area where the soil is markedly deficient in selenium. Children and young women from farm families, whose food is derived predominantly from products grown locally, are particularly prone to develop Keshan disease. Chinese physicians demonstrated that this disease can be prevented or ameliorated by selenium substitution. So that started me looking for animal-experimental data. I found that there is convincing evidence that selenium is very important for the homeostasis of the heart and perhaps also other organs. Since my case is a single case, the observation should be considered only suggestive and requiring confirmation. I now work with a group of cardiologists at Mt. Sinai Medical Center in New York

City. We are trying to determine whether selenium substitution has a beneficial effect in patients with arrhythmias.

KH: *Is there a trial going on with selenium?*

DL: There is a trial going on now at the Department of Medicine at Mt. Sinai Medical Center.

KH: *What dose of selenium are they using?*

DL: The dosage I suggested is 200 mcg per day.

KH: *And what type of selenium? I know there are different forms.*

DL: The preparation used in this trial is selenomethionine, manufactured by Solgar Vitamin Company of Lynbrook, New York. The company also supplied the placebo tablets. Selenomethionine is present particularly in meat and has been found to be well absorbed and distributed. One of the Mt. Sinai investigators has moved to the Medical School of the University of Pennsylvania and is continuing this study also at that institution. So we should eventually have pretty good data on this subject.

KH: *What causes the arrhythmia? What is selenium's role?*

DL: There are many different causes and mechanisms which may lead to the emergence of arrhythmias. It is quite impossible to outline them in this brief interview. Selenium is known to be an integral component of glutathione peroxidase, forming part of the active site of this peroxide destroying enzyme. The enzyme is apparently vital in the detoxification of lipid peroxides and hydrogen peroxide which are known to be damaging to the cellular membranes and subcellular structures. Therefore, in highly active organs, such as the heart, perhaps also the liver, kidneys and even some skeletal muscles, selenium deficiency could lead to cellular damage and increase calcium influx and may result in malfunction and death of the injured cells.

KH: *Are there any other nutrients that might work in synergy. For example, I know that vitamin E and selenium have a kind of a partnership?*

DL: They have a partnership. It has been demonstrated in animal-experimental studies that you can substitute vitamin E for selenium. There is evidence that the antioxidant effect is probably the most important if not the sole beneficial effect of selenium. This is, at the present time, still theoretical.

KH: *So there are, theoretically, some nutrients that may be valuable in arrhythmia control, obviously magnesium?*

DL: That is why I mentioned magnesium which is a true antiarrhythmic. Many people don't know that. If you inject a magnesium salt intravenously (it really works best intravenously) magnesium can, for a short time, completely eliminate most arrhythmias. Unfortunately, the effect is very short-lived, hence you have to continue injecting magnesium. It is therefore administered preferably by continuous intravenous infusion. Magnesium given by this route is not harmless. If you inject a high dose, you can induce a sudden drop in blood pressure or you may produce paralysis of respiration. It requires constant medical attention if one is to avoid such untoward effects. That is why antiarrhythmic therapy with magnesium cannot be given outside of the hospital setting. I think Dr. Brodsky correctly mentioned another reason why magnesium is not used more frequently. There are no patentable or trademark issues involved in the use of these generally available magnesium salts, hence pharmaceutical companies have no profit motive to promote the use of this form of therapy.

KH: *That is correct, though Dr. Brodsky uses large dosages.*

DL: It has to be used in large doses and intravenously. Therefore,

you have to watch the patient very carefully. If you find that the deep tendon reflexes begin to disappear, you are in a dosage range which may be toxic. If magnesium administration is not discontinued at this stage, there is danger of paralysis of respiration, probably due to peripheral neuromuscular blockade because consciousness is not lost. Yet, magnesium salt injections can be life-saving in many instances. As mentioned earlier, Zwillinger demonstrated convincingly that he could save victims of otherwise fatal digitalis poisoning by repeated injections of magnesium sulfate. We used both the sulfate and the gluconate salt of magnesium in our animal experiments and showed that severe, aconite-induced arrhythmias can be readily and repeatedly blocked by intravenous injections of magnesium salts with temporary return to normal sinus rhythm. Rabbits, pretreated with magnesium salts were found to survive with impunity a many times fatal, ventricular fibrillation-inducing dose of aconite.

KH: *How do you assess selenium status in a person?*

DL: One would certainly determine the blood level of selenium, but I think you will find in the literature that even with a normal selenium level, Keshan's disease can occur. This was reported by the Keshan Disease Research Group in China. There is actually not a single reliable way of assessing selenium status other than finding symptoms of Keshan disease in persons on selenium deficient diets. As I have mentioned, in my paper, patients suffering from anorexia nervosa probably have a very poor selenium intake and can readily develop selenium deficiency. This has not been thought of. It is well-known that most of the young women with this condition, who die suddenly, succumb to severe, intractable, ventricular arrhythmias. The reason why they develop these arrhythmias has so far remained unexplained. In the literature you might read about the mysterious sudden death of a patient with anorexia nervosa. The same applied to healthy young women who were overweight and put on a strict liquid reducing diet. Many of them also died suddenly with similar, intractable ventricular arrhythmias. I think that in 1 year 60 young overweight, but otherwise healthy women died suddenly while on a liquid protein reducing diet. This particular diet did not contain any selenium. We also know that patients on parenteral nutrition may develop a Keshan disease syndrome if selenium is omitted. There is thus much evidence which points to the essential presence of selenium. But because this evidence is relatively recent, it has as yet not been considered adequately. I think it is quite important to look at the available data. It is conceivable, moreover, that to enrich the diet with selenium may be beneficial even in the absence of a deficiency of this trace metal. This benefit may come from the availability of its potent antioxidant effect.

KH: *What would you say would be the upper level of safety for selenium in a dosage?*

DL: It has been shown that up to 800 mcg of selenium a day can be given without development of selenosis. The 200 mcg dose presently used in the Mt. Sinai Medical School Center study should therefore be considered perfectly safe for the planned 8 week exposure of individual patients. But even if some signs of selenosis were to develop after very prolonged administration at higher dose levels, one might see some loss of hair, loss of nails, discoloration of teeth, but nothing that is really dangerous.

KH: *Dr. Lehr do you have any preliminary results of this study at the Mt. Sinai Medical Center in New York City with selenium and arrhythmias?*

DL: The investigation at Mt. Sinai Medical Center is continuing in a double-blind fashion. For statistical reasons the key is still secret. ◆

Arrhythmias - Ventricular and Fish Oil

Dr. Jeppe Hagstrup Christensen, M.D.
Aalborg Hospital, Denmark
Section of Endocrinology
Department of Medicine/Section North
Postboks 561
DK 9000 Aalborg, Denmark
45 99 32 17 22 / 45 98 12 02 53 (FAX)

"N-3 Fatty Acids and Ventricular Extrasystoles in Patients With Ventricular Tachyarrhythmias," Nutrition Research, 1995;15(1):1-8. #22360

Kirk Hamilton: Could you please share with me your educational background and current position?

Jeppe Hagstrup Christensen (JHC): I studied medicine at the University of Aarhus, Denmark and qualified in 1987. After my internship I entered the residency program in endocrinology. At the present time I am senior registrar at the Department of Endocrinology, Aalborg Hospital, Denmark.

KH: How did you get interested in the role of omega-3 fatty acids and irregular heartbeats?

JHC: For the past years the evidence for an antiarrhythmic effect of omega-3 fatty acids has increased, although this evidence stems only from animal studies. After the publication of the DART Study (Burr, M.L., et al, Lancet, 1989;II:757-61), an obvious question was whether the 29% reduction in mortality among those patients advised to eat fatty fish was due to a reduction in sudden cardiac death (= reduction in the incidence of ventricular fibrillation). Dr. Burr and colleagues speculated in this theory. Together with Dr. E. B. Schmidt, we decided to pursue the hypothesis that omega-3 fatty acids have an antiarrhythmic effect in humans.

KH: What were the findings of your study?

JHC: In a double-blind, placebo-controlled study, patients with ventricular tachyarrhythmias were randomized to either supplementation with omega-3 fatty acids or a placebo (corn oil) daily for 16 weeks. The major endpoint was the number of ventricular extrasystoles (VE). We found a non-significant reduction in the number of VEs in both groups, but the reduction was most pronounced among those patients receiving omega-3 fatty acids.

KH: Even though there were not statistically significant differences between the corn oil group and the omega-3 fatty acid group, there was still a reduction in arrhythmias. Could you comment?

JHC: Our study could demonstrate a reduction of 42% in the mean number of VE after omega-3 fatty acids, but given a sample size as in our study, at least a 65% reduction in the mean number of VE was necessary to reach statistical significance at the 5% level. Thus, from the present study, it is not possible to conclude that omega-3 fatty acids reduce the number of VE in patients with ventricular tachyarrhythmias, although a trend was observed.

KH: How do omega-3 fatty acids and/or polyunsaturated fatty acids in general reduce arrhythmias?

JHC: Polyunsaturated fatty acids have proved efficient in reducing ventricular arrhythmias in animals, with those of the omega-3 family being superior to the omega-6 family. In general, these fatty acids reduce the incidence of ventricular tachycardia and fibrillation during ischemia caused by the occlusion of a coronary artery. The incidence of these arrhythmias also are reduced during reperfusion. The mechanism by which omega-3 fatty acids protect the myocardium against ventricular arrhythmias is not clearly understood although several mechanisms have been proposed.

KH: Is it related to arachidonic acid metabolism and the release of inflammatory mediators?

JHC: Alterations in the phospholipid composition of the myocardial membrane are observed after diets rich in omega-3 fatty acids. Eicosapentaenoic acid and docosahexaenoic acid are incorporated into the membrane, while a decrease in arachidonic content is seen. These alterations may stabilize the myocardial membrane, making it more resistant to arrhythmogenic stimuli. Furthermore, studies in animals support the view that the balance between local eicosanoids such as thromboxane A_2 (proarrhythmogenic) and prostaglandin I_2 (possible antiarrhythmogenic) may be involved in arrhythmogenesis. It looks like omega-3 fatty acids change this balance in a favorable way (Abeywardena, MY, et al, American J. Physiol 1991;260:375-85).

KH: Do you see a role in the future for omega-3 fatty acids as adjunctive agents to control ventricular arrhythmias?

JHC: Future clinical trials should clarify if omega-3 fatty acids really have an antiarrhythmic effect. If such an effect is shown, it is indeed an interesting thought to use omega-3 fatty acids as adjunctive agents.

KH: How would omega-3 fatty acids theoretically prevent sudden death?

JHC: Certain patients with ischemic heart disease have a high risk of sudden death partly due to an increased incidence of ventricular fibrillation. Omega-3 fatty acids might theoretically reduce the incidence of ventricular fibrillation and thereby reduce the incidence of sudden cardiac death in this group of patients. ◆

Arrhythmias - Ventricular Premature Complexes and Fish Oil

Alois Sellmayer, M.D.
Institut fur Prophylaxe und
Epidemiologie der Kreislaufkrankheiten
Klinikum Innenstadt
University of Munich
Pettenkoferstrasse 9, 80336 Munich, Germany
49 89 51 60 43 50 / 49 89 51 60 43 52 (FAX)

"Effects of Dietary Fish Oil on Ventricular Premature Complexes,"
The American Journal of Cardiology, November 1, 1995;76:974-977. #23513

Kirk Hamilton: Could you please share with me your educational background and current position?

Alois Sellmayer: I went to medical school at the University of Munich, and subsequently spent a postdoctoral fellowship at the Massachusetts General Hospital in Boston. After I returned to Munich, I did my German equivalent to an American residency program at the University Hospital and currently continue my specialization in internal medicine. I have a long interest in the physiologic and pathophysiologic role of polyunsaturated fatty acids and eicosanoids in cardiovascular disease which originates from my doctoral thesis on leukotriene metabolism in neutrophils.

KH: When did you get interested in the role of fish oil and arrhythmias?

AS: I got interested in the role of polyunsaturated fatty acids and arrhythmias during my postdoctoral fellowship at the Massachusetts General Hospital where I met Dr. H. Hallaq who was working with neonatal cardiac myocytes, which rhythmically contracted like a beating heart in primary tissue culture. In this model, we observe that only omega-3 fatty acids inhibited the proarrhythmic effects of the glycoside ouabain. Based on these observations and the well documented antiarrhythmic effects of N-3 fatty acids in animal models, it was of great interest to us to evaluate the effect of omega-3 fatty acids on ventricular arrhythmias in humans.

KH: What are the potential mechanisms of the antiarrhythmic effects of fish oil?

AS: There is strong evidence that the active antiarrhythmic compounds in fish oil are the omega-3 fatty acids. The underlying mechanisms have not been completely identified, but recent studies indicate that N-3 fatty acids directly modulate electrophysiologic processes in the isolated cardiac myocytes. They reduce the resting membrane potential and extend the duration of the refractory period. These effects are probably due to the modulation of ion fluxes gated by ion channels or transporter enzymes. In addition, N-3 fatty acids may also increase cardiac oxygen supply by their vasodilatory and antiaggregatory effects and thus reduce the proarrhythmic potential.

KH: What did you find in your study regarding fish oil supplementation and ventricular premature complexes?

AH: In a randomized, placebo-controlled study in 68 patients without organic heart disease, we found that supplementation with fish oil for 16 weeks resulted in a greater decrease in ventricular premature complexes as compared to the placebo sunflower seed oil. Mean frequency of ventricular premature complexes decreased by 48% after fish oil versus 25% after placebo. The proportion of patients with a more than 70% reduction in ventricular complexes, a criteria commonly used to evaluate antiarrhythmic effects of drugs, was significantly higher in the fish oil group (44%) as compared to the placebo group (15%).

KH: What was the dose of fish oil and was this a high dose?

AS: The patients were supplemented with a total of 2.4 gm of omega-3 fatty acids (.9 gm eicosapentaenoic and 1.5 gm of docosahexaenoic acid) per day. This is a moderate dose of omega-3 fatty acids equal to the consumption of about 150 gm of fatty fish (mackerel) per day.

KH: Do you see fish oil as an adjunctive therapy for the treatment of arrhythmias in the future?

AS: Given that the currently available observations on the antiarrhythmic effects of fish oil are confirmed in additional trials, supplementation with omega-3 fatty acids may become an adjunctive therapy to the treatment of ventricular arrhythmias in the future. But I want to emphasize that controlled trials have to confirm the antiarrhythmic efficacy and safety of omega-3 fatty acids, especially in patients with higher grade arrhythmias and/or organic heart disease. Right now, it is clearly too premature to recommend fish oil for the treatment of cardiac arrhythmias except in controlled trials. Given that the antiarrhythmic effects of fish oil are confirmed in humans, it is intriguing to speculate that increasing fish consumption could be a rather cheap and tasty approach to the prevention of cardiac arrhythmias and their fatal outcome.

KH: What are the adverse consequences of fish oil supplementation?

AS: In our study, as well as in many other studies conducted with fish oil, no severe adverse effects have been observed. The most frequent side effects were a fishy after-taste and fishy hiccups. Care must be taken in patients with gallstones as the oil contracts the gallbladder and may mobilize stones. In addition, some studies indicate that higher doses of fish oil or omega-3 fatty acids may increase serum cholesterol levels in normo and hyperlipidemic patients and serum glucose in diabetic patients. Negative effects on infectious diseases or the cardiovascular system including proarrhythmic effects have not yet been reported. ◆

Arterial Occlusive Disease and Hyperhomocysteinemia

Coen D.A. Stehouwer, M.D.
Department of Internal Medicine
Institute For Cardiovascular Research
Free University Hospital
De Boelelaan 1117
1081 HV Amsterdam, The Netherlands
31 20 4440531 / 31 20 4440502 (FAX)

"Hyperhomocysteinemia and Endothelial Dysfunction in Young Patients With Peripheral Arterial Occlusive Disease," European Journal of Clinical Investigation, 1995;25:176-181. #22112

Kirk Hamilton: What is your educational background and present position?

Coen Stehouwer: I studied medicine at the Erasmus University in Rotterdam, The Netherlands, and received my degree in 1985. After that, I trained in internal medicine for 5 years, during which period I became involved in research on vascular and renal complications of metabolic diseases. I wrote a thesis on endothelial dysfunction in diabetes mellitus. At present, I am an assistant professor of medicine at the Free University in Amsterdam, the Netherlands.

KH: How did you get interested in the role of homocysteine and peripheral arterial occlusive disease?

CS: In the late eighties it became increasingly clear that even mild hyperhomocysteinemia was associated with an increased risk of atherosclerotic disease. In addition, mild hyperhomocysteinemia appeared to be quite common, especially in patients with renal disease, who are also prone to develop atherosclerotic disease. So we decided to get involved. At the same time, the vascular surgeons at our hospital also got interested and started screening for hyperhomocysteinemia in their patients. The present article is a result of the collaboration that evolved from this mutual interest.

KH: How did you get interested in the role of folic acid and vitamin B6 and hyperhomocysteinemia?

CS: It is well known that folic acid and vitamin B6 are often effective in preventing arterial and venous thrombosis in patients with very severe hyperhomocysteinemia, so-called classic homocystinuria. These vitamins are thought to stimulate homocysteine remethylation and transsulfuration, respectively. Thus, both decrease the levels of homocysteine which is thought to be the toxic metabolite.

KH: How important is the methionine challenge in discovering hyperhomocysteinemia?

CS: A contentious issue! Originally, the methionine challenge was used to identify heterozygous cystathionine - beta-synthase deficiency, which converts homocysteine into cystathionine, and which was thought to be the major cause of mild hyperhomocysteinemia in patients with premature atherosclerosis. It now appears that this is not the case. Mild hyperhomocysteinemia is probably determined by genetic and environmental factors (such as vitamin intake), and the dissection of the contribution of each of these factors is an active area of research.

So can we do without the methionine challenge? I don't think so. About 30 to 50% of patients with abnormally high homocysteine after methionine challenge have normal fasting levels. Post-methionine hyperhomocysteinemia is strongly associated with premature atherosclerosis. I would speculate that hyperhomocysteinemia is a mixed bag of metabolic disorders, and that fasting and post-methionine hyperhomocysteinemia do not necessarily represent the same metabolic problem.

KH: Where did you come up with the dosages of 250 mg of vitamin B6 and 5 mg of folic acid?

CS: Studies in classic homocystinuria had shown that very high doses of these vitamins might be effective. There were almost no data in mild hyperhomocysteinemia. A small study by Brattstrom and coworkers (Atherosclerosis, 1990;81:51-60) suggested that dosages in that range might be effective. So we decided to do a fairly large study with the highest dose that is considered safe for long-term use (reported in The J. Vasc. Surg., 1994;20:933-940). For folic acid, which is generally considered very safe, the upper limit is somewhat unclear but 5 mg is known to be well-tolerated. The main theoretical concern is neurotoxicity in patients with a vitamin B12 deficiency. To exclude this, we measured vitamin B12 levels in all patients. For vitamin B6, the main dose-limiting side effect is neuropathy, which is probably rare below 1 gm/day but has been reported with dosages as low as 300 mg/day.

KH: Have these individuals that are treated and have normalization of homocysteine and endothelial dysfunction been followed long enough to see if there is any regression of atherosclerosis and improvement of clinical symptoms?

CS: No, they have not. We are currently engaged in a much larger study that addresses these questions. By the way, our paper showed improvement, not normalization of endothelial dysfunction.

KH: Do you think there will be a day when almost all cardiovascular patients will be routinely supplemented with vitamin B6, folic acid and also vitamin B12 for normalization of homocysteine levels?

CS: This is very speculative. The homocysteine story is just beginning. Much more data are needed. In addition, it must be emphasized that the dosages we use, although effective in lowering homocysteine, are not necessarily optimal. We do not really know what a normal homocysteine level is.

KH: *Do you think that homocysteine is a more significant risk factor than cholesterol levels?*

CS: This is unclear, mainly because lipid research is much more advanced than homocysteine research. I certainly think that hyperhomocysteinemia is an underestimated risk factor. Fully 30% of young patients (less than 55 years of age) with atherosclerotic disease have hyperhomocysteinemia. Hyperhomocysteinemia may be involved not only in atherosclerosis, but also in venous thrombosis, preeclampsia, hypertension and neural tube defects.

KH: *Do you see a day when homocysteine levels will be routinely screened as are cholesterol levels for cardiovascular patients?*

CS: Yes, definitely so. I would be surprised if we had not reached that stage within 10 years from now. However, vitamin therapy needs to be shown to be clinically effective. The great thing is that it promises to be an extremely safe type of treatment. ◆

Asthma and Oxidant Stress

Lawrence S. Greene, Ph.D.
Department of Anthropology
University of Massachusetts at Boston
100 Morrissey Blvd.
Boston, MA 02125-3393 U.S.A.
(617) 287-6850 / (617) 265-7173 (FAX)

"Asthma and Oxidant Stress: Nutritional, Environmental and Genetic Risk Factors",
Journal of the American College of Nutrition, 1995;14(4):317-324. #23054

Kirk Hamilton: Could you please share with me your educational background and current position?

Lawrence Greene: I received my Ph.D. in biological anthropology from the University of Pennsylvania and I am currently an associate professor and director of biology of The Human Populations Program at the University of Massachusetts in Boston.

KH: When did you get interested in the role of oxidant stress and asthma?

LG: I became interested in the relationship between oxidant stress and asthma about 5 years ago. As a biological anthropologist one of my main interests has been the population genetics of glucose-6-phosphate dehydrogenase deficiency (G6PD deficiency), and particularly the mechanism by which G6PD deficient erythrocytes are relatively protected against malarial parasitization. This is the selective advantage of G6PD (-) individuals and the reason why G6PD (-) allele frequency is high in many populations living in areas where malaria is endemic. It turns out that G6PD (-) erythrocytes are relatively protected against malarial parasitization because they are particularly vulnerable to the oxidant stress that is produced by parasites. The G6PD (-) erythrocytes tend to lyse and thus interrupt the parasitic cycle. For a number of reasons this led to me wonder whether oxidant stress was the primary etiologic factor in the development of asthma.

KH: Can you explain how oxidant stress effects asthma?

LG: The erythrocyte, and all cells in the body, have several enzyme-catalyzed metabolic pathways that help defend against oxidant stress.   Vitamins with antioxidant activity function in a similar fashion. If oxidant stress from exogenous sources (pollutants or chemicals) or endogenous sources (as a result of the inflammatory response) overwhelms the enzyme-catalyzed and vitamin-based antioxidant defense, then cellular damage may take place.   An exacerbated inflammatory response may lead to cell membrane and receptor damage and to the consequent predominance of bronchoconstrictive mechanisms. The chronic inflammatory process may also produce antigen modification of a number of macromolecules with secondary immune involvement that tends to dominant asthma symptomatology. I am arguing that the oxidant-induced inflammatory changes are the primary events in asthma etiology and should be the focus of preventive strategies.

KH: What role does dietary selenium play in asthma?

LG: Selenium is a co-factor that is a necessary component for the biosynthesis of the enzyme glutathione peroxidase (GSH-Px). GSH-Px catalyzes the final step in the glutathione pathway in which reduced glutathione (GSH) reduces endogenous and exogenous oxidants and thus defends the cell (especially the red blood cell) against oxidant stress. A number of laboratory and clinical studies have shown that dietary deficiency of selenium leads to diminished GSH-Px activity and increased tissue vulnerability to oxidant stress. Other studies have demonstrated that asthmatic patients have lower platelet GSH-Px activity compared to non-asthmatic controls and that dietary supplementation with 100 mcg of sodium selenite for about 3 months can increase serum selenium levels, GSH-Px activity, and ameliorate asthmatic symptomatology.

KH: What role do vitamin C and E play in asthma incidence?

LG: Vitamin C is a water soluble antioxidant that is the most abundant antioxidant in the extracellular fluids lining the respiratory system. Therefore, on theoretical grounds, vitamin C nutriture should have a significant influence on asthma risk if oxidant stress is indeed associated with the development of asthma. A number of studies do support this view, although there also have been consistent negative findings. Data from the National Health and Nutrition Examination Survey (NHANES) indicate that in the general population low dietary vitamin C intake is associated with decreased pulmonary function, and similar findings have been reported in a recent general population survey in Nottingham, England. In contrast, data from the Nurses Health Study did not find a relationship between dietary vitamin C intake and the incidence of physician-confirmed asthma in this sample of adults. However, the Nurses Health Survey is not a study of naive subjects, and there is a strong possibility that those nurses who had respiratory symptoms had self-medicated themselves with vitamin C through both diet and nutritional supplementation, thus biasing the finding of this study. A number of clinical studies have found vitamin C supplementation to be beneficial in the treatment of asthmatic symptoms, although there also have been negative findings. The short duration of the supplementation has been a common fault in these investigations. Nitrogen oxides and other substances in cigarette smoke create a major oxidant stress and vitamin C appears to be an important defense against this challenge as well as against the high levels of nitric oxide exhaled by asthmatic patients. Vitamin C also has an important role in maintaining vitamin E in the reduced state.

Vitamin E is fat-soluble and is mainly sequestered in cell membranes and in other lipid structures. As noted above, it is believed that vitamin C has an important role in maintaining vitamin E in a reduced state. Vitamin E is a powerful antioxidant with a well-demonstrated ability to protect red blood cells against oxidant stress.

Therefore, on theoretical grounds, vitamin E nutriture should have a significant effect on antioxidant defense in the respiratory system and on asthma risk. However, there are only a limited number of useful studies evaluating the role of vitamin E nutriture and asthma risk. Recent data from the Nurses Health Survey suggest that the high dietary vitamin E intake was associated with a reduced asthma risk, but that vitamin E supplementation was not effective (perhaps because it began <u>after</u> the onset of symptomatology). Data from Nottingham, England showed a positive association between vitamin E intake and lung function in a large population survey, but this relationship did not appear to be independent of the effect of vitamin C.

KH: *What is the role of iron in asthma?*

LG: There is no established role of iron in asthma. However, most oxidants are relatively innocuous by themselves and only produce their deleterious effects as a consequence of iron- and copper-mediated free radical production. I thus have suggested that high body stores of iron and copper are likely to augment free radical production and may be a risk factor for the development of asthma. In support of this view is the observation that high iron body stores are associated with elevated cancer rates.

KH: *What type of environmental factors can effect asthma incidence?*

LG: There are a number of pollutants, components of cigarette smoke, and chemical exposures that are strong oxidants (sulfur dioxide, nitrogen oxides, halides) which may increase asthma risk. Exposure to allergens such as those associated with dust mite and various plant pollens also may precipitate asthmatic episodes in atopic individuals. However, I suggest that two very common environmental exposures may have a particularly significant effect on asthma risk. Environmental lead exposure appears to compromise several-enzyme-catalyzed reactions within the glutathione pathway, and thus greatly diminish cellular reducing capacity and antioxidant defenses. A number of heavy metal exposures may produce similar effects. Also, as noted above, iron is extremely important in free radical production. I have suggested that iron contamination of drinking water from rusting pipes may significantly elevate asthma risk.

KH: *What kind of genetic factors in different metabolic pathways can increase asthma incidence?*

LG: I believe that genetically-based decreased activity of the enzyme glucose-6-phosphate dehydrogenase (G6PD) is particularly important. This enzyme catalyzes the first step of the pentose phosphate pathway, and through the production of NADPH it initiates the glutathione pathway - which is one of the main cellular antioxidant defense systems. The genetic locus coding for G6PD is on the X-chromosome and it is the most highly polymorphic genetic locus in humans. This is probably because G6PD deficiency protects against *Falciparum malaria*, and a large number of deficient alleles have been selected for in human populations derived from tropical and subtropical regions, including the Mediterranean. Since G6PD deficient individuals manifest a decreased ability to deal with oxidant stress, particularly in the G6PD deficiency erythrocyte, I believe that they are at increased risk for the development of asthma. Genetically-based diminished glutathione reductase and glutathione peroxidase activity should also increase asthma risk.

KH: *In review can you summarize the factors from your viewpoint that are involved in asthma risk?*

LG: As noted above, there are a number of factors which influence asthma risk in my model: lowered cellular reducing capacity due to genetically-based decreased activity in G6PD and/or other enzymes catalyzing the various steps of the glutathione pathway; environmental exposures, such as lead, which should produce the same depressive effect on the generation of cellular reducing capacity and the glutathione pathway; increased free radical production due to elevated body stores of iron; dietary deficiency of selenium which may compromise the last step of the glutathione pathway and lower cellular reducing capacity; and lowered dietary intakes of the antioxidant vitamins such as vitamin C and E and beta-carotene. Minimizing lead exposure from household and water sources and excess iron intake from drinking water from rusting pipes would be beneficial within the context of this model. For what it is worth, I take 100 ug of selenium and 200 IU of vitamin E daily and I rely on my diet for adequate intakes of beta-carotene and vitamin C. ♦

Asthma and Polyunsaturated Oils

Linda Hodge, Dietitian M.Sc. (Med.) Grad. Dip. Nutr. & Diet
Royal Prince Alfred Hospital
A.C.N. 002 198 095
Camperdown NSW 20505, Australia
61 2 516 7026 / 61 2 550 6115 (FAX)

"Increased Consumption of Polyunsaturated Oils May Be a Cause of Increased Prevalence of Childhood Asthma," Australian New Zealand Journal of Medicine, 1994;24:727. #21648

Kirk Hamilton: Can you please share with me your educational background and current position?

Linda Hodge: I received a Bachelor of Science from the University of New England, Armidale, N.S.W. with a major in biochemistry. I completed this in 1981 and in 1982 completed a post graduate diploma in nutrition and dietetics at the University of Sydney. In 1993 I completed a Master of Science in Medicine also at the University of Sydney which was a research degree with thesis entitled "Asthma and Food Chemical Sensitivity". This degree was conferred in 1994. I am presently employed at the University of Sydney on a research project to examine the effect of dietary intakes of omega-3 and omega-6 fatty acids on asthma in children. I also have several private practices in which I specialize in food intolerance for asthma and other respiratory related diseases such as chronic rhinitis and otitis media.

KH: When did you become involved in the role of polyunsaturated oils and asthma?

LH: In 1993 I was invited by Cheryl Salome and Jennifer Peat of the Institute of Respiratory Medicine at the Royal Prince Alfred Hospital to conduct a study investigating the diets of children aged 8-11 years with and without asthma. Previous epidemiological studies by the Institute had found that children who ate a meal containing fish more than once each week had ⅓ the prevalence of asthma. However, because the only dietary question in these studies related to fish consumption, it was possible that fish consumption was merely a marker for some other dietary characteristic. In order to investigate this finding, we used a well validated food frequency questionnaire which included questions on more than 200 foods commonly consumed in Australia. We received nearly 500 completed questionnaires which represented a return of 81%. These questionnaires were analyzed for 39 nutrients and 24 separate food groups. The study was completed in mid 1994 and a paper has been submitted for publication. The results of this research stimulated my interest in the role of various polyunsaturated oils in the diet of young asthmatics.

KH: How do polyunsaturated oils relate to asthma incidence?

LH: Although polyunsaturated fats have many roles in the body, the one relevant to asthma is that of the production and stimulation of inflammatory mediators. The polyunsaturated fatty acids of importance in inflammation fall into 2 classes known as omega-6 and omega-3 fatty acids. The omega-6 fatty acid, linoleic acid, is an essential fatty acid, i.e.; it must be derived from the diet because it cannot be manufactured in the body and it is necessary for normal body functioning. Desaturation and elongation of linoleic acid results in the production of arachidonic acid. Alpha linolenic acid is also an essential fatty acid but belongs to the omega-3 class. Desaturation and elongation of alpha-linolenic acid results in the production of eicosapentaenoic acid. All of these fatty acids are stored in cell membranes and both omega-3 and omega-6 fatty acids can be utilized via the same biochemical pathways to produce leukotrienes and prostaglandins. These chemicals are released after appropriate stimulation, such as allergen invasion. When arachidonic acid is used as the substrate the leukotrienes and prostaglandins produced are more pro-inflammatory than when eicosapentaenoic acid is used as the primary substrate. The extent of the use of both arachidonic acid and eicosapentaenoic acid appears to be dependent on the relative concentrations of each within the cell membranes. Altering the dietary intake of linoleic acid and alpha-linolenic acid can change the relative concentrations of arachidonic acid and eicosapentaenoic acid in the cell membrane. Since one of the features of asthma is inflammation of the airways, it is possible that higher levels of arachidonic acid and linoleic acid in cell membranes could contribute to more cases of asthma. Major sources of linoleic acid are safflower, sunflower, cottonseed and corn oils. In the past 25 years people have been encouraged to use more of these oils because linoleic acid was shown in the late 1950's and early 1960's to effectively reduce blood cholesterol. A consequence of the increased consumption of these oils, is that the ratio of omega-3 to omega-6 fatty acids in the diet of Australians has increased from approximately 1:8 prior to the late 1960's to 1:30 as measured in the most recent national dietary survey in 1993. There have been similar changes in the fatty acid consumption patterns in most westernized countries with high rates of heart disease. This reduction in the ratio of omega-3 to omega-6 could conceivably cause higher levels of inflammatory mediators in susceptible individuals and thus contribute to the increasing prevalence of childhood asthma in these countries.

KH: Is there evidence that fish oils, which are a source of omega-3 fatty acids, can benefit asthma?

LH: Fish oils are an excellent source of the omega-3 fatty acid, eicosapentaenoic acid. There have been several studies of the use of fish oils in asthma and, although they have shown that the ratio of omega-3 to omega-6 in cell membranes can be altered, this change is not generally reflected by a change in the severity of the disease. Possible reasons for this failure are the short duration of the studies and the age of the subjects. It has been shown that fatty acids are recycled in the body and turnover time can be very slow. One study showed that the maximum effect of supplementation with fish oils was reached at 18 weeks, 10 weeks after supplementation was ceased. There is also the possibility that once the disease has been established for a number of years that it cannot be easily reversed and thus fish oil supplementation in adults may be ineffective. All of the previous studies have been with adults. The theory that we have put forward relates to the prevalence and incidence of the disease, not the severity. Increasing the omega-3 and decreasing the omega-6 may only be effective in the prevention of asthma, not treatment.

KH: Are there any other nutritional trends over the last 10-20 years which may also have affected childhood asthma"?

LH: There have been many changes over the past 10 to 20 years in our diets. We eat more foods prepared outside the home and more packaged, manufactured and processed foods. This can result in increased consumption of preservatives, artificial colors, artificial flavors and processing aids as well as a higher intake of sugar, salt and fat. A considerable amount of the research has been done on the effect of food chemicals, such as those added to foods, as triggers for asthma. But sensitivity to these chemicals appears to be confined to a relatively small number of asthmatics and there does not appear to be a role for these chemicals in the pathogenesis of asthma. On the other hand, increased salt consumption has been linked epidemiologically to asthma and it is known that inhaled saline solutions can provoke bronchoconstriction. However, studies of the ingestion of salt have not shown any effect. Reduced intakes of antioxidant vitamins and cofactors have been hypothesized as a possible cause of increasing rates of asthma. In Australia, which has one of the highest rates of childhood asthma in the world, vitamin intakes and particularly vitamin C, are higher than they were 20 years ago due to the introduction of fruit juices and a broadening of the variety of fruits and vegetables available all year round. Reduced intakes of certain minerals such as magnesium which act as cofactors have been linked to increases in asthma and several studies have found variable results. Our research does not support links between any vitamin or mineral deficiency in childhood asthma.

KH: How does one alter the ratio of omega-3 to omega-6 fatty acids?

LH: It is not difficult to alter the ratio of omega-3 to omega-6 fatty acids in the diet. It involves a simple change in the types of oils used in cooking, and spreads on breads from polyunsaturated to monounsaturated which have higher levels of omega-3 and lower levels of omega-6 fatty acids.

KH: What dietary or nutritional recommendations can you make in general to help reduce the likelihood of asthma?

LH: I am reluctant to make general public health recommendations at this stage because our hypothesis needs to be thoroughly tested. We have begun a study in children which will be completed in 2 years. When the results of this study are available, I may be able to make some firm recommendations. Until then, I would suggest that people eat a variety of fats just as they should eat a variety of foods, and follow the dietary guidelines as set out by their dietitians association. ◆

Atherosclerosis and Antioxidant Vitamins

Howard Hodis, M.D.
Atherosclerosis Research Unit
Division of Cardiology
University of Southern California
School of Medicine
2250 Alcazar St., CSC 132
Los Angeles, CA 90033 U.S.A.
(213) 342 1478 / (213) 342 2685 (FAX)

"Serial Coronary Angiographic Evidence That Antioxidant Vitamin Intake Reduces Progression of Coronary Artery Atherosclerosis," JAMA, June 21, 1995;273(23):1849-1854. #22666

Kirk Hamilton: Would you please share with us your present position and educational background?

Howard Hodis: I am an assistant professor of medicine and preventive medicine, and the director of the Atherosclerosis Research Unit in the Division of Cardiology at the USC School of Medicine. My training as a medical student, resident and chief resident were done here at the University of Southern California. Then I did a fellowship for two years with David Blankenhorn, M.D., the "father" of the field in which I do investigation today.

KH: When did you get interested in the role of antioxidants and coronary heart disease?

HH: We have been investigating mechanisms and other basic aspects of free radicals and antioxidant activity in the laboratory ever since I have been part of the faculty here at USC. Our interest has been around for quite awhile, and since we have available data sets from our clinical trials, we decided to take a look at the clinical implications of supplemental antioxidant vitamin intake.

KH: What is the theoretical benefit of antioxidants with respect to coronary artery disease?

HH: We would like to believe that antioxidants can prevent the formation of atherosclerosis or plaque development in those individuals who have not yet developed clinical symptoms. In those who already have clinical symptoms, we would hope that antioxidants prevent further worsening of their disease process.

KH: Is the major theorized mechanism the prevention of LDL oxidation, or are there other mechanisms?

HH: This is a commonly held hypothesis. However, there is no real direct evidence that this is how these agents work *in vivo* in humans. Clinical trials to clarify these and other issues are badly needed.

KH: Do you have an educated guess?

HH: I don't because antioxidants (depending on what the product is) have other effects also. They can affect the blood coagulation system by making thrombosis less likely. Thrombosis is the end result of the atherosclerosis process which usually leads to the acute coronary event, to the heart attack or chest pain. They also

can prevent oxidation of the cells of the arterial wall itself. There is a lot of *in vitro* evidence that they may work by inhibiting LDL oxidation, but there clearly is no direct evidence that this is how they may work in humans. So there is a whole gamut of activity that these products exhibit, and specific antioxidants also have specific effects.

KH: Can you tell us a little bit about your study (JAMA 1995;273(23):1849-1854) regarding serial coronary angiography, antioxidant vitamins and the progression of coronary artery atherosclerosis?

HH: Basically, the information that we published in JAMA was derived from a study that was conducted here at USC and published in 1987 in which 162 subjects finished a serial coronary angiographic trial. The study showed a very favorable effect in those individuals who took colestipol and niacin versus those who just took placebo. What was basically shown was less coronary artery disease change or worsening of coronary atherosclerosis. What we did was study the dietary database of this study because within that database, we have an extensive amount of information about dietary intake as well as supplemental nutrient intake including antioxidant vitamins. We asked the question, did those individuals who had high dietary and/or supplemental intake of antioxidant vitamins have less coronary artery disease progression? We went into the data set and found the answer to be yes. Subjects who took supplemental vitamin E had less coronary artery disease progression than those who did not take supplements (vitamin E), and this effect was specific for those who also were randomized to cholesterol lowering with colestipol and niacin in a very specific class of coronary lesions - those less than 50% diameter stenosis or what we call mild to moderate lesions. In the placebo group, there was a trend in those who took supplemental vitamin E also to have less coronary artery disease progression than those who did not. This however, didn't quite reach statistical significance. The significance of the effect in the mild to moderate lesions is that these lesions tend to rupture or release their lipids and thrombose or clot off and cause a heart attack and coronary death. So it appears from our data, which is the first to show this with angiographic evidence, that antioxidant vitamin supplements (vitamin E specifically) may indeed prevent the worsening of coronary artery disease in the specific lesions which have also been related to coronary events such as heart attacks and coronary death.

KH: What was the dose range that you found or the minimum dose requirement?

HH: This study was not designed to specifically study vitamin E supplementation. In looking at the data, we found that an intake of 100 to 440 I.U. per day was associated with less coronary artery disease progression.

KH: Was there no added effect if you had 800 I.U. per day?

HH: None were really taking that high a dose. Remember, this study was conducted in the early and mid 1980s. Megadosing is more of a recent phenomenon.

KH: In your study you said there was no benefit from vitamin C supplementation. Does not vitamin C help regenerate the oxidized form of vitamin E?

HH: There was no significant association, but there was a suggestion that the supplemental intake of vitamin C greater than 150 mg per day in that group was associated with less coronary artery disease progression. Vitamin C does regenerate the oxidized form of vitamin E and therefore, perhaps makes it more available for further antioxidant activity. We don't really know, however, if this mechanism operates *in vivo* in humans.

KH: What makes vitamin E special as an antioxidant if there is anything for vascular disease?

HH: I am not sure that it is special. I think that there has been a lot of emphasis on vitamin E. If you look at the epidemiological data you will see associations with vitamin C, beta-carotene and green leafy vegetables in general. So I am not sure if there is anything specific about vitamin E. I just think that it has gotten a lot of research associated with it and a lot of press. So we need to keep an open mind in this whole area of antioxidants as a possible way of preventing coronary artery disease and perhaps even intervening once it is established. We need to conduct clinical trials to better understand antioxidants and heart disease.

KH: How do you as a health professional who does this research protect yourself from vascular disease?

HH: Well in terms of what I do for myself, it is predominantly lifestyle - eating the proper foods in proper quantities and the proper proportions, in addition to exercising.

KH: Could you be more specific?

HH: I follow the American Heart Association Step I Diet which is really the dietary recommendations for the general population - a cholesterol intake of less than 300 mg a day and total fat intake of less than 30% of total calories divided by approximately 10% of each of the major fats, saturated, monounsaturated and polyunsaturated fats, and then combining all that with regular aerobic exercise at least 3 times per week of about 30 to 40 minutes duration.

KH: Do you take a vitamin E supplement?

HH: I won't answer that. I will tell you that as a scientist I think that the proof is still needed in properly designed trials. This means they need to be randomized, double blind, placebo controlled trials. And we need good, hard endpoint evidence to tell us that yes indeed they do have some effect either at the arterial wall level or in preventing coronary events. We don't have that information yet. There is the possibility that some of the information will come out soon. Other trials are getting under way. So I think, over the next 5 to 7 years, we're going to have some very hard evidence saying whether these products are going to be efficacious or not and how

we would like to see them become useful in the field of preventing atherosclerosis. ◆

Atopic Dermatitis and Food

Harris A. Steinman, M.B.,CH.B.,D.Ch.
Department of Clinical Sciences and Immunology
University of Cape Town, Observatory Cape Town
7990 South Africa
021 471250 (FAX)

"The Precipitation of Symptoms By Common Foods in Children With Atopic Dermatitis",
Allergy Proceedings, July-August 1994;15(4):203-210. #21366

Kirk Hamilton: *What is your educational background and present position?*

Harris Steinman: I received my medical training at the University of Cape Town's Medical School and Groote Schuur Hospital in Cape Town, South Africa (where the first heart transplant was performed). Following my internship at Addington Hospital in Durban, I trained in pediatrics at the Red Cross Children's Hospital in Rondebosch, Cape Town. I am presently based at the allergy unit, Department of Clinical Sciences and Immunology, Medical School, at the University of Cape Town. I am investigating the effect of sulphite preservatives and sulfur dioxide on children, and the role in the urbanization and the development of asthma. This project is sponsored by the South African Medical Research Council and will contribute to a doctorate in medicine degree.

KH: *When did you get interested in foods and how they effect atopic dermatitis?*

HS: I became interested in this area by accident. Although I am aware of the discomfort of a child with atopic dermatitis, I was struck by their suffering when investigating the usefulness of a new blood test in determining sensitivity to food in a large group of children with this disease.

KH: *How important is breast feeding in the prevention or treatment of atopic dermatitis?*

HS: Very. There is clear evidence that breast feeding decreases the risk of atopic dermatitis or ameliorates its severity. Breast feeding's effectiveness is increased if the mother follows a partially restricted diet. However, whether a child benefits from a maternal-restricted diet before birth remains inconclusive.

KH: *What are your recommendations on the optimal program to prevent atopic dermatitis for the breast-feeding mother with regards to duration of breast feeding and diet?*

HS: These recommendations are particularly important to a family with an atopic background to follow. The mother should breast feed for as long as possible. If supplemental milk is required, this should preferably be a hypoallergenic formula, and at the very least, a soy preparation. During this time, the mother should attempt to avoid eating products containing eggs, milk, fish or nuts. Calcium supplementation may be required by the mother and the child during this period. Weaning should be delayed until 6 months of age and egg and nuts should not be introduced until at least 24 months of age. I also recommend not introducing fish until 12 months of age. Some clinicians would also recommend a delay in introducing wheat products until 12 months of age.

KH: *What is the role of the elimination diet in atopic dermatitis?*

HS: Elimination diets can be very useful if applied intelligently. Research has shown that the skin prick tests (SPT) and blood tests such as the RAST are not always useful in determining which foods are responsible for the symptoms in these children, and my experience bears this out. If these tests have already been performed, then a strongly positive test should be accepted as true. The only effective test appears to be an elimination diet and/or a food challenge. However, to test a variety of foods can be very time consuming. I believe we, as clinicians, should attempt to NOT make the treatment worse than the disease. *In the child with established atopic dermatitis and on a general diet, I would recommend an elimination diet of 2 to 4 weeks -- removing egg, fish, milk, nuts, wheat, tomatoes, oranges, pineapple, chocolate and foods containing preservatives and additives such as soft-drinks. In our patients, foods such as cola drinks, peach, potato crisps and bananas were reported to result in symptoms, and I would include these to the list.* This still leaves a great variety of foods that can be eaten. Following an elimination of these foods, one can reintroduce these excluded foods 1 by 1 probably starting with a food that the parent believes is important to the child. The reintroduction should preferably take place in the doctor's room when dealing with children who have severe allergy. Hugh Sampson has documented exacerbation of atopic dermatitis with various "innocuous" foods, and I have found that some children react dramatically to an introduction of green peas and beans following an elimination diet of these 2 foods. Interestingly, on taking a history, these children do not appear to be effected by the green beans or peas.

KH: *What other environmental factors effect atopic dermatitis?*

HS: It is always important to remember that atopic dermatitis is a multifactorial disease. There is clear evidence that house dust mite and passive smoking plays a great role in this disease, and elimination of these 2 has resulted in a great improvement in children with this disease. Other factors that are important and often overlooked include the type of washing detergents being used and the use of deodorants and strong antiseptics. Parents should avoid bioenzyme washing soaps at all costs, using a mild washing powder instead. Fabric softeners should be avoided at all times. Clothing should be light and "breathable" and clothing and bedding made from wool must be avoided. Excess sweating, even at night, can result in increased symptoms. Finally, stress can affect atopic dermatitis in many children and hence this should be minimized. This is why I have said that the treatment should not be worse than the disease, and thus removing a food item from a child who is particularly fond of that food should be handled with great consideration or not be removed at all in some. The same applies to pets, as not all pets may be responsible for increased symptoms in these children. At the very least, the pet should not be allowed in the child's bedroom. In severe allergy, there is a place for asking friends to look after the animal for 1 to 2 weeks to evaluate the effect of the animal on the disease, and then deciding thereafter.

KH: *What is the role of intestinal permeability in atopic dermatitis patients?*

HS: I wish I could give an answer to that question. The mechanisms resulting in this disease remains elusive and does not follow the traditional IgE mechanisms as with many of the other allergic diseases. There is clear evidence that increased intestinal permeability does play a role, but it seems certain that there are many other mechanisms also operating.

KH: *What is the role of fatty acid supplementation in atopic dermatitis?*

HS: Fatty acid supplementation remains a controversial issue. Studies which have avoided methodological and other faults, as in many of the earlier studies, have shown no benefit from these preparations. However, if a mother tells me that her child has benefited from these preparations, then I will be inclined not to disagree, as I will be happy with anything that helps -- including a placebo effect on secondary stress relief. As far as other nutritional remedies are concerned, there has been no uniform clinical acceptance of any, and as yet, I do not have faith in any.

KH: *Is there a problem in atopic dermatitis patients with the body's ability to metabolize fatty acids?*

HS: This is a paradox. There is clear evidence that the body is unable to metabolize these fatty acids appropriately, and there is in-vitro evidence that a variety of cells benefit from fatty acid supplementation. It is possible that a second component is required for fatty acid supplementation to be of benefit, but this part of the jigsaw has eluded us. As it is, we do not have a clear and certain hypothesis explaining the pathogenesis of atopic dermatitis.

KH: *What is the role of pathogens in the gut in atopic dermatitis?*

HS: This remains a controversial area and as such I cannot comment except to point out that any illness or infection can exacerbated atopic dermatitis. ◆

Atrial Fibrillation and Magnesium

Michael A. Brodsky, M.D.
University of California Irvine Medical Center
Division of Cardiology
101 The City Dr. South, Bldg. 53, Route 81
Orange, CA 92668-3298 U.S.A.
(714) 456-6545 / (714) 456-8895 (FAX)

"Magnesium Therapy in New-Onset Atrial Fibrillation",
The American Journal of Cardiology, June 15, 1994;73:1227-1229. #20387

Kirk Hamilton: Could give me some background information regarding your education and your present position.

Michael Brodsky: I went to medical school at the University of Illinois. I completed an internship, residency and part of a cardiology fellowship at UCLA Hospital. I then took fellowship in cardiology, specifically in cardiac arrhythmias at the Lown Cardiovascular Laboratory and Brigham and Womens Hospital. In 1982, I took a job at the University of California at Irvine initially as an assistant professor of medicine. My current title is associate professor of medicine in the Department of Medicine and Division of Cardiology. I am also director of the Cardiac Arrhythmia Service, which I initiated 12 years ago and continue to supervise.

KH: Before you discuss your research regarding atrial fibrillation and magnesium therapy can you describe what atrial fibrillation is?

MB: Atrial fibrillation is the most common cardiac tachyarrhythmia seen in elderly population. Approximately 1% of people under the age of 60 have atrial fibrillation, but upwards of 5% to 10% of the population over the age of 65 have it. Some of the people who have had atrial fibrillation include Presidents Nixon and Bush.

KH: Did either one of them get magnesium?

MB: I have no idea what the treatments were for either of them. Most doctors do not consider magnesium in this situation. We have done a questionnaire asking doctors how often they obtain magnesium levels. We asked 200 arrhythmia specialists, 350 cardiologists and 350 internists and found magnesium is not a commonly ordered test. Only about 20% of doctors recognize this test should be ordered with regards to atrial fibrillation.

KH: Serum levels are said to be relatively inaccurate as far as body storage of magnesium, but what other means of magnesium assessment would you recommend?

MB: Because I am a cardiologist, I am interested in the magnesium content in the heart. Short of a myocardial biopsy, one can get only estimates of the level of the heart by a whole range of different tests including magnesium levels in the serum, red blood cells, lymphocytes and in the skeletal muscle. The serum levels of magnesium have a very weak correlation with what is in the heart. However, it is easy to obtain a serum magnesium level so we rely upon it. The way to interpret a serum level of magnesium is if the serum level of magnesium is low, then the level of magnesium in the heart is almost certain to be low. If the serum level is high, you have

a reasonable chance the level of magnesium in the heart is at least adequate. The problem comes when the serum level is within the normal range. The way to tell more definitively is to give somebody a magnesium load (a couple of grams of magnesium intravenously) then measure how much is eliminated in the urine. If a great deal was retained then they were probably deficient.

KH: What is the problem with conventional digoxin therapy in new onset atrial fibrillation?

MB: In atrial fibrillation the top chambers (atria) are beating greater than 500 times per minute. The central electrical part (AV node) regulates impulses to the bottom part (ventricles). Most people with atrial fibrillation complain their heart rate is too fast. The goal is to slow the heart rate by blocking the AV node. The AV node is a complexed structure with different channels. Digoxin controls some of the activity through the AV node but it doesn't completely control all impulses through the AV node. For example, if the adrenaline level is very high, digoxin may not work. Most doctors are doing something in addition to digoxin. Recent research has shown digoxin by itself is not very effective. It takes a long time to work and when people look at it critically it has a narrow toxic therapeutic ratio. Alternative or additional therapy to digoxin includes drugs to block adrenaline or block the calcium channels. Beta blocker therapy blunts the effects of adrenaline and slows the heart rate. Another class of drugs are calcium channel blockers, notably verapamil or diltiazem. These drugs work in addition to digoxin and control the ventricular response to atrial fibrillation by slowing the activity in the calcium channel.

KH: Why did you even look at magnesium?

MB: We thought to try magnesium for a few reasons. First of all, magnesium might be nature's physiologic calcium channel blocker. The second reason is that magnesium has its own unique property which may be over and above the calcium channel blocker effect by stabilizing the heart muscle membranes. Thirdly, it is very easy to use, has a very wide toxic therapeutic ratio, and is very cheap. So, we attempted to use magnesium in addition to digoxin and we found it was superior to solitary digoxin therapy in terms of slowing down the heart rate, converting patients to their normal sinus rhythm and long-term 24 hour control of their symptoms.

KH: In your study in the American Journal of Cardiology, June 15, 1994 you talked about taking 18 patients with new onset atrial fibrillation of less than 7 days duration and your initial dose of magnesium (in addition to digoxin) was 2 gm over 15 minutes and then another 8 gm over the next 6 hours?

MB: I think it is important to tell your readers that I started with these numbers (magnesium dosage) in a prospective fashion. I was somewhat arbitrary. If I had this to do over again or if I had to advise clinicians, I would suggest being more selective and individualized in treatment. I think the dose was very appropriate for most of the patients, but it was probably a little too much for some of the elderly people. The second thing is when I mention the dose, I think the initial dose was no problem. It is the overall dose that was the problem. So I think 2 gm in 15 minutes is totally benign without any question. Up to 5 gm total over 5 hours is also usually benign. But once you start getting over the 5 gm total in 5 hours, you start to be a little concerned, particularly in the elderly and those with reduced renal function.

KH: *The 2 gm initial dosage of magnesium seems to be used frequently for heart attacks.*

MB: This dose of magnesium has been used in acute myocardial infarction, and sustained supraventricular and ventricular tachycardia. Magnesium is actually very well tolerated.

KH: *I would like to get into the side effects a little bit. Magnesium causes flushing, hypotension if you give it too quickly and you mentioned people with renal insufficiency. Are there any other concerns?*

MB: Flushing was uncommon in this study because we gave it very, very slowly. You only see flushing if you give it quickly such as 2 gm in less than 2 minutes. People feel a little fatigued when their level gets about 3.5 meq/L. If you get over a 3 meq/L, it is probably time to cut back. When you give magnesium, you have a tendency to reduce the level of potassium in the serum. You've got to be concerned about that. We made sure we continued to give potassium in all these patients and had an independent observer checking potassium to make sure it was more than 4 meq/L.

KH: *Maybe I am a little confused but I have read there are individuals with a low serum potassium level and when you replete them with magnesium, their potassium will go up. That is the opposite of what you just said.*

MB: Not the opposite. Once you give a large bolus of magnesium it has a transient tendency to cause a depression in serum potassium.

KH: *Does it go intracellularly?*

MB: Exactly where it is going I don't know. Magnesium is responsible for sodium potassium ATPase function. If people are deficient in magnesium, they are deficient in this enzyme, which may be associated with hypokalemia. If you replace their magnesium, you may normalize that enzyme, therefore restoring good potassium balance. This is not necessarily true with everybody.

KH: *Once these people are under control with the initial intravenous dose, do you ever give them oral supplements of magnesium when they go home?*

MB: That's a good question. There are very few people in whom the only reason they have atrial fibrillation is because of an electrolyte problem. I usually treat people with more than just magnesium supplements. Typically, people get digoxin chronically or they may get other treatments. But I will tell you up front that with most people, regardless of the basic therapy, I find that adding magnesium to their medical regimen helps control their arrhythmia problem. If, for example, they have recurrent atrial fibrillation, having them have an adequate magnesium level is always helpful to control their problem.

KH: *Can you highlight your concerns about diuretics? Are there any that really aggravate magnesium wasting?*

MB: Hydrochlorothiazide is probably the diuretic most likely to cause a low magnesium level. Unfortunately, it is in just about every combination drug such as all the ACE inhibitors or beta blockers connected with diuretics. What I also find is that when one is on a combination diuretic, the additional drug designed to prevent a low potassium like dyrenium or amiloride or aldactone, isn't strong enough to prevent the potassium and magnesium wasting occurring with the use of hydrochlorothiazide. What I commonly do in patients prone to low magnesium levels is I will stop their diuretics entirely or I will just give them dyrenium by itself. If I feel they need a regular diuretic, I would give them lasix. I think it is not as powerful as hydrochlorothiazide in causing magnesium wasting.

KH: *What is the oral magnesium dose you give?*

MB: Many people have a hard time taking any more than 6 magnesium tablets a day. There are two commonly available magnesium preparations. Mag Tab has about 7 mEq (86 mg) a tablet and Slow Mag has 5 mEq (62 mg). So the most elemental magnesium I have ever been able to get into anybody orally is about 42 mEq (517 mg) a day.

KH: *One of the most fascinating things in your article is the cost comparisons of magnesium with other medications. This is especially timely in light of the current debate regarding health care reform and expenditures. You share that a standard 24 hour therapy of 6 gm of Esmolol costs $400, 300 mg of diltiazem is $200, 10 gm of magnesium sulfate is $1 and 2 mg of digoxin is $2. The obvious question is why aren't more physicians open to using magnesium and why aren't the bodies that are concerned about health care costs encouraging the use of magnesium?*

MB: I would answer that in one word - advertising. There is nobody out there advertising magnesium's benefit because there is no money to be made on it.

KH: *And, that's why?*

MB: One reason is that companies advertise is because they want to make money. Why would anybody advertise Diltiazem? Because the company that owns it stands to profit every time there is some sold. But who is profiting when magnesium is sold? Nobody, because it isn't patentable. I believe magnesium is as safe and effective as those other drugs, as I pointed out in the article. You're asking me why magnesium isn't used more often and it is because doctors aren't being educated about it. Hopefully, that is one of the things that you will do.

KH: *You made a comment about the FDA clouding things with regards to nutrients. Do you want to elaborate on that?*

MB: There seems to be a trend for the FDA to regulate vitamins and supplemental agents such as magnesium, requiring people to do extensive scientific research to support claims which may end up reducing their availabilities to people. I think that might be a bad trend. I did this magnesium research myself. Nobody paid me to do this and hopefully I am giving people a sense that magnesium may have some value. Will the FDA look at this and suddenly approve this? Probably not. The only way the FDA will encourage labeling on a product is if there is extensive scientific study about it. There is no company or lobby to support that type of work on these compounds that are off patent.

KH: Yet there is enough in your mind to obviously use it scientifically?

MB: With this compound yes. I can't say there is enough out there to sanction giving anything what anybody wants. But, I think with magnesium there was enough evidence to support my completing this work and I felt that it was born out with the beneficial result. ◆

Back Pain and Exercise

Vert Mooney, M.D., Professor of Orthpedics

University of California San Diego
School of Medicine, Orthomed,
4150 Regents Park Row, Suite 300
La Jolla, CA 92037 U.S.A.
(619) 550-3494 / (619) 452-7135 (FAX)

"Why Exercise For Back Pain? Activity Reverses Biochemical Changes Caused by Injury?",
The Journal of Musculoskeletal Medicine, October, 1995:33-39. #23397

Kirk Hamilton: Could you please share with us your educational background and current position?

Vert Mooney: I graduated from Columbia University Medical School in 1957 and had training in orthopedic surgery at the University of Pittsburgh from 1960-1964. Since that time I have held various academic positions as an assistant professor at the University of Southern California, professor and chair of orthopedic surgery at the University of Texas Southwestern Medical School from 1977-1988, and finally here at the University of California, first at Irvine, and now at the University of California at San Diego. I am currently a Professor of Orthopedic Surgery and medical director of the University of California San Diego Spine and Conditioning Center.

KH: What is the current recommendation for low back pain as far as bed rest versus mobilization?

VM: The current recommendation for treatment of low back pain is gradual, progressive mobilization. All evidence points to the fact that bed rest prolongs the problem and offers no potential for therapeutic advantage.

KH: What is the actual physiology of an injured disc?

VM: The physiology of an injured disc is that the local metabolism is disturbed. Exchange of fluid within the disc is diminished. The disc is largely avascular and nutrition to the cells is only achieved by diffusion of fluid within the disc. The inflammation results in the diminished exchange of metabolic byproducts and thus an acid environment emerges.

KH: Why is mechanical movement so important in reducing pain?

VM: The mechanical movement is important in reducing pain within the disc as defined by the patient's description of pain location before and after repeated stretching exercises usually in extension. If the pain centralizes in the mid back from peripheral locations in the legs, this is an appropriate type of exercise. This is known as the McKenzie exercise program.

KH: What is the actual mechanism of pain within the disc?

VM: The mechanism of pain within the disc is increased intradiscal pressure and associated fall in pH due to swelling of the proteoglycans. This irritates the nerves at the periphery of the disc. The appearance of degenerative changes radiographically or even by discography does not necessarily indicate that the disc is painful. The only way one can determine that pain in the disc is created by local reactive inflammation is through pain response at discography.

KH: What is the role of pH in disc pain?

VM: Our research has indicated that in individuals who have no pain in the disc, even though the disc is degenerated, the pH within the disc is alkaline. In all patients who had painful discs, the pH was slightly acidic. This can be corrected for a short term by an injection of cortisone.

KH: Assuming that mobilization helps, could this in part explain the benefit of chiropractic or osteopathic care in early, acute back pain?

VM: It is clear that mobilization helps and obviously chiropractic and osteopathic care early offer a benefit for acute back pain. The assumption, although not established scientifically, is that mobilization of the tissues either in the disc or the facet joint creates a better environment for fluid exchange.

KH: What kind of stretching should be encouraged for back pain?

VM: The stretching for back pain patients should be the type of repeated gentle stretching which does not make the pain proceed further down the leg or does not become more intense. This usually is repeated extension exercise, although in about 10% of the people evaluated, flexion exercises are most appropriate. These stretching exercises should be repeated frequently to improve the end range.

KH: Have studies evaluated exercise and the return to work?

VM: Studies regarding rapid return to work after exercise have not been accomplished. There are many studies focused on exercise and the treatment of chronic back pain, but return to work is often a blurred criteria in that many other factors, other than pain reduction, correlate with an return to work under the worker's compensation system.

KH: Is there a point where exercise has a diminishing return if people wait too long before instituting the program?

VM: There is no point where exercise has diminishing returns. In most people tested with chronic back pain there is diminished strength in lumbar extension. Testing should specifically evaluate this and individuals should proceed with exercise until their range of motion and extension strength returns to normal. Flexibility and strength to the spine are always a favorable condition. In general, this can only be achieved and maintained by continued exercise focused at both flexibility and strength. ◆

Behavior, Cognition and Sugar (Con)

Mark L. Wolraich, M.D.
Vanderbilt University Medical Center
Child Development Center
Department of Pediatrics
426 Medical Center South
Nashville, TN 37232-3573 U.S.A.
(615) 930-0249 / (615) 936-0256 (FAX)

"The Effect of Sugar on Behavior or Cognition in Children: A Meta-Analysis,"
JAMA, November 22/29, 1995;274(20):1617-1622. #23659

Kirk Hamilton: Could you please share with me your educational background and current position?

Mark Wolraich: I am a developmental and behavioral pediatrician. I went to medical school in SUNY, the Syracuse Health Science Center, where I also completed my internship. I completed my residency at the University of Oklahoma Health Sciences Center and completed a fellowship in Developmental Pediatrics at the University of Oregon Health Science Center. I was a faculty member at the University of Iowa for 14 years. I am currently a professor of pediatrics, and chief of the division of Child Development at Vanderbilt University.

KH: When did you get interested in the role of sugar and behavior?

MW: I became interested in the role of sucrose, behavior and cognition in the early 1980's.

KH: Can you please share with me the general results of your study?

MW: I have actually been involved in 5 studies which have been reported in a total of 3 articles. The first involved 2 studies where we challenged children with Attention Deficit Hyperactivity Disorder with drinks that were sweetened with a large amount of sugar (sucrose) or with an artificial sweetener (aspartame) and then observed their behavior within a 5 hour period after ingestion. The first study entailed giving the drinks 1 hour after a standard lunch. The second entailed giving the drinks after an overnight fast. I was then involved in 2 studies where we actually kept the children on diets for 3 week periods -- one high in sucrose or two low in sucrose but sweetened with aspartame or saccharine. The first of these 2 studies entailed normal preschool children and the second study entailed children who were elementary school age and whose parents thought they were adversely affected by sugar. The most recent report was a meta-analysis of all existing controlled studies.

KH: Why would parents feel so strongly that sugar does have an effect on their children's behavior and yet this study does not bear this out.

MW: As we indicated in our last article, I suspect the parents have strong beliefs about the effect of sugar ingestion, despite the fact it has not been confirmed by rigorous study. Children generally receive large quantities of sugar at times of excitement such as Halloween or birthday parties, when there is a change in their routine and also at times when they are more likely to be fatigued.

In addition, suggestion can be a very potent force. There has been a great deal in the lay press about sugar affecting behavior. One study undertaken by Hoover and Milich demonstrated the effect of suggestion on belief about sugar. They took a group of children whose parents thought their children were adversely as affected by sugar and challenged them with artificial sweeteners, but half the parents were told their children were being challenged with sugar. The researchers found significant differences in the parents' ratings of children when the parents believed the child was challenged with sugar. They noticed their children as significantly worse and in addition, observations of the parents' behavior found the parents who thought their children received sugar, stayed closer to their children and were more demanding of the children. The effect size in this study was larger than the effect size in any of the studies of sugar we analyzed.

KH: Did these studies evaluate the immediate effect of sugar or did they evaluate whether children who consumed sugar might have a delayed effect which might even be depressive in nature?

MW: All but two of the studies were immediate challenges which measured the effects up to 3 to 5 hours after the challenge. The 2 studies that I completed, and described above, actually kept the children on diets high in sugar, or low in sugar with artificial sweeteners added, for 3 week periods each.

KH: Are you aware of the work by Dr. Larry Christiensen from the University of Southern Alabama showing that sugar and caffeine consumption appear to have a delayed effect of fatigue and depression days after ingestion?

MW: I am not aware of the work of Larry Christiensen.

KH: Have you ever empirically, in your clinical practice as a pediatrician, told children to remove simple carbohydrates such as added sugars, candies, fruit juices or other concentrated sources of simple carbohydrates to see what effect this might have in their behavior?

MW: In my clinical practice, I do not recommend dietary changes because I do not think the objective evidence has demonstrated that it is a worthwhile effort. In the clinical situation, where one does not control for expectation effects, it is difficult to evaluate actual effects.

KH: I understand that the results of your study are negative with regards to the fact that sugar might effect behavior or cognition in general, but from your experience as a pediatrician and/or parent, have you ever observed simple sugars in any way affecting behavior in a hyper or a somnolent manner?

MW: I have not been impressed that sugar has had any particular effect, or diet changes have any particular effect on children. My impression is, that many of the parents who report this phenomenon do not resolve their child's behavior problems with dietary changes alone, and these children require other intervention as well.

KH: Would you suspect that there is a difference in a behavioral response to a simple sugar when it is consumed in a whole food diet, rich in fruits, vegetables and whole grains, compared to a diet where there is lots of refined foods, soft drinks, pastries, refined flour products and lack of vegetables?

MW: Sugar such as glucose, fructose, or sucrose are essentially the same from a chemical standpoint, whether they are in fruits, vegetables or refined foods and soft drinks. Fruits initially contain fructose, but the quantity changes depending on the age of the fruit. In addition, many foods with supplemented sweeteners will be sweetened primarily with fructose from corn sweeteners.

KH: Do you think that there is enough interest in the topic of sugar and behavior to be studied further?

MW: With regard to children, it was a challenge for me to obtain funding for the studies that I did because the impression in the scientific community is that the phenomenon does not exist. In the face of the overwhelming evidence to date, that sugar does not seem to be related to behavior in children, I doubt that it will be possible to find further support for these type of studies.

KH: What changes in study design would you make if you could do a study?

MW: With regard to changes in design for the study of the behavioral effects of sugar it is always possible to come up with additional recommendations, but I think that the studies that have been completed to date have employed rigorous designs and have utilized the parameters suggested by the clinical reports of effects. ◆

Behavior, Cognition and Sugar (Pro)

Doris Rapp, M.D.
Associate Professor
State University of New York, Buffalo
Pediatric Allergist
Environmental Medicine Specialist
2757 Elmwood
Kenmore, NY 14217 U.S.A.
(716) 875-5578 / (716) 875-5399 (FAX)

8157 East Del Cuarzo
Scottsdale, AZ 85258 U.S.A.
(602) 905-9195 / (602) 905-8281 (FAX)

"Does Diet Affect Hyperactivity,"
<u>Journal of Learning Disabilities</u>, 1978;11:56-64. #24068
<u>Journal of Learning Disabilities</u>, 1979;12:42-50. #24067

Kirk Hamilton: Could you please share with me your educational background and current position?

Doris Rapp: I am a board certified pediatric allergist and environmental medical specialist. I have a bachelor's degree (magna cum laude), a master's degree and a medical degree. I practiced pediatric allergy exclusively for the first 20 years and then environmental medicine for the next 20 years.

KH: When did you get interested in the role of sugar and behavior?

DR: It all began when a youngster came into our office who was so hyperactive I could not examine her. I placed the child on a diet and there was a miraculous change within just 2-3 days. At that point I realized that foods could be a factor related to some individual's behavior and activity. I then worked with Buffalo Children's Hospital dietitians and they helped me devise a diet that excluded the foods which, according to the literature, were most apt to cause activity, behavior and learning problems. These were mainly the foods mentioned in Dr. Rowe's book published repeatedly between the late 1920s and the 1950s entitled, <u>Food Allergy.</u> In that book he clearly refers to many of the kinds of problems we are seeing today and relates it directly to various foods, and sugar is certainly one of them.

KH: Why would parents feel so strongly that sugar does have an affect on their children's behavior, yet most academic researchers feel there is no good evidence that this is the case?

DR: Parents certainly do believe that sugar affects their children's behavior because they can see that their children become wild on holidays (Halloween, Valentine's Day, large parties) after they eat too much candy. The problem is that the parents are not as discerning or as discriminating as physicians would be. They know that a candy bar or sugar dyed cereal causes hyperactivity, but they simply are not able to discern exactly what is causing the kind of reactions they are seeing. They assume it is sugar but don't consider the corn syrup, dyes, artificial flavor, wheat, nuts, chocolate, peanut butter, etc.

The academic scientists, however, are erring in the other direction when they say that sugar doesn't cause trouble. For example, in a study published in the <u>New England Journal of Medicine</u>, February 3, 1994;330(5):301-307 entitled **"Effects of Diets High In Sucrose or Aspartame on Behavior and Cognitive Performance in Children"**, errors in methodology appear to be present. First, the patients were said to be selected because the parents "believed" they were sensitive to sugar. These children could have been sensitive to any other food ingredient that was combined with the sugar and this should have been considered. By excluding sugar from the childrens' diet <u>in every single form</u> for about 1-2 weeks and then re-adding sugar in a large amount on an empty stomach (plain cane sugar, or any other kind of sugar the child usually eats) and then observing carefully. Only those who reacted to sugar should have been used as a subset of children for the evaluation of sugar sensitivity in this study. Secondly, the children were placed on 3 different diets for 3 weeks each. It appears that all 3 diets contain some sucrose and saccharine. One diet contained aspartame with low sucrose and low saccharine, the second diet contained high saccharine and low sucrose, and the third diet contained high sucrose and low saccharine.

The design stated that 1 diet is high in sucrose with no artificial sweeteners, but later in the article it stated, "small amounts of saccharine were used to sweeten items such as condiments . . . " during the nine weeks that the three different diets were administered. *It is not how much, but how sensitive,* children are to a substance that determines whether they have a symptom or not. Due to possible different levels of tolerance to these two various items (sucrose and saccharine), ihereforet would be very difficult to determine what is causing what.

There is another study published in 1978 which gave children 24 grams of food dyes. It is stated that most children eat much more food coloring than this each day. Some children need a minuscule amount and others need a large amount before they react adversely to a food. Challenging, therefore, needs to be quantified. You must know whether children are sensitive to a substance and how sensitive they are to a certain amount of that substance -- how much they can tolerate without difficulty.

In addition, children were watched for 15-60 minutes after eating. This does not take into account a child who has a delayed reaction. It is difficult for parents to get a global impression at the end of a week about a child's activity if the child became hyperactive on Tuesday and the parent didn't score the child until Saturday night. They might not remember much about the child being hyper on Tuesday. It is very difficult to rate violent outbursts if they happen repeatedly unless you are monitoring very, very carefully on a daily basis. Even then it can be a challenge. How would you rate the activity of a child who has one severe 5 minute episode on Tuesday and a mild to moderate reaction all day long on Thursday?

One must also ask who paid for any food-related research. I think it is somewhat interesting that the food industry paid for many of the studies that found sugar didn't cause trouble, while the food industry had no input in other studies that found sugar was a problem.

There is another study in which dyes were put into capsules but it wasn't mentioned in the methodology that the children would not swallow the capsules unless they were coated in chocolate. This immediately negates this study because you may have children who are possibly sensitive to chocolate used on the placebo, as well as the challenging item. I only found this out when I asked the investigator how does a five-year-old comply with swallowing capsules. It is a very practical question. The "Gold Standard" must be "Gold". Too many articles put the sample to be studied "substance A" in some "substance B", but never check to see if "substance B" causes any difficulty.

It is also of interest to note that most of the references in studies that are negative about foods causing hyperactivity and behavior problems neglect to mention a number of positive studies that indicate sugar can cause hyperactivity and behavior problems.

KH: Does sugar have an immediate or a delayed effect on behavior?

DR: It could be either. Some children will react within a few minutes and others might not react for about an hour. There's an occasional child who doesn't react for 6-8 hours after they ingest sugar. There is a marked individual variation and, once again, it depends upon a number of factors that aren't really controlled well in most studies. The child should ingest the sugar on an empty stomach. You should know how much sugar the child has to ingest before symptoms are noted. The sugar should be ingested at 5-12 day intervals as pointed out in Dr. Rinkel, Randolph and Zeller's book which was published in the 1950s. They found that you must not ingest a suspect food for 5-12 days prior to the challenge to detect a suspect food allergy. A reaction to a food therefore can depend on how much time has elapsed since the suspect food was eaten. If several weeks have elapsed a child might not obviously react to a food even though it is a problem. If, however, there is a short interval of time, 5-12 days, then you'll see a definite cause and effect relationship which is usually *exaggerated or worse* than the typical response that you see in an individual. If you eat a food that causes allergies every single day, you may not notice symptoms. This frequency causes masked food allergies so you won't spot or recognize the cause and effect relationships. I'm sorry to admit that I missed the detection of food allergies for 20 years because I did not realize the significance of the previous stated information. I must

also state that this is a persistent error which continues to be made in the design of studies which are taking place at the present time. Researchers also tend to neglect the importance of whether a substance is ingested on a full or an empty stomach.

KH: What are the effects of sugar on behavior and cognition and where is the evidence?

DR: In my mind, sugar can affect almost any area of the body, one being its effect on the brain, causing behavior and learning problems. There's a simple way to sort what it does and that is to eat the food in a large amount on an empty stomach after you haven't had it for 5-12 days. Before a child ingests the food: 1) Check the child's pulse, 2) Use a peak flow meter if asthma is a concern (800-787-8780), 3) Check the child's writing, 4) Check the child's appearance (Does the child have red ear lobes, wiggling legs and bright red cheeks or nose rubbing, which are made worse when rubbed?), 5) Check how the child feels (Is there a headache, a muscle ache, or a belly ache? Is there an urgent need to urinate? Can he or she concentrate? Is reading or writing a problem?), 6) Then check the child again in 15 minutes, 45 minutes and 1-1/2 hours after the suspected food has been consumed. Ingest a large amount on an empty stomach. Don't do this if you expect an anaphylactic reaction, since that is a life-threatening problem. But if there is a history of mild to moderate complaints, I certainly wouldn't hesitate to do it. The evidence is in the literature, but may not deal specifically with the relationship to sugar. If a mother says, "My child is hyperactive from sugar." I'd say, "Fine, show me. Don't give your child a speck of sugar in anything for 5-12 days, read every label, bring your child in, and on an empty stomach, when no food has been eaten for at least 4-6 hours, feed your child 6-8 sugar cubes. See what happens." Sometimes nothing happened. Other times we had a "whiz bang" within a few minutes and the mother said, "That's what I've been telling the doctors and they don't believe me."

KH: Do you routinely instruct your pediatric patients to avoid simple sugars, and what do you define as a sugar?

DR: Actually, there are different kinds of sugars and it's possible to be sensitive to cane sugar and not to beet sugar and visa versa. Dr. Randolph wrote about this years ago. There are corn, beet, date, turbinado and maple sugars and you really need to find out what kind of sugar a child eats. The bottom line is what bothers a specific child and not most children. So you check them with the kind of sugar that they ingest and you give it to them at a 5-12 day interval. I check for simple sugars along with a number of other foods by merely putting them on a diet for one week that excludes the major highly allergenic foods, and then we add these foods back (one at a time, one each day during the second week of the diet from the eighth to the fourteenth day). During that second part of the diet you can readily see which food causes what. If anyone wants a copy of that diet, all they have to do is contact (716) 875-5578 and we'll be glad to mail them one. I define sugar only as a sweetener. But once again, one could be more precise and I'm sure that these sugars are more different than most people realize. Some people will be sensitive to one type and not the other. Saccharine and aspartame need to be checked in a similar fashion.

KH: Do you feel these reactions to sugar are a true allergy or a metabolic response to the sugar?

DR: It depends on how you define allergy. I don't think it's always a true IgE-mediated allergy. I say this because sometimes they will not have an elevated IgE for sugar but a patient will have an elevated IgG. Sometimes they will not have an elevated IgG or IgE but I give them sugar, or a blinded skin test for sugar, and they have the typical allergy reactions (asthma or hay fever) or other symptoms such as hyperactivity. There is still much we don't know about food allergies and I suspect that cooking, digestion, and food processing of sugar alters it in a way that it would affect one person and not another. I think we need a tremendous amount of research with people who are very open-minded and we need studies that are not paid directly or indirectly by the food or sugar industry to try to figure out the answers. The one reason I think it is an allergy is that I can challenge a child who reacts to sugar cubes as follows: Feed sugar cubes on an empty stomach after no form has been ingested for 5 to 12 days. It is easy to show the reaction. Then I take the same child and wait 3-4 days, and put one drop of a stock-regular allergy extract for sugar in his arm. This is done single-blindedly. Only the nurse, not the mother or the doctor will know what was used for testing. If sugar is a problem, that child will react in some manner, usually in 3-8 minutes. Then progressively weaker dilutions of the same stock allergy extract are given every 8-10 minutes until the right concentration is found. It could be the 1:5 weaker dilution and it might be the 1:25, the 1:125, the 1:625 or the 1:3125 dilution that stops the reaction so the child is normal again in 6-8 minutes. We can turn it on and off like a light bulb. Now you can call that anything you want but to me it sounds very much like an allergy. The fact that their IgE isn't always elevated just means to me that the body is smarter than we are. As a board certified pediatric allergist I can't explain it. I think there's more to it than we presently understand and in time we'll know more.

The bottom line is - how we can help these children? You can take them off of sugar completely if that's a problem, but that's unrealistic. You can try to find the amount of sugar they can ingest without having symptoms, which means to quantitatively give only the amount that they can tolerate at a five day interval. You can allow them to eat that amount but only every 4 days. If you feed them sugar in that way you can actually desensitize them and in time they may be able to tolerate more and more sugar.

The other way you can do it, of course, is treat them with a sugar allergy extract. That's another discussion, but there's no doubt after 20 years of personally using Provocation/Neutralization allergy skin testing, it absolutely works! It's not equivocal in any way and anyone who ever goes to the office of an environmental medicine specialist can see someone's symptoms suddenly triggered within seconds. You can use a single-blinded injection of sugar versus a placebo to prove that it is not just a chance reaction.

KH: Do you see differences in children's behavior when they consume a refined Western diet versus a diet that is unrefined?

DR: I would say that there are extreme differences in children's behavior depending upon what they eat and that milk, wheat, eggs, chocolate, corn, sugar, orange juice and apple juice are frequent causes of hyperactivity and behavior problems. These foods are missed repeatedly, as they were by myself, for approximately 20 years until I started to realize that what we eat can affect various parts of the body. For example milk, apple juice, grape juice, orange juice and pineapple juice frequently cause bed-wetting after the age of 5 years. Wheat can cause muscle aches and some children can't even stand up if they eat a cookie or a slice of bread. But once again, everything has to be individualized. You can't give a stock answer. I think the biggest problem with so-called scientific studies is patient selection. They have to make sure that the patients have the problem they are trying to investigate and not some other confounding problem of which they're not aware.

KH: What is the best evidence or way to share with your pediatric colleagues that sugar has an effect on behavior if they are "non-believers"

at present?

DR: Well, all I can say to my colleagues is that I wouldn't have believed it at all for the first 20 years in practice, because that's the way I was trained in pediatric allergy and, in retrospect, I was trained incorrectly. At this point, I regret that I was told that Rowe and Rinkel did not know what they were talking about. If any of you find a copy of Rowe's book, Food Allergy, and Rinkel's book, Food Allergy, read them. You will be astounded by what you read. You will realize you're seeing it, and you have seen it every day in your offices and have probably missed it. I think the best evidence is to try the one week diet that's been so successful. It's not difficult. They can eat any number of meats, fruits and vegetables. Then, the second week add the previously omitted foods back, one at a time, and you will find not only not only what affects their behavior, but how their physical well-being is affected. Certain foods will cause headaches. Others, such as milk, in particular, will cause leg aches and ear problems. (The ear problems, incidentally, occur about two days after their ingestion of dairy products at 5-12 day intervals). You will also see other cause-and-effect relationships and you'll say, "How could I have missed it so long?" It's because we, as physicians, were not trained correctly. We were told that foods don't cause these kinds of problems and the only way to prove it to yourself is take 20 patients who are hyperactive and put them on the diet. That's the way I did it in the Journal of Learning Disabilities, in 1978. I merely asked 20 some children who were on Ritalin to try a one week diet and two-thirds of them were markedly improved within 3-7 days. If you do this with the children who have a multiplicity of complaints that you really cannot help except with medications, you might be pleasantly surprised. You can figure out the specific cause of chronic bed-wetting, belly aches, headaches, behavior problems, learning problems, high IQ children who can't remember, and recurrent ear infections. You won't need a double-blind study to confirm what parents have been telling you. When parents add the foods back that they think caused the difficulty at a 5-12 day interval, but you'll be able to quickly confirm their observations.

Let me give you one other tidbit test that has not been scientifically documented. That is, you can buy Alka-Aid at the health food store or Alka-Seltzer in the gold foil at a drug store, which is called, "Alka-Seltzer Antacid Formula." If you give this type of alkali before a child eats a problem food you can **prevent** a food sensitivity reaction in about two thirds of the patients. If child is already reacting to a food, an alkali can stop a reaction in 10-20 minutes.

I hope what I have said has been helpful. If anyone has any questions they should feel free to call me and I would be glad to discuss any aspect of this in more depth. Better, go visit the office of an Environmental Allergy Medical Specialist. See for yourself and base your conclusions on your personal observations. ◆

Blood Pressure and Nutritional Factors

Claude K. Lardinois, M.D.
Veterans Affairs Medical Center, Reno, NV
Department of Medicine (111E)
1000 Locust Avenue
Reno, NV 89520 U.S.A.
(702) 786-7200 / (702) 328-1769 FAX

"Nutritional Factors in Hypertension",
Archives of Family Medicine, August 1995;4:707-713. #23022

Kirk Hamilton: Can you please share with me your educational background and current position?

Claude Lardinois: I received my M.D. from George Washington University in 1975. I completed an internal medicine residency with the United States Air Force in 1978. Upon completion of my military obligation I did a combined fellowship in endocrinology and gerontology at Stanford Medical Center in Palo Alto, California. I am currently a professor of medicine and physiology at the University of Nevada School of Medicine and the Director of the Endocrinology Division at the University and at the Affiliated Veterans Affairs Medical Center.

KH: How did you get interested in nutrition and blood pressure?

CL: I have always been interested in diabetes mellitus and nutritional approaches to the management of subjects with the disorder. Since many of my patients had hypertension in addition to their diabetes, I wondered if there was an association. The demonstration of insulin resistance in subjects with hypertension in 1988 strongly suggested that insulin resistance not only contributes to diabetes but to hypertension as well. Healthy nutrition, especially weight loss, improves both diabetes and hypertension. It was only "natural" for me to expand my diabetic nutritional recommendations to subjects with hypertension with or without diabetes.

KH: What role does weight loss play in hypertension?

CL: There is no question that weight loss lowers blood pressure. In my review article I have sighted numerous studies that show reductions in both systolic and diastolic blood pressure with even modest weight loss. Many subjects are able to discontinue their antihypertensive agents with weight loss.

KH: What is the role of calcium and magnesium in hypertension?

CL: Calcium supplementation in pill preparations probably does not lower blood pressure. What I found was very interesting in that calcium intake by means of dietary change (i.e.; dairy products) did lower blood pressure. Dairy products provide in addition to calcium, magnesium and potassium, which may help reduce blood pressure. If one has to supplement with calcium I would do so with non-fat dairy products. The role of magnesium is still unclear.   At the present time there is no evidence that magnesium supplementation has much effect on blood pressure. I only recommend magnesium when serum magnesium is low. Given that only 1% of magnesium is in the serum this makes it very hard to interpret what a low serum magnesium concentration means.

KH: What is the role of potassium in hypertension?

CL: Potassium supplementation may play a role in the prevention of hypertension, but making clear recommendations regarding ideal potassium intake is difficult. Potassium should be supplemented if hypokalemia occurs during diuretic therapy. There is some evidence to suggest that the black individuals with hypertension would benefit most from potassium supplementation. The risk of hyperkalemia with potassium supplementation probably outweighs the benefits.

KH: What really does salt restriction do as far as blood pressure reduction?

CL: It is difficult to know which subjects respond best to sodium restriction at the bedside. Many people eat salt well in excess of physiologic need and do not get hypertensive while other subjects eating the same amount of salt get hypertension.   I recommend that daily sodium chloride intake be limited to 6 g/d or 100 mmol of sodium which is about 1 teaspoon of salt. In subjects with hypertension not well controlled on multiple drugs, a 24 hr. urine sodium should be collected and if over 100 mmol aggressive sodium restriction should be instituted.

KH: How does "restricted" breathing effect hypertension?

CL: It is well known that obese patients are often hypertensive. Their obesity impairs their ability to take a "full" respiration and would "restrict" their work of breathing. The mechanism of the hypertension is unclear but it is interesting to speculate that the insulin resistance and associated hyperinsulinemia well described in hypertension are contributing factors. Insulin enhances renal tubular reabsorption of sodium and this could result in elevation of blood pressure.

KH: What roles do fatty acids play in hypertension?

CL: In my review I could not find an important link between fatty acids and hypertension with the exception of the omega-3 fish oil fatty acids. Three meta-analyses suggested a dose response effect of omega-3 fatty acids on blood pressure. The role of proinflammatory products like arachidonic acid (AA) is interesting but vegetarians consume a lot of 18:2 (linoleic acid), the precursors of arachidonic acid and tend to have lower blood pressures. Fish oil increases prostacyclin, a very potent vasodilator without much change in blood pressure.   I speculated that it is the micronutrients i.e., magnesium, potassium and not the macronutrient fatty acids that exert the blood pressure lowering properties.

KH: *Have you seen any role for food hypersensitivity in blood pressure?*

CL: I am not aware of any association. Many people test "positive" for food allergies without expressing anything clinically making it difficult for me to make any corrections. Except in a handful of people, food allergies are probably insignificant. I get upset when I hear people explain all their life problems on food allergy.

KH: *What role does exercise play in hypertension?*

CL: Although my article focused on nutritional factors, there is no question that exercise independent of weight loss lowers blood pressure. Exercise decreases insulin levels and improves insulin action with a lowering of blood pressure. Catecholamine levels are also decreased which helps benefit blood pressure as well.

KH: *What effects do diuretics have on blood pressure?*

CL: There is no question that hypokalemia and hypomagnesemia caused by diuretics can adversely effect blood pressure. What is less clear is what effect diuretics have on changes in both potassium and magnesium that remain within the normal range. Diuretics increase insulin and catecholamine levels which may have a negative effect on blood pressure.

KH: *Are there any other nutritional factors that can effect blood pressure?*

CL: Caffeine may increase blood pressure temporarily but tolerance to the pressor effect occurs rapidly. As a general rule caffeine does not elevate blood pressure. One exception is in borderline hypertensive subjects with other risk factors, i.e., family history of hypertension, higher percentage of body fat. In this subgroup caffeine restriction may be prudent. Garlic has also recently been shown to lower blood pressure. Given the beneficial effects of garlic on lipoprotein metabolism, hypertensive subjects with dyslipidemia may benefit from long-term garlic supplementation.

Consumption of black licorice in excess can elevated blood pressure through impairment of cortisol degradation. It is very important to question patient's consumption of licorice which may be contributing to the hypertension. Nonsteroidal antiinflammatory drugs can negate the beneficial effects of many antihypertensive agents and their use should be limited in subjects with hypertension. Central acting agents and calcium channel blockers are less affected by nonsteroidal antiinflammatory drugs. Other important drugs that can elevate blood pressure include nasal decongestants, oral contraceptives, corticosteroids, antidepressants, cocaine, cyclosporine and erythropoietin. ◆

Bone Density, Calcium Intake and Teenagers

Jeri W. Nieves, Ph.D.
Regional Bone Center
Helen Hayes Hospital
Rt. 9 W.
West Haverstraw, New York 21849 U.S.A.
(914) 947-3000, ext. 3833 / (914) 947-2485 (FAX)

"Teenage and Current Calcium Intake are Related to Bone Mineral Density of the Hip and Forearm in Women Age 30-39 Years,"
American Journal of Epidemiology, 1995;141:342-51. #21849

Kirk Hamilton: Could you please share your educational background since college and your present position?

Jeri Nieves: I received a BS in nutrition and food science from the University of Rhode Island, a Master of Science in Nutrition from Cornell University, and a Ph.D. in Epidemiology from the graduate school of arts and sciences at Columbia University.

KH: And your present position?

JN: I am a research scientist with the New York State Department of Health at Helen Hayes Hospital. I am also an adjunct assistant professor of Public Health and Epidemiology at Columbia University.

KH: When did you get interested in calcium intake and bone loss?

JN: When I was working on my doctorate my advisor came to me and said that they were doing a study on osteoporosis and diet and they wanted someone with a background in nutrition to try and gather the data as accurately as possible. So that is really when I started back in the mid 80s.

KH: Could you describe your study about teenage and current calcium intake and their relationship to bone mineral density at the hip and forearm in women age 30 to 39 years?

JN: We recruited women between the ages of 30-39 from the community around Helen Hayes Hospital, in Rockland County New York. They completed a very extensive interview that included questions on several variables that can affect bone mineral density such as menstrual function, pregnancy, lactation, oral contraceptive use, disease and medication history, physical activity, occupation and drinking water history. One other component of it was a dietary intake questionnaire which was self-administered and it took a half an hour to complete. Because we were interested both in current and teenage dietary intake we structured the questionnaire so they would be asked about foods such as milk correct consumption (one year preceding) and also between 13 and 17 years of age. We did this for each of the foods which was one of the novel things for this study. One of our concerns was whether or not the data was actually being gathered reliably. We called back 15 of these women and asked them to complete the questionnaire again. We had as good agreement between the 2 tests with the teenage diet as we did with the current diet.

KH: What did you measure in this study?

JN: When these people came in they also had several physical measurements. One of them was a bone mineral density scan of the spine, hip and forearm. They also had a measurement of body composition and grip strength.

KH: What was the technique for bone density assessment?

JN: We used a dual photon absorptiometer. Right now that technology has been improved to be a dual x-ray absorptiometer. But during the time that we started the study it was the best technique that was available.

KH: What did you find with this group?

JN: The higher the calcium intake the higher the bone mineral density was in the hip and also in the forearm. However, we did not see any relationship between any nutrient consumption and bone mineral density of the spine. Teenage phosphorous intake was related to bone mineral density and that could be just because it varies so highly with calcium intake. What we also found in this group of 30-39 year olds is that they were already losing bone from the hip. It appears that the loss of bone mass probably occurs in the 20s.

KH: You basically were following what this group of 30-39 year olds said their diets were then and now, compared to their bone density now?

JN: Exactly.

KH: And the results were?

JN: Dietary factors such as calcium and phosphorous were positively associated with bone mineral density of the hip and possibly with the forearm. We had a slightly smaller sample size for the forearm measurement because of machine problems. Then there is no association at this point with the spine and dietary intake of any nutrients.

KH: What role does fiber play in bone density?

JN: We evaluated fiber basically because of its ability to bind to calcium in the intestine, and therefore decrease the absorption of calcium. The fiber intake, at least in terms of this study, appears to be detrimental to the calcium absorption. If we control statistically for fiber intake you actually see increases in the strength of the association between calcium and bone mineral density.

KH: *What were the most common sources of calcium in foods?*

JN: For the most part it was dairy products. Milk and cheeses. We had some tofu and alternative sources. There was a little bit less consumption of the dark green leafy vegetables that are particularly high in calcium. So for the most part the women in this study consumed dairy products. There was only moderate use of calcium supplements. About 40% of the population used supplements.

KH: *What is your recommendation for maintenance of bone health starting in your teenage years?*

JN: You need to try and consume as much calcium as you can. The optimal daily intake for calcium was just increased for women and for teenagers. Between ages 11 and 24 you should be having at least 1200 mg of calcium a day.

KH: *What is your recommended way to get this amount?*

JN: For the most part dairy is your best source. If you're concerned with fat intake you can use the low fat alternatives. But dairy products have the advantage of being more highly absorbed than any other group. The lactose in milk and other dairy products actually helps to increase the calcium absorption. Cost wise it is one of the least expensive ways of actually getting the calcium.

KH: *Are there any other risk factors for bone loss other than calcium intake that you would include in your bone loss prevention program?*

JN: Definitely include physical activity particularly activity that is weight bearing. Somewhere around 30 minutes a day at least 3 or 4 times a week would be the minimum that you would want to do. With bone it is "If you don't use it you lose it."

KH: *Are you ever concerned about things such as high protein diets, high salt diets, caffeinism as aggravants of bone loss or calcium spill?*

JN: There has been some data on each of those showing a negative impact on calcium. For the most part if you're getting your calcium intake from dairy products you'll have less of a concern of the protein because the protein in there does not have the sulfites that have been shown to be detrimental to calcium absorption. It is the same thing with the caffeine content. Caffeine can increased urinary excretion of calcium. However, there was a recent study from California that showed that if you have at least a glass of milk a day, that 2 cups of coffee a day was not detrimental.

KH: *Enter your cafe late'. I'll remember that one.*

JN: Another risk factor is vitamin D deficiency. With everyone being so sensitive to the detrimental effects of the sun they're putting on a lot of sunscreen and basically stopping the body from manufacturing enough vitamin D. That is another reason I would say that the dairy products might be better as a means of getting adequate vitamin D. Vitamin D is one of the nutrients that experts are starting to feel is almost as important as calcium. If you don't have enough vitamin D you're not going to absorb the calcium that is in your diet.

KH: *Any other trace elements important for bone loss prevention?*

JN: There is nothing else that has been proven.

KH: *If you don't take diary products - do you have any*

recommendations on a type of calcium?

JN: Well there is really 2 alternatives to do. One is to consume different foods. Calcium fortified foods are coming out like calcium fortified orange juice and breads. So you could choose those alternatives. Then there is broccoli, kale and the dark green leafy vegetables that have a fairly high content of calcium. In addition some of the beans like lima, kidney or snap beans are good calcium sources.

KH: *If somebody takes a calcium supplement do you have any bias towards a particular form?*

JN: For the most part the forms that seem to give you the most calcium are calcium citrate and calcium carbonate (40%). These can be found in different sources. Almost any manufacturer makes a lower cost brand of calcium carbonate like TUMS. ♦

Bone Loss, Boron and Risk Factors

Susan L. Meacham, Ph.D., R.D.
Department of Human Nutrition
College of Arts and Sciences
Winthrop University
Rock Hill, SC 29733 U.S.A.
(803) 323-2101 / (803) 323-2347 (FAX)
E-Mail: Meachams@Winthrop.edu

"Effects of Boron Supplementation on Blood and Urinary Calcium, Magnesium, and Phosphorus, and Urinary Boron in Athletic and Sedentary Women," The American Journal of Clinical Nutrition, 1995;61:341-345. #21766

Kirk Hamilton: *What is your present position and educational background since college?*

Susan Meacham: Currently, I am an assistant professor at Winthrop University in Rock Hill, South Carolina. I have been doing research with the USDA Grand Forks Human Nutrition Research Center in North Dakota. Prior to that I was a research associate after completing a doctorate degree in human nutrition at Virginia Polytechnic Institute and State University.

KH: *How did you get interested in boron and bone loss?*

SM: In 1989, while a doctoral candidate at Virginia Tech, I was asked to work on a proposal that was being submitted to study the effect of boron supplementation in young female athletes.

KH: *In your article in The American Journal of Clinical Nutrition mentioned above what were you initially trying to do with this study?*

SM: The recommendations for calcium supplementation and vitamin D have not shown positive results universally with regard to nutritional preventive therapy for all osteoporotic patients. There may still be some other nutritional factor, in addition to exercise and hormones, that influences bone metabolism. We started looking at boron after reading the work of Nielsen and Hunt in Grand Forks.

KH: *When you talked about vitamin D and calcium having "not universally shown positive results," what did you mean by that?*

SM: It seems to prevent or treat osteoporosis in some people and not in others, and varies with the types of calcium supplements and the addition of vitamin D.

KH: *You mean in preventing bone loss or actually adding bone?*

SM: The literature reports are mixed regarding the effectiveness of calcium and vitamin D supplementation for both pre-and postmenopausal women with the picture being complicated by types and amounts of exercise, types and amounts of minerals added, and hormonal status of the individuals being studied. Our attention was focused on college female athletes where adequate bone deposition and stress fractures were the primary concern. In such special cases as females with amenorrhea, we were concerned with preventing premature bone loss. Thus, our objective was to look for a nutritional approach to maximize bone deposition in these young women to prevent stress fractures and to provide a "savings account" of calcium for later in life.

KH: *Please tell me the essence of your study. What did you find?*

SM: Twenty-eight individuals completed the study, 17 athletes and 11 controls. The 17 female athletes were supplemented daily for 10 months with a 3 mg supplement of boron or a placebo.

KH: *Was that a particular type of boron?*

SM: We ordered a commercial supplement that contained boron citrate, aspartate and glycinate chelates. Before and after supplementation with boron or cornstarch placebos, physical fitness, hormonal status, mineral status and bone mineral density were compared between sedentary controls and athletes. The athletes were more aerobically fit and had lower body fats. Exercise diminished the effects of supplementation.

KH: *Negatively or positively?*

SM: Sometimes we wouldn't see as much change in the athletes as we did in the controls, for example, serum magnesium concentrations would be greater in our sedentary control group when they were supplemented with boron. Our exercise group didn't show the same magnitude of increase in serum magnesium with supplementation.

KH: *What did you find looking at calcium, phosphorus, magnesium and boron supplementation in this group?*

SM: Serum phosphorus concentrations were lower in boron supplemented subjects than in placebo supplemented subjects. Compared with all other subjects, serum magnesium concentrations were greatest in the sedentary control subjects supplemented with boron and increased with time in all subjects. Calcium excretion increased over time in all boron supplemented subjects, counter to what was being reported by Grand Forks.

KH: *With the boron supplementation?*

SM: Boron excretion increased over time in all boron supplemented subjects.

KH: *As I read your study, it doesn't really give us anything to put* *our finger on.*

SM: No, it just stirs our curiosity.

KH: *What are the main changes again?*

SM: Boron supplementation very modestly affected mineral status, and exercise modified the effects of boron supplementation on serum minerals and urinary calcium.

KH: *What recommendations do you give to female athletes to maintain bone status?*

SM: I recommend exercising at competitive levels that are not obsessive levels because we did find female athletes who were exercising at extreme levels had altered hormonal status, they were becoming amenorrheic. I also recommended a varied diet that supplies a balanced mineral intake with emphasis placed on achieving the recommended amounts of calcium. The varied diets help assure that even the trace and ultratrace minerals are consumed at levels that are adequate. We do not have recommendations for most of these lesser known minerals to date.

KH: *And the boron supplementers had lower bone density or increased urinary calcium?*

SM: In one situation low bone density was observed and in a young female who had altered hormonal status. Overall, exercise promoted a significant increase in the change of bone mineral density over time as compared to the sedentary controls.

KH: *What other life-style recommendations can you make regarding bone maintenance?*

SM: The best nutritional preventive factor we have right now for bone fractures in young athletes, particularly women, and for preventing osteoporosis in elderly individuals is to maximize the bone calcium stores starting in infancy or even preconceptually. By starting at infancy and then continuing well into the 25 to 35 year age bracket, pushing the intakes of calcium and the less well known minerals, we might make a difference in maintaining an optimal bone mineral density well into the later years of life.

KH: *And that is when your peak bone mass is?*

SM: Peak bone mineral density continues long after bone height is reached.

KH: *So even though you were teased a little bit to the fact that there were some alterations with boron supplementation with these minerals, there is no other recommendation that you would give for oral intakes of minerals besides calcium at this moment?*

SM: Well, a varied diet is going to provide the boron and the other minerals that we are not aware of, including ultra trace minerals and the major minerals such as calcium, phosphorus and magnesium. I would not recommend any type of supplementation that would provide intakes above the RDA's. However, a vast majority of individuals, particular females, are not getting the recommended levels of calcium. Therefore, we might also assume that there are other minerals, the more obscure ones like boron, that may not be at optimum intake levels.

KH: *Given the fact that somewhere between 9% and 20% of the U.S. population eat 5 servings of fruits and vegetables every day, we have quite a dilemma.*

SM: That's right. Boron in particular is one mineral that people don't ever think about, but it may be playing a very critical role. We don't have the evidence to concretely say that, only indications that keep us looking at the ultra trace minerals such as boron in relation to optimal bone metabolism.

KH: *What foods are rich in boron?*

SM: Green leafy vegetables and pulpy types of fruits such as apples, peaches and grapes are good sources of boron. So the "5-a-day" recommendation covers boron, too.

KH: *What have you found about your dietary surveys of boron?*

SM: Not having a good data base for boron and the other ultra trace minerals in our food supply is a major problem. We can't alter or even make recommendations on what high or low intakes are until we know what is currently being consumed. So that is why we are going back to a very basic level, simply analyzing the most commonly consumed foods and then estimating the boron intakes in the typical American diet. From chemical analysis we determined the daily intakes of boron to be 1.5 ± 1.3 mg and 0.7 ± 0.3 mg in female athletes and sedentary controls, respectively.

KH: *Do you have a comment about vitamin B12? It stimulates osteocalcin and therefore may have a positive effect on bone.*

SM: No. But I have been following some of the reading on B12, folic acid (primarily the folic acid) and neural tube defects (closure of the spinal cord). This may be a folic acid, bone and mineral interaction. We might find a need to increase folic acid and minerals to improve proper development.

KH: *I didn't even think about the bone formation component of neural tube defects. Thank you! How about a high protein diet - any comment?*

SM: Typically the American diet is too high in protein, and there are reports of associated calcium losses through excretion. An adequate amount of protein is recommended. In bone, the protein matrix is embedded with the mineral crystals and this might also include the ultra trace minerals whose structure and or enzymatic roles, if any, have yet to be determined.

KH: *Do you have any concern about the American high protein diet aggravating bone loss?*

SM: I know that has been a concern. I haven't been involved in the work directly, but I think sometimes we err to the extremes, whether it be too high or too low. And our safest bet at the moment is still to maintain an adequate (not maximum and not minimum) intake of protein to maximize (particularly in young individuals) bone and lean body tissue development without compromising calcium nutriture.

KH: *Is there a theoretic mechanism by how boron may enhance bone metabolism?*

SM: Boron may compensate for deviations in energy utilization in vitamin D deficient bone. Boron may possibly enhance the major mineral content of bone. It also may enhance indices of cartilage formation. Boron is also being looked at in a lot of different ways in relation to energy and substrate utilization. Most of this work is being done by Drs. Forrest Nielsen and Curtis Hunt at the USDA Human Nutrition Research Laboratory in Grand Forks, North Dakota. ◆

Bone Loss, Calcium and Caffeine

Susan S. Harris, MSc.
Calcium & Bone Metabolism Laboratory
USDA Human Nutrition Research Center on Ageing
Tufts University
711 Washington Street
Boston, MA 02111 U.S.A.
(617) 556-3073 / (617) 556-3344 (FAX)

"Caffeine and Bone Loss in Healthy Postmenopausal Women,"
American Journal of Clinical Nutrition, 1994;60:573-578. #21095

Kirk Hamilton: *Would you be so kind as to start off and tell me your educational background from college and your current position?*

Susan Harris: I was a teacher for a number of years and went back to school at Tufts University where I got a Master of Science degree in nutrition. I am now at Boston University School of Public Health in the Department of Epidemiology where I am writing my doctoral dissertation.

KH: *What is your dissertation on?*

SH: Relationships of body composition to bone and change in bone density in several different populations.

KH: *How did you get interested in caffeine's effect on bone mineral density?*

SH: The women who were assessed for caffeine were enrolled in a larger study of calcium and vitamin D supplementation. Since caffeine is one thing that may influence bone loss, we collected information on caffeine intake.

KH: *Can you share with us what effects caffeine does have on bone density?*

SH: When you see lists of risk factors for osteoporosis or bone loss, sometimes you see caffeine or coffee intake on that list and sometimes you don't. The effect of caffeine hadn't been looked at in a prospective study of older women, and we were able to do that. We followed 205 women for 1 year. We had all kinds of information about dietary intakes not only of caffeine, but of calcium, vitamin D and other nutrients. We had information on exercise, anthropometric and other variables related to bone loss. We looked in the group as a whole and did not see any relationship between caffeine intake and bone loss. It had been suggested previously that caffeine's effect on bone might depend on calcium intake, so I divided the group according to their calcium. The group with the lower calcium intake had average intakes around 600 mg which is somewhat lower than the RDA of 800 mg. The women in the other group had calcium intakes of around 900 mg which is slightly above the RDA. What I found was that in the women with the lower calcium intakes, those who also had the highest caffeine intakes, had greater rates of bone loss than the other women. However, among the women with the higher calcium intakes, caffeine intake didn't matter.

KH: *So if you had your cappuccino or your latte with the milk in it that might be protective?*

SH: Yes, it might. In fact we did see a correlation in this study between caffeine intake and calcium intake. Not everyone reports that. In younger women I think it may go the other way because they are getting more of their caffeine from sources other than coffee, like soda, that you don't put milk in. I think there are really two conclusions here. One is that if you're getting your calcium requirement, which many women in this country are not, then caffeine is probably not something you need to worry about. If you're not getting enough calcium - first of all get it. The answer isn't just to lower your caffeine intake but it is to increase your calcium intake. Secondly, if for some reason you won't or can't increase your calcium intake, you should probably limit your caffeine intake.

KH: *The 450 mg of caffeine per day was the highest group. Can you give me an estimate of how many cups of coffee that is?*

SH: In the Boston area among our women the most common type of coffee was brewed coffee. A large cup of coffee would probably have about 219 mg of caffeine.

KH: *We are talking about greater than 2 or 3 cups of coffee per day.*

SH: Well, I think in some parts of the country instant coffee is much more commonly consumed and it is much lower in caffeine. It is less than half as much. So you could double the number if you are talking about instant coffee.

KH: *The message from your work is that if the calcium intake is adequate, then coffee is really kind of an irrelevant risk factor for bone loss. If your calcium intake is low, then those people should not only increase their calcium intake, but they might also want to cut down their coffee intake a little bit. Is that what you are saying?*

SH: Well, maybe. If they increase their calcium intake they may not need to worry about the caffeine. We don't have a lot of 15 cup per day drinkers in this group. I think the highest caffeine intake for any individual in this study was 1896 mg which would be 9 cups of coffee. So out of 205 people, that was the biggest intake. You know, if you were talking about some other group like college students who were drinking coffee all night to write papers it might be a more serious problem.

KH: *What is the theoretic mechanism of caffeine's effect on bone if there is one?*

SH: That's a great question and we had hoped to find

something about that. One of the things that we had to look at was urine calcium excretion, the idea being that caffeine increases urinary output of calcium. There is no good evidence from the literature that this is sustained beyond the couple of hours after you drink the coffee. Right after you drink the coffee you definitely excrete more calcium in your urine, but whether you make that up later in the day we don't know. And in our group we saw no increase in urinary calcium excretion with increasing caffeine intake. On the other hand, a very small increase could have an important effect on bone, and we would not have been able to detect a very small increase. So we still don't know, and that is people's best guess so far as to the mechanism. But it is also possible that caffeine may increase the amount of calcium that is lost in the sweat or in the feces.

KH: *What are the risk factors that you think are important in sharing with the female about protecting bone?*

SH: It changes with age. If we're talking about postmenopausal women, not taking hormone replacement therapy is a risk factor. I am not implying that everyone should take it, but women who do take it do not lose bone at the rate that women who don't take it do. Calcium intake is important and is low in this country. Postmenopausal women consume around 600 mg per day when the RDA is 800 mg. Of course many women would be far below that. So calcium intake, exercise (especially weight bearing exercise) and then smoking are important risk factors. There are other things like caffeine and alcohol that we are really not quite sure about. Many medications affect bone loss. Thiazide diuretics are commonly used in this population and actually protect bone.

KH: *Are there any minerals besides calcium that can affect bone positively?*

SH: Researchers for the Framingham Osteoporosis Study recently reported that elderly women with low dietary magnesium had modestly lower hip and spine bone density than women who consumed at least two thirds of the RDA for that mineral.

KH: *As you look at the literature, you see those classic three or four risk factors. You hardly ever see much on any other mineral or nutrient and I am not sure if that is because there isn't research or the question hasn't been asked. Substances like boron and silicon all have little bits of suggested evidence, but no one seems to do in-depth research with these agents.*

SH: I think there are two reasons for this. One is that the food contents of nutrients like boron are not readily accessible to researchers. Also it's hard to look at one single thing because nutrients don't travel alone. You need to consider each nutrient in the context of related nutrients that may also affect bone loss. It is hard to tease out singular connections.

KH: *If you look at the human being in an evolutionary sense, it is the only animal species that attempts to consume milk after weaning, and yet that (milk) is what you hear about constantly as your main source of calcium. It is hard for me to imagine that if we were foragers with occasional carnivorous habits and we evolved without dairy products, that dairy products are so necessary for our bone health. If we were truly foragers consuming the paleolithic diet (consumers of roots, tubers, berries, etc.), there would be a tremendous amount of chlorophyll, magnesium, folate and other trace elements in it.*

SH: A lot of calcium also.

KH: *Calcium more than magnesium?*

SH: I don't know what the ratio would be.

KH: *Calcium seems to be a little over blown, and we have a lot of diseases that are related to abnormal calcium metabolism. Otherwise calcium channel blockers wouldn't be so frequently used in cardiovascular disease.*

SH: On the other hand, osteoporosis isn't a disease that paleolithic people suffered from.

KH: *They didn't live long enough?*

SH: Maybe we do need a somewhat different approach since we are living so long. I agree that there are probably all kinds of changes that have come with our change in diet that we don't know the health consequences of yet. ◆

Bone Loss, Calcium Metabolism and Vitamin K

Cees Vermeer, Ph.D.
Associate Professor of Biochemistry
Leader, Division on Vitamin K Research
Department of Biochemistry
University of Limburg
P.O. Box 616
6200 MD Maastricht, The Netherlands
31 43 3881 682 / 31 43 3670 992 (FAX)

"Role of Vitamin K in Bone Metabolism",
Annual Review of Nutrition, 1995;15:1-22. #23088

Kirk Hamilton: *Could you please share with me your educational background and current position?*

Cees Vermeer: I studied biochemistry at the University of Leiden where I received my bachelor degree in 1969 and my Ph.D. degree in 1973. In 1973 and 1974 I worked at the central laboratory of the Netherlands Red Cross Blood Transfusion Service, and in 1975 I initiated the Division on Vitamin K Research at the University of Limburg, Maastricht. I was chairman of the biochemistry department from 1987 through 1990 and board member of the Faculty of Medicine from 1991 through 1993. Currently I am an associate professor of biochemistry.

KH: *When did you get interested in the role of vitamin K and bone loss?*

CV: In 1974 it became clear that vitamin K is involved in the posttranslational formation of gammacarboxyglutamate (Gla) residues in proteins. These Gla-residues are unique products of vitamin K action and can be detected rapidly. Initially, Gla was found in a number of blood clotting factors, but it did not take long before the abundant presence of Gla-proteins in bone was established. So from that time on we knew that vitamin K played a role in bone metabolism. Remarkably, the precise role of these proteins has never been elucidated. Therefore, we have started investigations concerning the correlation between nutritional vitamin K intake and markers for bone metabolism as well as bone mass.

KH: *What physiologic mechanism connects vitamin K with bone loss?*

CV: First vitamin K functions as a cofactor in the formation of Gla-residues in at least 3 bone proteins: osteocalcin, matrix Gla-protein and protein S. All three proteins are synthesized by the bone forming cells, the osteoblasts. Since Gla-residues are calcium-binding groups, the presence of the three Gla-protein substantially increase the calcium-binding capacity of the organic matrix of the bone. Second, recent developments show that vitamin K may stimulate osteoblast differentiation and diminish osteoclast activity (bone resorption). The mechanism underlying this regulatory role in cell growth and function is unclear at this moment but we cannot exclude, for instance, the presence of vitamin K receptors at the surface of these cells.

KH: *What are the main types of vitamin K and what are they derived from?*

CV: The two main types of vitamin K are phylloquinone (also known as vitamin K_1) and menaquinone (vitamin K_2). Phylloquinone is exclusively synthesized by green leafy plants, where it functions as an electron carrier in the photosynthetically active thylakoid membranes of the chloroplasts. Green vegetables are a main nutritional source of phylloquinone. Menaquinone is a group name for a number of related compounds which are produced in microorganisms. Nutritional menaquinones are found in fermented products like yogurt. Animal food is often fortified with menadione (vitamin K_2), which is converted into menaquinone in a number of animal tissues. This explains the variable presence of menaquinone in most dairy products and meat. The biological activities of phylloquinone and the most abundant menaquinones are of the same order of magnitude. Also, the intestinal flora produces menaquinones, but the extent to which this fraction contributes to human vitamin K status has remained a matter of debate.

KH: *Is vitamin K deficiency a problem in Western civilization?*

CV: The answer to this question depends on how vitamin K deficiency is defined. According to the classical definition, vitamin K-deficiency is a state in which the hepatic vitamin K supply is so poor that spontaneous bleeding will occur. I would like to call this clinical vitamin K deficiency. In healthy subjects this phenomenon is extremely rare, we only find it occasionally in newborns and in a limited number of patients, (i.e. those with fat malabsorption). We define a biochemical vitamin K deficiency as a state in which the Gla-content of the bone protein osteocalcin is below normal, and in which vitamin K supplementation corrects this abnormality. If defined in this way vitamin K deficiency is found among a fairly large fraction of the western population, notably among postmenopausal women.

KH: *Can supplementation of vitamin K retard bone loss or enhance bone accretion?*

CV: It has been reported by several independent groups that vitamin K supplementation may result in an increase in the biochemical markers of bone formation and in a number of cases a decrease in the biochemical markers of bone resorption. It has also been reported that women with a biochemical vitamin K deficiency had a reduced bone mass of the femur neck, and a 6-fold enhanced risk for hip fracture. Circulating vitamin K levels were extremely low in those who had fractured their hip. Thus far the only study claiming a positive effect of vitamin K-supplementation on bone mass comes from Japan. It is not clear whether this interesting data may be extrapolated to the western, caucasian population. Therefore, a clinical trial concerning the effect of vitamin K supplementation on bone mass in caucasian women is badly needed.

KH: *What are the dosages of vitamin K that might be used and in what form?*

CV: In our studies we have used phylloquinone at a dose of 1 mg per day. This is 10-fold the recommended daily allowance (which is based on blood coagulation data). The standard preparation used was Konakion, which is available in dropper bottles. Clinical studies in Japan were made with menaquinone (Menatetrenone) in a dose of 45 mg/d. I would like to make it clear that I don't recommend any particular dose before the clinical trial mentioned above has been completed.

KH: *What markers of bone loss is vitamin K associated with?*

CV: Our data demonstrates that increased vitamin K intake results in an increase of circulating osteocalcin and the bone-derived alkaline phosphatase. Both are markers of bone formation, and the increase was found in nearly all subjects tested (postmenopausal women only). In parallel we have also found that vitamin K administration resulted in a decrease in 2-h fasting urinary hydroxyproline/creatinine and calcium/creatinine ratios. Both are markers for bone resorption, but the changes were only significant in women with a high initial urinary calcium loss. Obviously this is also the group at risk for bone loss. ◆

Breast Cancer and Fatty Acids

Masakuni Noguchi, M.D., Ph.D.
Kanazawa University Hospital
Operation Center
Takara-Machi
13-1 Kanazawa, 920, Japan
81 762 62 8151 (ext. 3394) / 81 762 34 4260 (FAX)

"The Role of Fatty Acids in Eicosanoid Synthesis Inhibitors in Breast Cancer",
Oncology, 1995;52:265-271. #22879

Kirk Hamilton: *Can you please share with me your educational background and current position?*

Masakuni Noguchi: I trained as a surgeon and received my doctoral degree from the Department of Surgery (II), School of Medicine, Kanazawa University. I am presently an associate professor at Kanazawa University and a vice manager of Operation Center, Kanazawa University Hospital.

KH: *When did you get interested in the role of essential fatty acids and breast cancer?*

MN: In 1985, I studied breast cancer at the Memorial Sloan-Kettering Cancer Center in New York. When I participated in the breast cancer conference and breast services, the physicians discussed a clinical trial investigating whether dietary intervention might improve the survival of breast cancer patients. I had recognized that a reduction in dietary fat intake may be effective as an adjunctive treatment for breast cancer patients. Since then, I have been interested in the role of essential fatty acids in breast cancer.

KH: *What role do omega-3 fatty acids play in breast cancer?*

MN: An inverse relationship has been found between the incidence of breast cancer and the level of fish consumption, suggesting a protective role for omega-3 fatty acids in human breast cancer. Several experimental studies have confirmed that dietary eicosapentaenoic acid (EPA) and docosapentaenoic acid (DHA) reduce mammary tumorigenesis and tumor growth.

KH: *What role do omega-6 fatty acids play and how well does linoleic acid get converted to arachidonic acid in humans? I was under the assumption that there was a poor conversion in humans.*

MN: Although linoleic acid cannot be synthesized *de novo* in the human body, it is derived from plant sources or meat. In humans, linoleic acid can be converted to arachidonic acid, which gives rise to the 2 series of eicosanoids (prostaglandins). Also, in an *in vitro* study of a human breast cancer cell line (MDA-NB-231), it has been shown that the addition of linoleic acid resulted in significantly increased cell growth, thymidine incorporation, and prostaglandin E and leukotriene B secretion (Oncology, 1995;52:458-464).

KH: *What role do preformed arachidonic acid products such as dairy products and red meat have on the levels of arachidonic acid metabolites and breast cancer risk?*

MN: The distinction between animal and vegetable fats is quite misleading, and it is more adequate to distinguish omega-3 and omega-6 fatty acids rather than animal and vegetable fats. There have been several reports that dietary linoleic acid in either animal, meat or vegetable oils is associated with breast cancer risk. Proposals have been made for controlled trials investigating a reduction in dietary fat intake to influence breast cancer risk. I think that dietary intervention can decrease breast cancer risk. The balance of fatty acids may be more important than the total quantity.

KH: *Could inhibitors of lipoxygenase and cyclooxygenase be beneficial in breast cancer prevention and/or treatment?*

MN: In order to prevent and/or treat breast cancer, it is important to inhibit both lipoxygenase and cyclooxygenase pathways. While indomethacin at lower concentrations stimulates cell proliferation via the synthesis of lipoxygenase products, at a higher concentration it inhibits both the lipoxygenase and cyclooxygenase pathways. We have reported that a low dose of indomethacin significantly reduces tumorigenesis in rats fed either high- or low-fat diets but significantly promotes tumor proliferation in rats fed either diet (Cancer Research, 1991;51:2683-2689). Therefore, a high dose of indomethacin might be beneficial for prevention and treatment of breast cancer. On the other hand, EPA is a competitive inhibitor of both the cyclooxygenase and lipoxygenase pathways, whereas DHA is a strong inhibitor of prostaglandin but not leukotriene synthesis. However, both EPA and DHA significantly reduce the secretion of prostaglandin E and leukotriene B (Oncology, in press), at least in part by the phenomenon of conversion of DHA to EPA. It has been reported that the growth-inhibiting effect of omega-3 fatty acids was apparent when the omega-3/omega-6 ratio was close to one. Therefore, a large amount of dietary omega-3 fatty acids will be required for breast cancer prevention and treatment. This would be a food rather than a drug.

KH: *Are we really talking about prevention when we talk about essential fatty acids, or could these essential fatty acids be used as adjunctive treatment?*

MN: Omega-3 fatty acids are effective not only for breast cancer prevention but also for adjuvant treatment of breast cancer. It has been shown that both EPA and DHA inhibit the growth and metastases of mammary tumors transplanted into mice and also improve the survival of transplanted mice (In Vivo, 1994; 8:371-374). On the other hand, it also has been shown that switching from a high-fat diet to a low-fat diet decreased the proliferation of mammary carcinoma (Oncology, 1992;49:246-252).

KH: *What role does lipid peroxidation play in these essential fatty acids in breast cancer development?*

MN: Inhibition of the growth of breast cancer by dietary omega-3 fatty acids may be via the accumulation within the tumor or cytostatic and/or cytolytic lipid peroxidation products. Under certain conditions, secondary products of lipid peroxidation can decrease cell proliferation and tumor cell survival. However, the exact mechanism by which lipid peroxidation products retard or inhibit tumor growth processes is not certain.

KH: Could the omega-6 family, particularly gamma-linolenic acid, be converted to arachidonic acid? Could it have an adverse effect or be converted to dihomogamma-linolenic acid and then to prostaglandin E1, which may have an anti-inflammatory effect?

MN: There are several hypotheses to explain the possible mode of action of essential fatty acids. The essential fatty acids are obligatory precursors of prostaglandins of the 1, 2, 3 and 4 series, and it is well recognized that prostaglandins can influence malignant cell behavior. Many cancers produce excessive amounts of the 2 series prostaglandins and yet are unable to manufacture prostaglandin E1, which is itself tumoricidal to DMBA-induced mammary tumors *in vitro*. However, prostaglandin E2 as well as leukotrienes B4 and C4 directly stimulate the growth of malignant cells, in addition to their effects on cell-mediated immunity. While the action of essential fatty acids may be expressed via derived prostaglandin products, it is difficult to predict or control which of the many prostaglandin classes would be gained by simple provision of additional dietary substrate.   ◆

Breast Cancer Risk Reduction and Mammography

Harold Sox, M.D.
Department of Medicine
Dartmouth-Hitchcock Medical Center
One Medical Center Drive
Lebanon, NH 03756 U.S.A.
(603) 650-7684 / (603) 650-6122 (FAX)

"Screening Mammography in Women Younger Than 50 Years of Age,"
Annals of Internal Medicine, April 1, 1995;122(7):550-552.

Kirk Hamilton: Can you please share with me your educational background and current position?

Harold Sox: I received my medical degree from Harvard Medical School and did my internal medicine training at Massachusetts General Hospital and as a chief medical resident at Dartmouth. I spent two years doing basic research at the National Institutes of Health before becoming interested in research on medical decision making, which I pursued first as a faculty member at Dartmouth and then for 15 years as chief of general internal medicine at Stanford University at the Palo Alto VA Medical Center. I took my present position as chair of medicine at Dartmouth in 1988.

KH: Why did you get interested in the optimal age to begin mammographic screening?

HS: My interest in breast cancer screening derives from a general interest in analyzing the best way to use screening tests through work I did with the American College of Physicians. Mammography became an interest when I became chair of the U.S. Preventive Services Task Force in 1990.   Age is one of many controversial aspects of screening that I find interesting.

KH: How have mammographic screening practices changed over the past 20 years?

HS: The evidence that mammography can reduce the death rate from cancer began with the Health Insurance Plan of New York randomized trial in the 1960's. This evidence, together with increased emphasis on early detection of disease, public concern about breast cancer, and a real increase in the incidence of breast cancer has lead to an increasing proportion of physicians who perform mammography on their women patients and an increasing number of women who expect regular mammographic screening.

KH: What are the health risks of mammography?

HS: The radiation received during mammography is small, but theoretical calculations based on the effect of high doses of radiation on cancer incidence indicate that mammography should increase the risk of breast cancer, albeit only slightly. Of course, the mammogram itself would detect most radiation-induced tumors very quickly. The benefits of early detection, at least in women age 50-70, far outweigh any increased risk of breast cancer due to radiation. The other risks are those due to evaluation of an abnormal mammogram and include the anxiety experienced while waiting to find out if the abnormality is cancer or not and the discomfort and costs of breast biopsy.

Women under age 50 undergo twice as many follow-up tests to detect one cancer as women over the age of 50.

KH: Are there any differences in the way that radiologists interpret mammograms? Is significant training required?

HS: Studies which compared 2 radiologists' interpretations of the same radiographic image almost always have shown different interpretations of a small percentage of the films. Mammography is no exception.   All radiologists receive extensive training in interpreting mammograms. Some radiologists choose to specialize in mammography and confine their practice to mammography.

KH: Are all mammographic machines and technicians created equal?

HS: The equipment used to perform mammography has improved over the years and is more accurate and requires less radiation than 10 years ago. Radiology departments undergo a periodic accreditation process, during which the reviewers evaluate each radiologist, each piece of equipment, and each technologist. Mammographic programs must keep up with the times in equipment and in monitoring of the performance of the technicians who actually take the radiographs.

KH: Is there evidence of the effectiveness of mammographic screening before age 40 years?

HS: There is wide consensus that the form of evidence that is least likely to be misinterpreted is a clinical trial of screening, in which a large number of women are assigned at random to either undergo periodic mammographic screening, often with annual breast examination, or to receive "usual care." In these studies, the period of follow-up observation for death from breast cancer is typically 10 or 15 years, which is required to accumulate enough outcome events to make an unequivocal interpretation of the results. The outcome measure is death from breast cancer. All of the large-scale studies that I am aware of enrolled women starting at age 40 or later. I know of no major studies that included enough women under age 40 to draw any meaningful conclusions.

KH: Is there proven benefit in mammographic screening after the age of 50?

HS: Mammographic screening, often in association with breast physical examination, reduces the rate of breast cancer death by 30%. It took studies involving over 100,000 women to prove this point unequivocally, but there is no doubt whatsoever that women in the 50-69 year age group do benefit substantially. In the largest study of women age 40-74, the breast cancer death rate after an average of 12 years of screening and follow-up was 3.9 per 1000 women in the screening group and 5.1 per 1000 in the control group. Most of the women in this study were between 50 and 69 years of age and the only group that showed a statistically significant reduction in death rate.

KH: *What are the risk factors for breast cancer that might encourage women under age 50 to seek breast cancer screening? Is there good evidence that these factors are important?*

HS: There are a number of factors of proven risk for breast cancer. Many benign conditions of the breast increase the risk of breast cancer. Women who have had breast disease should check with their physician to see if they have had one of the conditions that increase the risk of breast cancer. There are also familial and genetic factors as well. Breast cancer in a first degree relative (especially more than one first-degree relative) is an important risk factor for breast cancer as is a personal history of breast cancer. The risk is especially high when breast cancer occurred in one's mother, and particular if the mother had cancer in both breasts or was premenopausal when the cancer developed. Other risk factors include a long period between menarche and menopause, first pregnancy after age 30 years, exposure of breasts to radiation, and nulliparity. Estrogen replacement after menopause increases the chance of breast cancer by a small amount and is a factor in deciding whether to undergo this treatment.

KH: *What are the psychological risks to the patient from overuse of mammograms?*

HS: The news of an abnormality on a mammogram can cause great anxiety in many women. Some findings usually require follow-up tests, such as repeat mammography, breast ultrasound scans, or breast biopsy in order to resolve concern about cancer. The period between learning of an abnormal finding and undergoing the followup diagnostic procedure is often a very difficult time. Women under age 50 undergo almost four times as many followup diagnostic procedures in order to detect one breast cancer that do women aged 50 and older.

KH: *Are younger breasts more difficult to interpret with mammography?*

HS: The answer is not simple. The breasts of many younger women have less fat and are, therefore, more radiodense than the breasts of older women. Greater radiodensity means that smaller tumors are harder to detect. It is then harder to be sure that a mammographic image is normal and that there is no need for a follow-up mammogram or a biopsy. However, the majority of women aged 40 to 50 years do not have significantly dense breast.

KH: *After age 50 should a woman have yearly mammograms if a baseline mammogram is normal?*

HS: Women between age 50 and 70 should have mammograms at regular intervals. The usual recommendation is a mammogram every 1-2 years. The studies which prove the effectiveness of mammography did mammograms at intervals that varied between 18 and 33 months. There have been no good studies that compare the breast cancer death rate with annual mammography, to the death rate with mammography performed every other year.

KH: *Can estrogen replacement therapy have an adverse effect on reading mammograms of postmenopausal breasts?*

HS: In one-third of women, estrogen replacement therapy makes the breast more radiodense and more like the breast of premenopausal women.

KH: *Should mammography hurt?*

HS: Mammography involves flattening the breasts between two flat surfaces in order to get a good image of the breast and reduce exposure to radiation. This process causes pressure on the breast itself and some pulling on the skin near the breast. Some women find this experience uncomfortable.

KH: *What is the cost of mammography under the age of 50?*

HS: The charges for mammography range between $70 and $100 in most centers.

KH: *What about breast implants and mammograms?*

HS: Breast implants do obscure breast tissue and make the early detection of breast cancer more difficult. Silicone obscures more than saline implants. Mammographers take additional views of the breast in women who have breast implants. The recommendations for mammography are the same in women who have had a breast implant.

KH: *What are your basic recommendations for starting mammograms and frequency?*

HS: My recommendations are the 1995 recommendations of the U.S. Preventive Services Task Force, which as are follows:

> "Routine screening for breast cancer every 1 or 2 years, with mammography alone or mammography and an annual clinical breast examination (CBE) is recommended for women ages 50-69. There is insufficient evidence to recommend for or against routine mammography or CBE for women aged 40-49 or aged 70 and older, although recommendations for high risk women age 40-49 and healthy women > than 70 may be made on other grounds."

In addition, I believe that women aged 40-49 should discuss with their physician whether or not to undergo mammographic screening. Women in this age group need to understand the risk of false-positive mammograms, the number of breast biopsies required, and frequency with which breast biopsy shows cancer. They also need to understand that past studies of the effect of screening mammography in women aged 50 and older. Because mammography in young women has known downstream risks and costs and, as yet, unproven benefit, physicians and their patients need to engage in a thorough discussion prior to testing. ◆

Breast Feeding and Toxin Exposure

Janna G. Koppe, M.D.
Academic Medical Center
Department of Neonatology
Meibergdreef 9
1105 AZ Amsterdam, The Netherlands
31 20 5663969 (of) / 31 20 6965099 (of-FAX) / 31 294 291589 (h - Phone/FAX)

"Nutrition and Breast Feeding,"
European Journal of Obstetrics & Gynecology & Reproductive Biology, 1995;61:73-78.   #23706

Kirk Hamilton: Can you please share with me your educational background and current position?

Janna Koppe: At the University of Amsterdam I trained as an M.D. and became a pediatrician and neonatologist at the Academic Hospital of the University of Amsterdam.   At present I am a full professor in neonatology at the University of Amsterdam.

KH: When did you get interested in the role of environmental pollutants and breast feeding?

JK: In 1985 I became interested when dioxins were found to be present in breast milk collected in my department for the first time in Holland.   Leo Stern, a late professor in pediatrics at Brown University, stimulated me to investigate this environmental pollution problem.   In 1987, I hypothesized that PCBs and dioxins play a role in late hemorrhagic disease in the newborn by interfering with vitamin K metabolism.   This has been confirmed in animal experiments.

KH: Why is breast milk such a concentrated source of contaminants such as PCBs and dioxins?

JK: Because of the long half-life of these chemicals (more than 7-14 years) you accumulate them during your life.   They are difficult to metabolize and the body stores the chemicals in the body fat for safety reasons.   For making breast milk body fats are mobilized and the chemicals are dissolved in the fats and then excreted in the milk. The concentration in human breast milk is related to the age of the mother (more when the mother is older) and how many babies she breast fed before.   While producing breast milk the mother is losing the pollutants, but intoxicates her baby.

KH: What are food-sources of PCBs and dioxins?

JK: The main sources of PCBs and dioxins are animal fats in food products, especially fish and dairy products.   The fish are polluted by manufacturers that dump chemicals into the rivers polluting lakes and the sea.   Milk is contaminated by waste incinerators. Incinerating waste especially plastics with chlorine, like PVC, generates dioxins and PCBs. The chemicals are present and partly formed in the smoke and spread over the pastures where cows are grazing. Burning of the chemicals is even worse. In cow's milk the chemicals are stored and unfortunately the most toxic ones. Another source can be open fires where wood treated with pentachlorophenol is burned and the smoke is inhaled.

KH: At what levels of PCBs and dioxins are found in human milk with regard to exposure of infants? Are there any clinical symptoms that have been shown to manifest themselves?

JK: Subclinical symptoms are found in babies of mothers with high levels of PCBs and dioxins.   The symptoms are immunosuppression, abnormal neurologic development and a thyroid hormone disregulation.   For the future we are afraid of problems with reproduction and cancer.

KH: What foods do we need to be careful of with regards to dioxins and PCBs?

JK: Food must be controlled for levels of dioxins and PCBs so that every citizen knows what he/she is eating. Now it is difficult to tell whether you should eat fish or not.   It depends on the region where you live.   The same holds true for milk and milk products.   In general, animal fats are contaminated but the levels differ considerably.

KH: How do we lower concentrations of PCBs and dioxins in these foods?

JK: To lower levels of dioxins and PCBs in foods it is first necessary to measure the levels continuously.   This is at the moment not routinely done globally.   Governments claim that dioxin levels will be lower because of better and cleaner ways of incinerating. Levels in cow's milk must be lower than 1.5 pg TEQ/gr milk fat. TEQ (toxic equivalents) is a way to measure toxicity.   At the moment the situation with PCBs is that 1.5 million tons of PCBs have been produced on a global basis since 1930.   The production is now forbidden.   Calculations suggest that about 20-30% of all produced PCBs in one way or another have found their way to the environment, accumulated in dump sites or in the sediments of lakes and coastal zones.   This portion of PCBs is beyond control and a certain portion will gradually be found in organisms. Seventy percent is still in use, or in stock, and could reach the environment in the future. This very large pool of PCBs must be located and destroyed in a proper way, otherwise serious ecotoxicological effects will happen.

In foods the levels can be lowered by cleaning the fish oils used for consumption.   Levels in fish differ widely.   Cultivated salmon, for instance, is free of contamination.   Also fish from the oceans have lower levels than coastal fish.

KH: Is there a point where you would say to the mother not to breast feed due to toxin exposure?

JK: If the levels in the breast milk of a mother are higher than 80 pg TEQ/gr milk fat then one might consider to restrict breast-feeding for a few weeks. Prenatal control in blood is necessary for that purpose. Methods to do that in a simple way have to be developed. This is at the moment not yet possible. ◆

Breast Feeding Benefits and Physician's Knowledge

Elizabeth Williams, M.D., M.P.H.
Emory University School of Medicine
Department of Family and Preventive Medicine
478 Peachtree Street, Suite 818
Atlanta, GA 30308 U.S.A.
(404) 686-7619 / (404) 686-4366 (FAX)

"Breast feeding Attitudes and Knowledge of Pediatricians-in-Training",
American Journal of Prevenive Medicine, 1995;11;26-33. #21844.

Kirk Hamilton: Dr. Williams could you please share with us your educational background and current position?

Elizabeth Williams: After college I pursued graduate study in 19th century American english and history. I received my master's from Cornell University. I graduated from the University of Virginia School of Medicine in 1984 and did my internship in family medicine at the University of California San Francisco. I then switched to preventive medicine completing my residency at the University of California Berkeley, including a Masters of Public Health in Maternal and Child Health in 1988. I was a fellow in preventive medicine at Stanford from 1989-92 and then research associate and attending physician in preventive cardiology untill 1995. I have recently returned to training as a second year resident in family medicine in the Department of Family and Preventive Medicine at Emory University School of Medicine.

KH: When did you get interested in breast feeding as an important health promotion activity?

EW: For me breast feeding was really the intersection of my training in family medicine, preventive medicine and maternal and child health. I first really got interested in doing research in this area as a byproduct of doing another study. I observed some of what was going on in the well baby nursery and realized that it wasn't optimal breast feeding practice that was being encouraged and supported. I started asking myself some questions about why that was because it was contrary to what the research indicated was really best for mothers and babies. I did a study on what mothers knew and what information they were basing their feeding choice on. I also got some information about what they had found out from their physicians. I decided to find out directly from physicians what they were being trained in terms of breast feeding. So one study lead to another study.

KH: What did you find out about physicians' attitudes and knowledge toward breast feeding?

EW: This study was done at Stanford, which has an excellent pediatric training program and is representative of pediatric training programs. I found there was poor knowledge. There was a generally positive attitude about breast feeding, but the residents simply weren't being trained at the time when the study was done. It has improved quite a bit since this study was done, but they simply were not being given the knowledge and given the skills to translate that attitude, if you will, into the care they were providing to breast feeding mothers.

KH: How important is breast feeding when put it into the context of total preventive care, especially with respect to cost effectiveness?

EW: Dr. Miriam Labbok at Georgetown has evalutated this question and found that it would save our health care system on the order of billions of dollars using very conservative assumptions in various models. In fact, with respect to cardiovascular disease, there are studies in Britain that indicate that breast feeding as a child may actually lower your risk of atherosclerosis as an adult. More and more of what we are finding out, in terms of the benefits of breast feeding, point to considerable benefits in the geriatric age group.

KH: What are the benefits of breast feeding for the infant that the average person could understand and talk to their doctor about?

EW: There is a clear dose-response relationship -- the more a baby is exclusively breast fed in the first 6 months, the greater the protection against ear infections. What isn't generally understood among physicians is that many of the benefits extend beyond the period of the breast feeding. For example, in terms of ear infections and urinary tract infections, the protection persists for a significant period of time beyond the time that breast feeding stops.

KH: What is the optimal length of time to breast feed?

EW: The term, "optimal breast feeding practice" is actually a term from the World Health Organization, which states that looking at the benefits to mothers and babies, the optimal practice is 6 months of exclusive breast feeding. Actually, the current printed recommendation is 4 to 6 months of exclusive breast feeding. But more and more the research is indicating that we should be exclusively breast feeding longer, not shorter. Then the gradual introduction of solid foods at that 4 to 6 month period - not so much for nutrition as for the baby to start learning how use the complex muscle actions that are necessary to chew the food. The World Health Organization recommends continued breast feeding for a minimum of two years. The American Academy of Pediatrics says a minimum of one year. There is no recommendation that a baby should be weaned from the breast at a certain period. Worldwide, the average age at weaning is 4.2 years.

KH: How about breast feeding benefits to the mother?

EW: When mothers are making their choice, too often they don't realize that there's really any medical benefit to them. Usually we talk about how it's going to be more convenient to them. I'd like to talk about breast feeding purely from a medical viewpoint. Premenopausal breast cancer is something that most women, even young women who are having their babies, are very concerned about now. Several studies have now documented a significant decrease in the risk of premenopausal breast cancer for mothers who breast feed. There is probably some minimal amount of time that is necessary before that protection starts to occur. If you breast feed for two weeks, you probably aren't going to experience that particular benefit, although your baby will have the benefit of being breast fed for two weeks. There are some animal studies that indicate that receiving breast milk as an infant may lower the risk of that girl's baby's risk of breast cancer later in life.

KH: *One of the things I wanted to get into is how can you get a mother off to a good start breast feeding start? From the time she is pregnant, what can the obstetrician, pediatrician or family practitioner do?*

EW: Many women make their decision before they even conceive, so there are lots of interventions that we could be implementing preconception. During the prenatal visits, it is very important that the breasts be examined not just with a view toward is there an abnormal lump here, but is there any potential problem with respect to breast feeding that we could start working on during the prenatal period. That might mean flat nipples or truly inverted nipples, which for most women are not a problem, but they may be worrying about it. Simply to hear that it probably is not going to be a problem can be very reassuring. In short, the practitioner gives a breast examination from the viewpoint of breast feeding and starting a dialogue. How do you plan to feed the baby? What are the issues for you? Are you planning on going back to work? These are some basic questions. In the hospital, it's very important for the mother to understand how to get off to the best start, particularly since we have such short hospital stays now. The mother needs to know, and the hospital needs to know, that the best start for breast feeding is for babies to be allowed to nuzzle at the breast immediately after birth. This is the time when they're most alert. In fact, they're more alert than they are ever going to be during most hospital stays now. The mother needs to know if breast feeding is truly going to be an option for her. The best thing she can do is breast feed exclusively until her milk supply is well established.

KH: *How long does it take for the "milk to come in ?"*

EW: Days 3 to 5 are when the "milk comes in" for the first time mother - sooner for women who have had a child previously.

KH: *I understand you can be very uncomfortable during that period when the breasts become full.*

EW: The best way to prevent really painful engorgement is for the baby to be breast feeding frequently. That can often times prevent that painful engorgement from ever really being a problem for the mother. The first few weeks are when the milk supply is getting well established. The best practice is to avoid using other artificial nipples until the milk supply is well established. Because if the baby is sucking on a pacifier she is not nursing. She's not at the breast. The mother's body needs to know there's a baby there who needs to be fed and that milk supply gets stimulated by the baby being at the breast.

KH: *We have a lot of moms working. I wonder if you could give them some positive strokes on how they can breast feed going to work.*

EW: First mothers need to know that breast feeding is an option and that there are a lot of different ways of incorporating breast feeding into a working mother's schedule depending on the situation. Generally, the best start is to get the mother's milk supply well established in those early weeks. When mothers start going back to work even part-time, if the milk supply has never been adequately stimulated, they are more vulnerable to losing their milk or seeing it decrease which makes it harder for them to keep on breast feeding. The older the baby is when they go back to work, the easier it will be. It's much more difficult if you're going back to work at three weeks than if you are able to delay that and go back, say, when the baby is two months old and initially working 20 hours a week.

KH: *Are there any organizations in San Diego that people could call with breast feeding questions. Was there a resource?*

EW: Wellstart in San Diego deals with educating and developing curricula for health professionals. The La Leche League is a wonderful organization to provide help to mothers. Their number is 1-800-La Leche. ◆

Breast Milk, Antiinfective Factors, Additives and Intestinal Permeability

Richard Quan, M.D.
University of Nevada Medical School
Department of Pediatrics
Associate Professor Clinical Medicine
411 W. 2nd Street
Reno, NV 89503 U.S.A.
(702) 784-6170 / (702) 784-4420 / (702) 784-4828 (FAX)

"The Effect of Nutritional Additives on Antiinfective Factors in Human Milk",
Clinical Pediatrics, June, 1994:325-329. #20482

Kirk Hamilton: *Can you give me your educational background since college and then your present position?*

Richard Quan: I went to Stanford University as an undergraduate, majoring in human biology. I went to the University of South Alabama in Mobile, Alabama for my medical education and did my internship and pediatric residency at Children's Hospital in Birmingham. I then went to Stanford University for my pediatric gastroenterology fellowship. I did 2 clinical years and then did 3 years of research with the Department of Internal Medicine in the Division of Gastroenterology at Stanford University under the mentorship of Dr. Gary Gray. I received my first faculty position in 1987 with the University of Texas Southwestern in Dallas. I was recently appointed as division head of the Pediatric/GI Nutrition Department at the University of Nevada.

KH: *How did you get interested in breast milk, antiinfective factors and antioxidants?*

RQ: It stems from a discussion with Dr. Sunshine, a neonatologist at Stanford University, who had done some previous work looking at antiinfective factors in breast milk in the nursery and the practice of freezing and thawing. He had observed that there was a practice of thawing frozen breast milk using a microwave in the nursery, but there was no evidence to show that this was safe. He felt "all" modifications that we make to breast milk ought to be studied.

KH: *What are the antiinfective factors in breast milk that we're concerned about?*

RQ: There are a variety of factors (i.e. lysozymes, immunoglobulins, lactoferrin, nucleotides) that help to prevent infection in the breastfed infant, as evidenced by a reduced incidence of diarrhea and respiratory infections. Some people have proposed that lactoferrin is an antiinfective agent, in addition to its accepted role as an iron transport vehicle. Lactoferrin activates certain lymphocytes and perhaps prepares them to respond to bacteria.

KH: *After reading your article, I thought why doesn't the mother separate the consumption of her breast milk at a different time than the Similac or other supplemental formulas?*

RQ: There was at least one study supporting that idea. I think the reason additives were combined with breast milk was the fact

that mature breast milk may not be optimal nutrition for the premature infant. Infants accumulate certain elements during their time in utero, especially in the last trimester. Premature infants are deprived of these nutrients, and must assimilate them outside the womb. In a perfect world, what one would do is simply take human breast milk and remove some of the water, thereby concentrating everything including calcium and protein and all the antiinfective factors and give that to the premature infant.

KH: *Are you discovering which "additives" have what effect?*

RQ: I think we're still at the point of trying to decide which nutrients are most important to the premature infant.

KH: *What is your solution now for a premature infant? Do you feed them the breast milk and formula at different times, or do you mix them accepting the trade off between suppression of the antiinfective factors versus the increased need for specific nutrients?*

RQ: I think what most people do is accept the fact that you get some lowering of immune function and go ahead and add whatever is needed for growth.

KH: *There really isn't a problem in a term infant?*

RQ: There are very few mothers who have insufficient quantities of breast milk for their term infants. Most of those occur because of an absence from the baby and lack of stimulation. Let's say a mother was in a motor vehicle accident or is taking medications that might suppress her breast milk, causing an interruption in the breast milk supply. Then there might be a need for supplementation with formula.

KH: *Even if you freeze the breast milk - you wouldn't mix it?*

RQ: Correct.

KH: *You give the breast milk at a different time than the formula?*

RQ: Yes.

KH: *Are there any other things that suppress these antiinfective factors?*

RQ: Certainly, microwaving is another aspect. In the process of thawing by microwaves, we showed how it really isn't good for the breast milk.

KH: *Are there things the mother consumes or lifestyle factors that affect these antiinfective factors that you know of?*

RQ: If a mother were malnourished, there is a tendency to decrease her immunoglobulins in breast milk and would probably affect the amount the baby would receive.

KH: *What about adding water to breast milk? Does that reduce these factors?*

RQ: We actually tried that in the pilot study of the article and it did not seem to have any adverse effect.

KH: *You are a pediatric gastroenterologist?*

RQ: That is correct.

KH: *Do premature infants have enhanced intestinal permeability? If so, is this increased permeability to help them absorb immunoglobulins from the mother?*

RQ: Yes, in some animal species, immunoglobulins are absorbed intact. If they didn't have those, they would probably catch infections very easily. The role of early enhanced intestinal permeability in humans has not been determined.

KH: *Theoretically, if we gave a foreign protein during this period of increased intestinal permeability such as cows' milk, egg or wheat gluten, could you create an immunologic reaction?*

RQ: Correct.

KH: *In normal infants, isn't there an early period where there is increased intestinal permeability - such as the first couple of days?*

RQ: The "increased intestinal permeability" probably is longer than the first couple of days. There is some suggestion in the literature that "gut closure" may not occur until 6 to 8 months of age. From a clinical standpoint, we see some children develop cows' milk and soy protein allergies and have to be placed on either hydrosylated formulas or even defined formula such as Tolerex in order to avoid these antigens. Their manifestations include diarrhea, blood in the stool or vomiting. Somewhere around 6 to 8 months of age, gut closure occurs where few of these large antigens cross the intestinal wall surface. You can then switch the babies back to a regular formula and sometimes even to plain cows' milk.

KH: *If you created an inflammatory condition, could that prolong the intestinal permeability? For example, if you were consuming cows' milk or wheat gluten in the first months and years of life, could that theoretically prolong the intestinal permeability problem?*

RQ: Yes, that could prolong it or may be the cause of food allergies in some children. Viruses can cause a break in the barrier because of gastroenteritis, and these macromolecules (such as casein) get across the intestinal barrier and then the infants become sensitized.

KH: *If you have increased intestinal permeability which allows for larger molecules to be absorbed, can you in the same breath have malabsorption of basic nutrients?*

RQ: Sure. The idea is that if you have macromolecules being absorbed this can cause an immunologic reaction with release of cytokines that stir up the intestines and cause the intestines to secrete fluid. When there is more flow through the intestine, increased peristalsis and decreased transit time, then the intestinal flow doesn't allow the nutrient sufficient time to get across the enterocyte and there is malabsorption. ◆

Calcium Balance and Caffeine

Janet Barger-Lux, M.S.
Creighton University Osteoporosis Research Center
601 North 30th Street, Suite 5766
Omaha, NE 68131 U.S.A.
(402) 280-4470 / (402) 280-5173 (FAX)

"Caffeine and the Calcium Economy Revisited,"
Osteoporosis International, 1995;5:97-102. #22386

Kirk Hamilton: *Can you please share with me your educational background and current position?*

Janet Barger-Lux: I earned a bachelors of science in medical technology from Creighton University in 1964. I received a Masters in Pathology and Laboratory Medicine from the University of Nebraska in 1982. I was appointed to the faculty as a senior research associate in medicine, Creighton University School of Medicine, Omaha, Nebraska and currently I am a co-investigator and project manager in the Creighton University Osteoporosis Research Center.

KH: *Why did you decide to look at the role of caffeine in calcium metabolism?*

JBL: Calcium balance is daily calcium input less daily calcium output at the level of the whole organism (person). Positive calcium balance is required during periods of skeletal growth and consolidation (until about age 30 in healthy women). Negative calcium balance means loss of skeletal mass, itself an imperfect surrogate for skeletal strength.

In 1982, Heaney and Recker of our group reported a small negative association between caffeine-containing coffee intake and calcium balance. Since that time, caffeine has regularly been listed as a risk factor for osteoporosis, both in scientific papers and in articles in the popular press.

In 1993, I was asked to present a review on caffeine's effect on calcium balance at an international symposium. Heaney and Recker's 1982 paper presented early data from a study of women who were followed for many years thereafter. We were able to update and expand the caffeine part of the paper by examining data from 560 balance studies. Our 1995 publication in *Osteoporosis International* was derived from that symposium presentation.

KH: *What are the effects of caffeine's ingestion on calcium balance?*

JBL: Our 1995 paper reported a small negative effect of caffeine on calcium balance - for every 6 fl oz serving of caffeine-containing coffee, calcium balance was more negative by 4.6 mg. It has been presumed that caffeine affects calcium balance mainly by increasing calcium output in the urine. However, our data show caffeine effects on calcium intake rather than output. Caffeine intake was inversely associated with both calcium intake and calcium absorption efficiency. This means that, among the women we studied, those who consume larger quantities of caffeine tended to have lower calcium intakes, and vice versa. Also, those who consumed larger

quantities of caffeine tended to absorb calcium slightly less efficiently, and vice versa. Coffee supplied about 93 percent of all the caffeine consumed by our subjects.

KH: *What are the strategies for offsetting the adverse effects of caffeine on calcium?*

JBL: It is hard to maintain a generous calcium intake if one consistently chooses to drink coffee, tea or soft drinks (whether they happen to be caffeine-containing or not) rather than milk.

Caffeine also increases one's individual requirement for calcium. About 40 mg of additional calcium (as contained in about 1 fl oz of milk) would offset the negative effect of 6 fl oz of caffeine-containing coffee.

KH: *What is the effect of sodium ingestion on calcium balance?*

JBL: Both sodium and protein exert well-known effects on calcium balance. On average, for every 2,300 mg of sodium ingested, 52 mg of calcium is lost in the urine, and for every 1 gm of protein ingested, about 1 mg of calcium is lost in the urine. Our 1995 paper presents an example to put this all together. An ordinary hamburger sandwich contains about 15 gm of protein, 525 mg of sodium and 60 mg of calcium. An overall calcium balance effect of -22 mg can be estimated as follows: -14.5 mg from the protein, -13.7 mg from the sodium, and +6 mg from the calcium (at a net retention of roughly 10 percent). High intakes of sodium and/or protein cause us to need more calcium than we otherwise would.

KH: *What are the effects of trace nutrients on bone maintenance?*

JBL: Vitamin D is vital to bone health, and we believe that vitamin D insufficiency is widespread among persons with little sun exposure. I believe that deleterious effects of deficiencies of vitamin K and zinc are also suspected.

KH: *What are the risk factors for osteoporosis and their order of importance?*

JBL: Because there are many paths to osteoporosis, it is also difficult to arrange risk factors in rank-order. It is important not to limit ourselves to bone loss. Some persons fail to gain a high enough peak bone mass in early adult life. Here is my personal list of risk factors that lead to osteoporosis-related fractures: Among adolescents and young adults: low intakes of calcium, high sodium intakes, excessive thinness, and cigarette smoking. In adults: low calcium intake, a high sodium intake, cigarette smoking, abuse of alcohol, certain diseases that can produce gonadal hormone deficiencies, impaired physical activity, endocrine problems such as hyperthyroidism, over-treatment of hypothyroidism, and treatments with corticosteroid drugs or antiseizure medications. In older adults: physical inactivity, vitamin D insufficiency, low calcium intake and impairments (e.g. in balance, vision, gait, or level of consciousness) that may lead to falling. Any of these factors can be critical, but they often occur in combination.

KH: *What is your comment on hormone replacement therapy in the prevention of bone loss?*

JBL: Maintenance of bone mass of both women and men is, after adolescence, dependent upon gonadal hormones. Estrogen withdrawal (in association with natural or surgical menopause, or with ovarian failure at any age) leads to the loss of roughly 15 percent of skeletal bone over a 2 or 3 year period, as well as slightly less efficient calcium absorption. Estrogen replacement postpones this loss until the estrogen is discontinued.

KH: *What sources of calcium do you recommend?*

JBL: In the United states the wide prevalence of low calcium intake, especially among girls and women, constitutes a serious public health problem. NHANES II data show that the average calcium intake among U.S. females peaks at age 8. Although we often say that nutritional needs should, preferably, be met from food sources, this strategy has limited utility. I believe that serious studies should be made of calcium fortification of selected, widely-consumed items in the food supply, such that ample calcium would be consumed without particular individual effort.

KH: *What are the crucial periods of calcium need?*

JBL: An adequate calcium intake is important throughout life, but I would identify 3 particularly crucial times:
Adolescence: About 50% of adult bone mass is acquired during adolescence. Optimal skeletal build-up during this time probably requires a daily calcium intake of about 1,600 mg per day. However, 2 of 3 U.S. girls and half of the boys in the 9 to 14 age group have calcium intakes less than 1,000 mg per day.

Pregnancy and Lactation: As early as the 12th week of pregnancy a woman's skeleton begins to "load up" on calcium. If she maintains an ample calcium intake, she will be prepared for the weeks and months of lactation, when some bone loss probably always occurs. The pregnant woman contributes about 25 gm of calcium to mineralize the baby's skeleton, but she will contribute 4 times that much to carry out 9 months of breast feeding.

Older Adulthood: In older adulthood no one yet knows how much age-related bone loss is really inevitable and how much is due to the interactive effects of poor nutrition and declining physical activity. Several recently-published studies have shown the remarkable effectiveness of calcium and vitamin D in reducing the number of fractures occurring among older adults, even those 85+ years of age and/or living in nursing homes. ◆

Cancer Chemoprevention, Antioxidants and N-Acetylcysteine

Boudewijn J.M. Braakhuis, Ph.D.
Research Scientist/Section of Tumor Biology
Department of Otolaryngology/Head and Neck Surgery
Free University Hospital
P.O. Box 7057
1007 M.B. Amsterdam, The Netherlands
31 20 444 0905 / 31 20 444 0983 (FAX)

"Antioxidant-Related Parameters in Patients Treated for Cancer Chemoprevention With N-Acetylcysteine", European Journal of Cancer, 1995;31A(6):921-923. #23078

Kirk Hamilton: *Could you please share with me your educational background and current position?*

Boudewijn J.M. Braakhuis: I trained as a biologist with a doctoral degree in life sciences (immunology and pharmacology). I joined the Department of Otolaryngology/Head and Neck Surgery of the Free University in Amsterdam. In this department I obtained my Ph.D. degree in cancer chemotherapy. I am presently an associate professor with research interests in the field of risk factor assessment and chemoprevention of head and neck cancer. I am head of the section of prevention research within the laboratory of tumor biology of the Department of Otolaryngology/Head and Neck Surgery.

KH: *When did you get interested in the role of N-acetylcysteine and cancer chemoprevention?*

BJB: Within our department we have a close cooperation between the physicians and the researchers in the lab. Since 1988 our clinicians started to prescribe drugs to patients who had been cured for head and neck cancer. These patients were at high risk (between 10 and 20%) to experience another primary tumor within 5 years after the diagnosis of the first carcinoma. Those so-called multiple primary tumors can develop in the whole respiratory and upper digestive tract, including lung and the esophagus. The drugs chosen were N-acetylcysteine, retinyl-palmitate or a combination of these drugs. A no-treatment group was included. Our efforts are part of the European trial called Euroscan. To date over 2,500 patients have entered this trial from all over Europe. The trial is initiated by the "Lung" and "Head and Neck" group of the EORTC (European Organization For Research in the Treatment of Cancer). From the early 90s on, we have directed laboratory research on chemoprevention and one of the compounds used in this respect was N-acetylcysteine.

KH: *What was the theory behind evaluating antioxidant parameters in these individuals with cancer?*

BJB: In fact, the patients that were treated had no detectable cancer. N-acetylcysteine was tested in patients who were cured from their carcinoma. The aim was to prevent second primary tumors and about 10 to 20% of these patients would have another carcinoma within 5 years. The choice of N-acetylcysteine was based on the preclinical work of Dr. De Flora and his group from Genoa, Italy. They showed that N-acetylcysteine was an active anti-mutagen and anti-carcinogen. The aim of our clinical trial was to protect the DNA from reactive free radicals. N-acetylcysteine itself has such function or can be metabolized to glutathione. N-acetylcysteine is thought to be active in the first (initiating) steps of carcinogenesis. Since it was not known whether the dose was high enough to alter plasma and tissue levels of glutathione this study was undertaken. A part of this study was to see whether supplementation with N-acetylcysteine could alter the TRAP-value of the blood plasma. TRAP stands for total radical trapping-ability parameter. This assay reflects the synergistic protection of various antioxidants against biological damage caused by peroxyl radicals.

KH: *What was the dosage of N-acetylcysteine used and what was the desired effect?*

BJB: The doses of N-acetylcysteine was 600 mg per day for 2 years. This dose was based on experience using N-acetylcysteine as a mucolytic drug. Toxicity should be very low, because most people eventually will not develop cancer. The ultimate aim is to prevent the occurrence of a second primary tumor in the respiratory and upper digestive tract. Since it will take a long time for the end points of the trials to be reached, the occurrence of such a second primary tumor in the Euroscan trial will be evaluated three years from now at the earliest.

KH: *What did you find out with regards to N-acetylcysteine supplementation in these "cured" cancer patients?*

BJB: Administration of N-acetylcysteine did increase the blood plasma level of glutathione by 38%. No change in blood-plasma levels were observed for the other antioxidants ascorbic acid and urate. Also the non-protein-thiol concentration (consisting predominantly of cysteine, glutathione, N-acetylcysteine) in erythrocytes did increase by 31%. Glutathione levels in exfoliated cells of the buccal mucosa were too low to measure. The TRAP-value did not show any change either. *In vitro* incubations of blood plasma with an antioxidant showed that N-acetylcysteine prevents early damage, while glutathione functions over a longer time period.

KH: *Is it better to give N-acetylcysteine or glutathione to enhance glutathione levels?*

BJB: Oral administration of glutathione did not lead to higher glutathione plasma levels. However, good results are seen with lung fibrosis if glutathione is inhaled in an evaporated form. With this method of administration glutathione levels increased in the epithelium of the lung.

KH: *Is there any data yet from the trials to show benefit?*

BJB: We do not know yet. As described earlier, we have to wait a few years before the answer of the Euroscan chemoprevention trial is known.

KH: *Would it be reasonable to give N-acetylcysteine in cancer treatment to prevent secondary tumors at present?*

BJB: I think the results of this Euroscan and other trials have to be completed before any conclusion can be drawn. The fact that glutathione levels increase after administration of N-acetylcysteine is encouraging and points to a possible beneficial effect. ◆

Cancer, Sleep and Melatonin

Russel J. Reiter, Ph.D.

Department of Cellular and Structural Biology
The University of Texas Health Science Center
7703 Floyd Curl Drive
San Antonio, TX 78284-7762 U.S.A.
(201) 567-3859 (of) / 210 567-3805 (sec)
(210) 567-3900 (dept) / (210 567-6948 (FAX)

"Melatonin Suppression by Static and Extremely Low Frequency Electromagnetic Fields: Relationship to the Reported Increased Incidence of Cancer," Reviews on Environmental Health, 1994;10(3-4):171. #21990

Kirk Hamilton: What is your educational background since college, and what is your present position?

Russel Reiter: My college degree is in biology. I received my Ph.D. in endocrinology in 1964 at Bowman Gray School of Medicine at Wake Forest University, Winston-Salem, North Carolina. For two years I was a captain in the Medical Service Corp, where I did research at the Army Chemical Center in Maryland, and I was at the University of Rochester School of Medicine for 5 years. Since 1971, I have been here in San Antonio at the Department of Cellular and Structural Biology. I am currently a professor of neuroendocrinology, and I advanced to the rank of professor in 1973. I recently authored a book with Jo Robinson on the subject of melatonin. It is published by Bantam Books and is titled Melatonin: Your Body's Natural Wonder Drug.

KH: How did you get interested in melatonin?

RR: In 1964, after I obtained my Ph.D., I was at the United States Army Arsenal. It was about 5 years after Sputnik. At the time, there was a very aggressive program for putting people into outer space and traveling to distant planets. There was also interest in having the placed in suspended hibernation. To travel to Mars, it may take 6 months. For people to live in a capsule, have sufficient food and water, there just would not be sufficient space. So the Army, at the time, was interested in hibernation. If we could isolate the "hibernatory factor" and identify it in animals, then maybe we could use it to produce a state of hibernation in humans and have them, "sleep" for the 6-month period and arouse them when they arrived. This would greatly reduce the resources needed on board. So we were asked to work with hibernation. At about the same time, it was shown that the pineal gland might produce a hormone called melatonin, and we thought maybe melatonin was that "hibernatory factor." Initially we linked melatonin to reproduction and later to cancer. Within the last two years its antioxidant properties and its ability to reduce the possibility of cancer has been shown.

KH: Please elaborate on melatonin's antioxidant capabilities?

RR: We knew for many years that melatonin had effects that couldn't be explained on the basis of what we conventionally knew about melatonin. In other words, in every organ melatonin had some subtle effects. We deduced that maybe melatonin was a free radical scavenger, an antioxidant that neutralizes free radicals. We set up a series of experiments to test this. Much to our surprise, melatonin proved to be about a 5-fold better scavenger of the most toxic free radical.

KH: Is that hydroxyl radical?

RR: Mainly. Melatonin seems to be 5 times better than glutathione, which is a very good intracellular free radical scavenger, and 15 times better than mannitol. Mannitol is one we get from foods. Subsequently, it was shown by a group in Italy that melatonin is also a better peroxyl radical scavenger than is vitamin E. Vitamin E was felt to be the best of the best against lipid peroxidation. Now it appears that melatonin is as good as vitamin E in that capacity.

KH: Why aren't we hearing more about melatonin as an antioxidant in conditions like the prevention of LDL oxidation?

RR: You have to realize that the information on the antioxidant properties of melatonin was first published in May 1993. It is not uncommon for research knowledge amongst physicians and textbooks to lag years behind. There is considerable interest in melatonin in reference to LDL oxidation and there is a group in Dusseldorf, Germany working on this very problem.

KH: How is melatonin affected by light?

RR: During the daytime, in all individuals, melatonin levels are low because light inhibits melatonin production. Melatonin production increases at night in the pineal gland, a small gland in the brain. In your case, for example, your melatonin levels may go up 5-fold higher at night than they are during the day. In somebody else's case, they may go up 15-fold over daytime levels. If you get up at night and expose yourself to light, melatonin levels immediately plummet. In other words, melatonin production is shut off and it disappears from the blood. This is unfortunate and also unhealthy in the sense that you are depriving yourself of antioxidant protection against free radical damage. The bottom line is, we were not meant to have light at night. We evolved from animals where it was either light or dark. The pineal gland only produces melatonin at night. Light is good, of course, but light at the wrong time of the 24-hour period is bad because it inhibits melatonin. The same thing happens in jet lag. You fly, for example, from Seattle to Frankfurt, Germany eastwardly overnight and experience a very short night. You get off the plane in Frankfurt at 8 a.m., but in Seattle, it is midnight. The bright light in Frankfurt depresses your melatonin, and then for about 5 to 6 days your melatonin tries to resynchronized the new light-dark cycle. This contributes to the phenomenon of jet lag.

KH: *Then do people who sleep less -- let's say they are working a lot -- have an increased risk to all the free radical diseases?*

RR: Those surveys have not been adequately done. There is considerable interest in blind individuals who cannot perceive light (they are in essence in darkness all the time). There is some evidence that they have a lower cancer risk than nonblind subjects. However, they have some other associated problems because their melatonin rhythm is not in synchrony with their sleep\ activity pattern because it is not synchronized by the light-dark cycle.

KH: *How about the role of electromagnetic fields in altering melatonin secretion and the possible increased risk of breast cancer? before?*

RR: There is a great interest in this. There are a number of epidemiological studies, claiming that people who live near or are exposed to unusually high electromagnetic fields (and it appears to be the magnetic field that is harmful, if anything is) may have a slightly higher incidence of cancer. Not only breast cancer, but various types of leukemia and brain cancer as well. These fields in experimental animals, under the right conditions, do act somewhat like light in reducing the amount of melatonin the pineal gland produces. So, theoretically, there could be a link between the reduced melatonin that is a consequence of electromagnetic field exposure and the alleged higher incidence of cancer. There are 2 caveats. First of all, it has never been definitively proven in humans, that the fields to which we are exposed from conventional instrumentation or high powered lines are sufficient to reduce or significantly alter melatonin levels. If they are, whether in fact it would cause cancer or lead to a higher incidence of cancer is unknown. Also, whether in fact the epidemiologic studies are correct in claiming there is a higher incidence of cancer is highly debated.

KH: *Are there lower levels of melatonin in cancer patients? Has anybody ever studied that?*

RR: Yes. Individuals with various types of cancer have been reported to have an inherently lower melatonin rhythm. In the early 1980s, a group of scientists at the National Institute of Health published a report showing that women with estrogen receptor positive breast cancer have a lower nighttime rise in melatonin than women who do not have cancer. The implication was that possibly the lower than normal melatonin was causative. But that conclusion is premature. It is unknown whether the lower melatonin was a cause or effect or even related to the cancer. Subsequently, in terms of prostate cancer in males, similar associations were made. In experimental animals if the source of melatonin is removed by doing a surgical pinealectomy (the origin of the melatonin), these animals may develop cancer faster than they would if their pineal gland was intact and they had adequate melatonin.

KH: *You triggered a question in my mind going back to "light at night concept." Is it any type of light? We talk about full-spectrum light having some kind of positive benefit. What about working at my computer with a lamp on from 11 p.m. to 2 a.m.? Is that suppressing melatonin?*

RR: Very likely. The most important feature about light seems to be how bright it is. Different wavelengths, in other words colors, also impact melatonin levels slightly differently, with those in the blue-green range being the most inhibitory. What is important mostly seems to be how bright the light is. If you are working, for example, at your computer and you have a desk lamp beside you and the light is relatively bright, in many individuals this would cause a partial or total suppression of their melatonin at night. Moonlight experienced outdoors, or from a skylight in your bedroom, will not affect melatonin rhythm levels. What is generally considered to be bright light, such as an office light, would likely partially suppress melatonin in many individuals at night. If we are worried about electromagnetic fields depressing melatonin (and I am not saying they do) and possibly increasing the incidence of cancer, a much greater danger is the exposure of light at night because there is no doubt that bright light at night depresses melatonin.

KH: *It sounds like melatonin should be taken by all these entrepreneurs working late at night. I am thinking about myself.*

RR: As a matter of fact, melatonin is a good sleep aid. One reason it is sold is for jet lag and now as an antioxidant, which implies melatonin as an anticancer agent as well. There are a many people taking it. When you do take melatonin (I am not telling you to or not to), you should always take it at night because it also gives a timing signal. It signals night to your body, and if taken during the day the body interprets this message as night and it gears down as if to go to sleep.

KH: *I just interviewed a breast cancer surgeon who believed strongly that a plant-oriented diet decreases the risk of breast cancer. He worked in developing countries and saw a low incidence of breast cancer. I am thinking that in addition to the diet, because there is little artificial light in developing countries and people go to sleep when it gets dark, this could reduce the breast cancer risk further?*

RR: We've always assumed that light and the use of artificial light was totally innocuous. Many people who work night shifts have terrible difficulties sleeping. It is very disruptive to many circadian rhythms in the body. We have always taken light absolutely for granted and said, "Oh it's just fine." It is not just fine. It causes biochemical changes in the body which alter circadian rhythms as well. In reference to plants, I am glad you brought that up because we have just published our first paper showing that melatonin also occurs in some plants.

KH: *And which plants are those?*

RR: We only looked at edible plants. It is highest in rice and corn products. In Japan, where they eat a lot of rice, epidemiological studies have shown that there is a lower incidence of certain kinds of cancer, particularly breast cancer. I am not implying that eating of rice is the cause of the lower cancer incidence, but you get the gist of the way scientists think. We feel some people ingest more melatonin than others and this may be beneficial to them.

KH: *Do you know if the melatonin is removed during the refining process of rice (white rice)?*

RR: This has not been investigated. It is important to know whether the processing of foodstuffs removes the melatonin. To date, this information is not available.

KH: *In the future, where do you see melatonin? What clinical uses would you use melatonin in?*

RR: There are many. We now think melatonin is a very good antioxidant. Vitamin E, vitamin C and beta-carotene are the ones seen advertised on television as the antioxidant combination. They are limited in the sense that they do not go into all parts of the cell. Vitamin E confines itself primarily to lipid, which makes up the membrane of the cell. Vitamin C is primarily in the cytosol because it is a water-soluble vitamin. Melatonin goes into the nucleus of the cell, into the cytosol, and into the plasma membrane. It is both a lipid and water-soluble compound. There are many free radical-based diseases. For example, after a heart attack or stroke when the tissue is reperfused with blood after the blood vessels are reopened, the tissue is reoxygenated and large numbers of free radicals are produced. This is called ischemia-reperfusion injury. There has been great interest in uncovering antioxidants to protect against this. Melatonin gets into the brain very easily. Parkinsonism is believed to be related to free radicals. We envision melatonin will have utility in treating a variety of free radical-related diseases. Porphyrias are another example. Myasthenia gravis and many of the neurodegenerative diseases of aging are free radical-based, as is cancer. We think melatonin may be important in advanced age. As you age, the rate at which you age accelerates. A primary cause of aging is accumulated free radical damage. If this is really true, then giving antioxidants should delay aging. Many attempts have been made rather unsuccessfully to do this with the exception of melatonin. Animals live longer, and they live healthier longer when given melatonin. What normally happens in humans is, as we age, the melatonin rhythm becomes more and more attenuated. We lose some protection against free radical-related diseases as we age. Other antioxidants may be elevated, but they are insufficient to overcome oxidative damage, which possibly melatonin can protect against. Not only will melatonin be taken as a factor to delay certain diseases, but it may also be taken as an antiaging agent. I doubt whether just taking melatonin will solve the problems of aging, but it may be a significant component in delaying aging. The secret is not to live to be 120 -- I don't think many people want to live to be 120. But they would like to live to be 90 and be in good health until near the time they die. What you want to do is die young as late as possible. That is what melatonin may assist in doing.

KH: *That is called rectangularizing the death curve.*

RR: Exactly. That is what it is called.

KH: *It makes me remember the saying, "Early to bed, early to rise, makes a man healthy, wealthy and wise." Life could be so simple if we would just follow some basic rules.*

RR: That's a very good axiom that I think we should actually follow it. Before artificial light sources, that is pretty much the way it was. If we still utilized that program, we would probably be more healthy. Using light at inappropiate times and jet lag are terrible punishments to the body.

KH: *Is the best time to take meltonin before you sleep at night?*

RR: Yes. What you want to do if you are 70 years old is to maintain the melatonin rhythm of a 20 year old. Since melatonin is normally high at night, that's when melatonin should be taken.

KH: *What dosage of melatonin is reasonable for sleep disorders and for antioxidant effects.*

RR: This is a difficult question to answer because the experimental data are incomplete. For sleep disorders, nightly doses of .2-10 mg have been mentioned. It is recommended that the lowest effective dose be taken. For antioxidant protection, in some cases the effective doses may be higher.

KH: *Do you take melatonin? If so how much and when? And for what reasons?*

SS: I do take melatonin for a very specific reason. I take medications which prevent my pineal gland from producing melatonin. So I take melatonin nightly (1 mg or less) to give myself a nightly melatonin increase. I encourage all of you to read my book (Melatonin: Your Body's Natural Wonder Drug) to see what drugs altered your melatonin rhythm and how to preserve your own melatonin production. ◆

Carcinogenicity of Lipid-Lowering Drugs

Thomas B. Newman, M.D., M.P.H.
University of California at San Francisco
Box 0626, Department of Laboratory Medicine
San Francisco, CA 94143-0626 U.S.A.
(415) 476-6451 / (415) 476-2796 (FAX-O) / (415) 697-3724 (FAX-H)

"Carcinogenicity of Lipid-Lowering Drugs,"
JAMA, January 3, 1996;275(1):55-60. #24021

Kirk Hamilton: *Can you please share with me your educational background and current position?*

Thomas Newman: I have a bachelor's degree in chemistry from the University of California Santa Cruz, and a MD degree from the University of California San Diego. I did my pediatric internship and residency at the University of California San Francisco School of Medicine and a 2 year fellowship in clinical epidemiology at the University of California San Francisco which also included a Masters in Public Health in epidemiology from the University of California Berkeley. My current position is associate professor of laboratory medicine, pediatrics tand epidemiology and biostatistics at the University of California San Francisco.

KH: *Why would a pediatrician become interested in lipid-lowering drugs and their association with cancer risk?*

TN: I became interested in the risks and benefits of cholesterol lowering when people began recommending screening and treatment of children for high blood cholesterol levels. About that time a meta-analyses of primary prevention trials of cholesterol reduction by Muldoon and colleagues showed a significant (P=.01) excess of cancer deaths among those randomized to cholesterol-lowering interventions. Although in subsequent, larger meta-analysis this effect was diminished and no longer statistically significant, it remains a concern. We know that chemical carcinogenicity may take 20 or more years to become evident, and that in cohort studies low cholesterol-levels are associated with a higher risk of cancer death that probably cannot be entirely explained by pre-existing cancer.

KH: *Can you describe the findings of your study with regards to the suggestion of increased cancer risk of lipid-lowering medications?*

TN: We tabulated the results of rodent carcinogenicity studies of lipid-lowering drugs, and compared these with carcinogenicity results for antihypertensives. We found that all members of the two most popular classes of lipid-lowering drugs (the fibrates and the statins) cause cancer in rodents, in some cases at levels of animal exposure close to those prescribed to humans. In contrast, few of the antihypertensive drugs have been found to be carcinogenic in rodents. Evidence of carcinogenicity from clinical trials in humans is inconclusive, due to the inconsistent results and insufficient duration of follow-up.

KH: *How is it possible to extrapolate the animal data regarding carcinogenicity and have relevancy to humans with respect to lipid-lowering medications?*

TN: Rodent carcinogenicity studies can provide only a suggestion of carcinogenic risk to humans. However, the consistent carcinogenicity of cholesterol-lowering drugs, coupled with their intended pattern of long-term use, is a matter of concern. If this were not so, there would be no point in requiring that drugs be tested for carcinogenicity in rodents. As stated by the World Health Organization's International Agency for Research on Cancer (IARC), ". . . in the absence of adequate data on humans, it is biologically plausible and prudent to regard agents and mixtures for which there is sufficient evidence of carcinogenicity in experimental animals as if they presented a carcinogenic risk to humans."

KH: *What is the theoretic mechanism by which these specific classes of lipid-lowering drugs increase the risk to cancer?*

TN: The two classes of drugs for which carcinogenicity is the greatest concern are the fibrates (clofibrate, gemfibrozil) and statins (lovastatin, simvastatin, etc.). The mechanisms of carcinogenicity are not clear. Neither class is mutagenic. The fibrates' tendency to induce proliferation of peroxisomes (an organelle in the liver) is associated with their carcinogenicity across species, and such proliferation occurs less in primates than in rodents. However, the exact mechanism of carcinogenesis is not understood for either class of drugs.

KH: *In your conclusion, you suggest that "lipid-lowering drug treatment, especially with fibrates and statins, should be avoided except in patients at high short-term risk of coronary heart disease." Can you describe the type of patient that is "at short-term risk of heart disease?"*

TN: The most attractive candidates for lipid-lowering therapy are men at high short-term risk of coronary heart disease (CHD) death, such as those who already have evidence of CHD (angina or past myocardial infarction), and those whose high cholesterol level and risk factors (age, smoking, diabetes, hypertension, family history) put them at high risk. Benefits of treating women are much more uncertain, though it is probably reasonable to treat those at very high risk of CHD. For most young people (men <40 and women <50) it is hard to justify drug treatment in the absence of known CHD or extraordinary levels of risk factors.

KH: *Do you feel that lipid-lowering medications are being overused?*

TN: Lipid-lowering medications are not just being *overused*, they are being **misused**. Some patients like those mentioned above, in whom the benefits are likely to outweigh the risks may not have been offered these medications, whereas others, in whom risks and costs very likely outweigh benefits are being told they need to take them.

KH: *Can you explain why these cholesterol lowering drugs were approved despite their animal carcinogenicity?*

TN: I believe the drugs were approved by the FDA because their short-term benefits, in the appropriate patients, were felt to outweigh the long-term, uncertain risk of cancer. In the case of statins, I believe the current evidence suggests that this is indeed the case. The fibrates look a lot worse, because of the clinical trial evidence of increased mortality. In any case, the key is to treat the appropriate group of patients.

KH: *Since the lipid hypothesis has been so heavily promoted for atherosclerosis might it not be more prudent to work on preventing LDL oxidation by the antioxidant approach, rather than the reduction of LDL cholesterol by these lipid-lowering medications?*

TN: I am not a basic scientist, so I'll answer as an epidemiologist. The prudent thing to do is to wait until there is good clinical trial evidence of treatment benefit before recommending treatment with any drug. This applies to antioxidants as well as other lipid-lowering agents. This evidence did not exist for the statins until last year, but we were lucky, and it looks like they are beneficial in selected patients.

KH: *Do you have any data on the long-term effects of niacin with regards to carcinogenicity and lipid-lowering since niacin is a model medication that is cheap, lowers LDL cholesterol, triglycerides, lipoprotein (a) and increases HDL cholesterol?*

TN: The most recent edition of the PDR suggests that niacin does not cause cancer in rodents. This and the fact that it is inexpensive and has been around for decades makes it an appealing choice for lipid-lowering. ◆

Cardiac Surgery and Alternative Therapy

Mehmet C. Oz, M.D.
Division of Cardiothoracic Surgery
College of Physicians and Surgeons of Columbia University
630 West 168th Street
New York, NY 10032 U.S.A
(212) 305-4434 / (212) 305-2439 (FAX)

"New Age Therapies Put to Double-Blind Test,"
<u>Family Practice News</u>, November 13, 1995;9. #23672

Kirk Hamilton: Dr. Oz, could you please share with me your educational background and current position?

Mehmet Oz: I was educated at Harvard University and the University of Pennsylvania Medical School prior to receiving my surgical training at Columbia Presbyterian Medical Center in New York. I am presently an attending surgeon and assistant professor of surgery at Columbia University and the director of The Mechanical Circulatory Assist Program at Columbia Presbyterian Medical Center.

KH: When did you become interested in the role of nutrition and eastern approaches in your traditional cardiac surgery evolution and why?

MO: Alert clinicians who work with surgical patients recognize that the mental outlook of the patient is often a determinate of how well they will do in the postoperative period. This becomes even more evident with extremely ill patients who are receiving mechanical hearts and this is a population on whom I first started working. These patients, who had survived extremely high risk surgery, were especially aware of the roles that their mind had played in their recovery. They were interested in changing their lives and were willing to use non-traditional approaches to expedite this regeneration.

KH: When was the Columbia Cardiac Complementary Care Center Established?

MO: The Columbia Cardiac Complementary Care Center was established approximately 1 year ago.

KH: What is the goal of this Cardiac Complementary Care Center?

MO: The goals are to broaden the modalities which were available to the mechanical heart patients and make them a part of care of all patients undergoing open heart surgery.

KH: How have you felt so far in working intraoperatively with energy healers in the 20 plus cases noted in the article?

MO: I have been impressed by the professional approach of the energy healers who have worked on patients in the operating room. More importantly, patients themselves have been very receptive to these modalities. It is difficult to objectively demonstrate the role these energy healers have had on the improvement of these patients. However, I can safely say that there is no harm done by the incorporation of these individuals into the health care delivery system.

KH: What has been the benefit in the 50 patients or so that have undergone the Columbia's Cardiac Complementary Care Center Hypnotherapy Protocol?

MO: The patients that have undergone the hypnotherapy prior to open heart surgery have demonstrated a significant reduction in anxiety levels and in pain medication requirements in the postoperative period. Some patients have taken <u>no</u> pain medications after surgery.

KH: The article in <u>Family Practice News</u> talks a lot about energy medicine. Which energy medicine modality appears from your observations to have the most efficacy?

MO: I have been impressed by the effect of therapeutic touch on patients. The practitioners have a consensus on how their approach works and this is reassuring to the patients.

KH: I am curious as to what utilization of nutrition you use in our patients?

MO: Nutrition is a major obstacle for patients in the hospital due to major financial constraints.   All patients are given very rigorous nutritional guidelines to which they are asked to adhere following discharge. However, to truly be successful in this area, strong follow-up in the postoperative period is required.

KH: Recently I interviewed Dr. Karmy-Jones from Henry Ford Hospital who utilizes magnesium during cardiac surgery and notes a reduction in ventricular arrhythmias. Can you comment on this?

MO: Magnesium has been demonstrated to be valuable in the reduction of ventricular tachyarrhythmias after cardiac surgery. I use 2 gm of magnesium intravenously immediately after separating from cardiopulmonary bypass in the operating room and often request the patients take 300 mg 3 times a day of magnesium following their hospitalization. Hypomagnesemia is a very common problem in the postoperative period and is associated with malignant arrhythmias.

KH: Have you used any of the following agents in your cardiac patients which include coenzyme Q10, magnesium, L-carnitine, thiamine, tocopherol and/or vitamin C either intravenously or by mouth.

MO: I will often recommend coenzyme Q10, L-carnitine, thiamine and vitamin C to my cardiac patients. Of these, the only ones that are commonly administered in the hospital are vitamin C and magnesium.

KH: *In what directions do you see the Columbia's Cardiac Complementary Care Center going in the future to further clarify the role of these alternative therapies?*

MO: I see the Cardiac Complementary Care Center playing a major role in demonstrating the efficacy of alternative modalities for patients undergoing open heart surgery.   Likewise, we have an obligation to identify modalities which are ineffective in this setting. Being a large academic institution, I believe a fair and objective review of complementary medicine could enhance the reputation of the field and bring it more into mainstream medicine. ◆

Cardiovascular Risk and Homocysteine

Meir J. Stampfer, M.D., Dr.P.H.
Harvard School of Public Health
Brigham & Women's Hospital
75 Francis Street
Boston, MA 02115 U.S.A.
(617) 432-2747 / (617) 432-0335 (FAX)

"Can Lowering Homocysteine Levels Reduce Cardiovascular Risk"?
The New England Journal of Medicine, February 2, 1995;332(5):328-329. #21740

Kirk Hamilton: *Would you be so kind as to share with me your educational background and your present position?*

Meir Stampfer: I went to college at Columbia Medical School at New York University, and I did my internship at Maimonides in Brooklyn and a year of residency at Mt. Sinai in New York. Then I got a master's and doctorate in public health at Harvard. I stayed here and am now a Professor of Epidemiology and Nutrition at Harvard School of Public Health and an Associate Professor of Medicine at Harvard Medical School.

KH: *What have been your general areas of interest in the last 5 years of study?*

MS: My main areas of interest have been two-fold. One is diet in relation to risk of cardiovascular disease and cancer. The second area concerns hormones, cardiovascular disease and cancer.

KH: *How did you get interested in homocysteine as a potential risk factor for cardiovascular disease?*

MS: There had been some cross sectional and case-control studies that found that people who had already been diagnosed with cardiovascular disease of one form or another seemed to have higher levels of homocysteine than did controls. That was the background that led to my work in the Physician's Health Study, which was the first prospective demonstration that blood samples drawn at a time when people were healthy could be used to predict a higher risk of myocardial infarction among people who had elevated homocysteine at baseline.

KH: *What exactly did you find in the Physician's Health Study?*

MS: We found that the men who were in the top 5% of the distribution for homocysteine had about a three-fold excess risk of myocardial infarction compared to men who were in that first 90% of the distribution. There was a statistically significant increased risk in the group with higher values, even though for the most part the values were generally considered to be in "normal" range.

KH: *How important in your opinion, is homocysteine as a risk factor when compared to cholesterol?*

MS: Well it's a tough question to answer because it really depends on the individual pattern of risk factors and on population distribution of risk factors. I think as a global issue in the U.S., cholesterol is more important than homocysteine. But I think they are in the same ball park. I don't think homocysteine is going to turn out to be an obscure risk factor that only matters for a very small fraction of people. I think it will matter to a lot of people but not as much as cholesterol.

KH: *Do we know how elevated homocysteine might cause atherosclerosis or be associated with it?*

MS: Well, it is not clear. There are several theories with some data to support them. One is that homocysteine can be directly toxic to endothelial cells that line the vessel wall, and this can impair their function in terms of maintaining the proper ability to dilate and contract. It also can impair their function to promote prompt thrombolytic activity or prevent thrombosis from forming at the wall of the vessel. Another theory is that homocysteine stimulates smooth muscle cell proliferation which can be important in the development of atherosclerosis. And the third mechanism, related to the first, is that it may work on stimulating coagulation. So it's not completely worked out what the mechanism is, but there are several theories that . . . well I shouldn't keep calling them theories, there are several proposed mechanisms that do have some data to back them up.

KH: *What makes homocysteine as a model, so intriguing as a modifiable risk factor for cardiovascular disease?*

MS: Well, I think the main thing about it is that it is so easy to treat. In most instances elevated homocysteine can be reduced with folate, which has very little in the way of adverse effects. So we have an association with a risk factor that is very easily modifiable compared to some of the other risk factors such as hypertension, which of course can be treated but at a cost. So I think that is an intriguing aspect. I think another intriguing aspect, for which there is less supportive evidencet, is the possibility that some people may have a genetic predisposition to high homocysteine, which is affected or modified by their folate intake.

KH: *What other nutrients are involved in homocysteine metabolism that are worth looking at?*

MS: The other main ones are vitamin B6 and vitamin B12.

KH: *And are there models where we have lowered homocysteine with these 3 nutrients?*

MS: Yes. There have been a number of experimental studies where people with high levels of homocysteine can lower their levels with supplements of these vitamins. Typically folate is the key one. But B6 probably also is important. B12 is important as well, but deficiency from B12 is a lot less common than folate.

KH: *What are the ball park dose ranges of these nutrients that have been shown in this study to lower homocysteine?*

MS: Well for folate, the lowest level that I know of that has really been studied properly is 650 mcg. But in observational studies, it looks like 400 mcg may even be enough in some instances. However, people vary so there are individuals who need considerably more. But on a population level, probably 400 mcg of folic acid would be enough to make a difference. It probably would not be enough to get everybody to the lowest level of homocysteine that they could be, but on a population level it would make a difference.

KH: *How about B6 and B12?*

MS: It is a lot more variable there, and it depends on the specific situation so I wouldn't want to give a number for those.

KH: *Now as we look at this, let's say the homocysteine theory proves to be correct. What does that say about the American diet? Is it that we're not eating enough folate, vitamin B12 and B6 rich foods? Or is there just a need for supraphysiologic dosages?*

MS: Well no. I think we're not eating enough folate for sure. Only about 40-50% of the population is eating enough folate. So around half of the population is eating less than 400 mcg.

KH: *What kind of study would you like to see to confirm this suggestion of homocysteine being a modifiable risk factor for cardiovascular disease?*

MS: What we really need is a randomized trial whereby individuals either in the general population, people at high risk or people who have already had cardiovascular disease would be randomized to homocysteine lowering therapy or placebo to confirm the homocysteine hypothesis. Although we can see an association with homocysteine and high risk and we know how to lower homocysteine, we don't know for sure that lowering homocysteine will in turn lower risk. I think it is a good bet that it might. But to make public health policy recommendations, I think we need that final link to be solidified just as was done for cholesterol lowering. For a long time people knew that high cholesterol was associated with higher risk of heart disease. We knew how to lower cholesterol, but we needed a trial to show that lowering cholesterol did lower risk before launching a massive campaign for education and treatment. That is what I think we need here.

KH: *Homocysteine is elevated in other conditions, not only cardiovascular disease but recently neural tube defects?*

MS: Yes, because we know that folate nutrition is important to prevent neural tube defects. It is not clear that it is the homocysteine that is causing the problem or whether it is just a reflection of inadequate folate.

KH: *The picture that is being drawn for me is a new way of assessing risk factors in individuals. In other words, elevated homocysteine has been associated with not only heart attacks, but coronary artery disease, cerebrovascular disease, neural tube defects, neuropsychiatric disorders and actually recurrent abortions. There are a variety of conditions where this one element has been elevated. A new, more functional model of health care would be one in which one screening test might affect four or five different disease states. Do you see a day where homocysteine is used as frequently as a CBC?*

MS: No, I doubt it. I don't think it will be as frequently used as a CBC, but it might be. If the trials are definitive, it might be used like cholesterol.

KH: *That would be a much utilized test!*

MS: Yes. You know, I don't think we're there yet. As far as neural tube defects, that is proven beyond any doubt now, and certainly any woman who is considering conceiving needs to be on supplements to be sure that she's getting enough folate.

KH: *I agree. I can just see a day where a gynecologist, as part of a blood screen, includes homocysteine levels.*

MS: I wouldn't even measure homocysteine. I would just say to any woman considering conceiving, "Take a supplement." I don't think you need to do the measurement. Just take the folic acid...just do it. ◆

Cardiovascular Risk and Homocysteine

M.R. Malinow, M.D.
Laboratory of Cardiovascular Diseases
Oregon Regional Primate Research Center
505 N.W. 18th Avenue
Beaverton, Oregon 97006-3499 U.S.A.
(503) 690-5258 / (503) 690-5563 (FAX)

"Can Lowering Homocysteine Levels Reduce Cardiovascular Risk?"
New England Journal of Medicine, February 2, 1995;332(5):328-329. #21740

Kirk Hamilton: Can you please share with me your educational background and current position?

M. Rene Malinow: I received my medical degree from the University of Buenos Aires Medical School, Buenos Aires, Argentina. I became a cardiovascular fellow at the Michael Reese Hospital in Chicago, Illinois. I am a professor of medicine at The Oregon Health Sciences University and a research scientist at the Laboratory of Cardiovascular Diseases, the Oregon Regional Primate Research Center in Beaverton, Oregon. Currently I am a research associate at the Heart Institute at Providence St. Vincent Hospital, Portland, Oregon.

KH: When did you get interested in the role of homocysteine and cardiovascular disease?

RM: About 8 years ago when I consulted on a 30-year-old woman who was having her second myocardial infarction (MI), and without major risk factors. It turned out that she was my first case of hyperhomocysteinemia and probably the first diagnosed adult, nonhomocystinuric case in the Pacific Northwest.

KH: What is the risk of elevated homocysteine?

RM: Hyperhomocysteinemia is a common risk factor for arterial occlusive disease, which is easily treated with supplemental vitamins.

KH: How do elevated homocysteine levels compare to elevated cholesterol as a risk factor for cardiovascular disease?

RM: Both are important risk factors, but knowledge on cholesterol has accumulated for about 100 years, but data on homocysteine has only occurred during the past 2 or 3 decades.

KH: What is the mechanism by which homocysteine may cause atherosclerosis?

RM: The mechanism is unknown, but is probably mulitfactorial. Several have been demonstrated such as damage of endothelial cells *in vitro* and changing a normally anticoagulant state into a procoagulant state.

KH: What cardiovascular diseases are at risk with elevated homocysteine?

RM: Myocardial infarction, stroke, intermittent claudication and preclinical carotid artery atherosclerosis.

KH: What are the nutrients that can lower homocysteine levels and what are the therapeutic dose ranges?

RM: Folic acid at .4 to 2 mg, vitamin B6 at 10 to 25 mg and vitamin B12 at 100 to 500 ug per day.

KH: What are the risks of treating homocysteine at these levels?

RM: The main risk is masking a pernicious anemia with high dose folic acid.

KH: How common are elevated levels of homocysteine?

RM: About 5% in the general population and 15 to 30% in arterial occlusive diseases.

KH: How could the general public reduce their risk to hyperhomocysteinemia?

RM: By taking over-the-counter vitamin supplements.

KH: How do you test for homocysteine and do you use a methionine challenge?

RM: I test for homocysteine in the blood. I do not use a methionine challenge since basal levels are adequate in most but not all cases.

KH: Is the test becoming more prevalent and the cost coming down?

RM: Yes. Interest in developing a relatively inexpensive test is increasing and it is likely that it will be available in the near future.

KH: Do you take vitamin supplements and if so in what dosage?

RM: Yes. I take multivitamins plus 1 mg of folic acid per day.

KH: Do you think it is reasonable, if an individual has confirmed coronary artery or cerebrovascular disease, to take the above mentioned doses of folic acid, vitamin B6 and B12 while we are awaiting the confirmatory supplemental trials?

RM: Pending clinical trials, it is reasonable in patients with confirmed coronary or cerebrovascular disease, to request measurement of homocysteine levels, folic acid, vitamin B6 and B12 and treat accordingly by a physician. ◆

Cataracts and Antioxidants

William Christen, ScD.
Brigham & Women's Hospital
900 Commonwealth Avenue E.
Boston, MA 02215-1204 U.S.A.
(617) 278-0795 / (617) 734-1437 (FAX)

"The Use of Vitamin Supplements and the Risk of Cataracts Among U.S. Male Physicians",
Journal. of Public Health, May 1994;84(5):788-792. #20777

Kirk Hamilton: *Thank you again for being here and could you please tell me your educational background and your present position.*

William Christen: I was trained originally as a basic researcher in visual development and received my Ph.D. from the University of Miami, Florida. I then spent about 5 years studying abnormal visual development in cats. While we were able to get some insight into visual pathology, it became obvious that in order to understand what goes on in humans, you have to study humans. So for the past 8 years I have been involved in vision epidemiology studies. I am currently instructor in the Division of Preventive Medicine, Department of Medicine, Brigham and Women's Hospital, Harvard Medical School.

KH: *How did you get interested in diet and cataracts?*

WC: In trying to understand the causes and possible preventive agents for cataracts, there is quite a bit of basic research which suggests antioxidants are at least worthy of investigation in human populations.

KH: *Can you tell me some of the causes of cataracts or the basics of cataract development?*

WC: Typically, we study "age-related cataracts," which are cataracts that have no obvious cause such as trauma or congenital cataracts, steroid-induced cataracts, cataracts resulting from intraocular surgery and so on. I think the term "age related" implies that we don't know specifically the mechanism involved with these cataracts, although a growing body of research suggests oxidative mechanisms are involved in the etiology of age-related cataracts.

KH: *From the study in The American Journal of Public Health entitled, "The Use of Vitamin Supplements and the Risk of Cataract Among U.S. Male Physicians" the general finding, if I interpret it right, is that those who took multivitamins tended to have a lower risk of cataract and the reduction was not related to those who took vitamin C and/or E supplements individually.*

WC: That is correct. Let me just briefly describe the study. We investigated this hypothesis in the Physician's Health Study, which was a randomized trial designed to study aspirin and beta-carotene in cancer and cardiovascular disease prevention, and involved more than 22,000 male physicians in the U.S. We limited the analysis to the approximate 18,000 physicians who did not report a cataract at baseline, but did provide complete information on other potential risk factors for cataract. These physicians were followed-up for 5 years for the development of newly diagnosed cataracts. At baseline, based on self report, we found that about 12½% of the physicians reported taking multivitamins only. About 7½% reported taking

multivitamins and C and/or E supplements, and about 4% reported taking vitamin C and/or E supplements only. And, as you said, we found that after the 5 years of follow-up, those who reported taking only multivitamins had a statistically significant 27% reduction in the risk of new cataract.

KH: *Did that include vitamins C and E with the multivitamin or just the multivitamins by themselves?*

WC: Physicians who reported taking vitamin C and/or E supplements in addition to multivitamins had a nonsignificant 23% reduction in the risk of cataract. So there was no additional benefit for those who were taking multivitamins of also taking C and/or E. And, in the group that took just C or E alone we found no reduction in risk.

KH: *So is there the possibility that there are other antioxidants in the multivitamins that may be of benefit, or nutrients such as vitamin A, vitamin B2 or selenium . . .?*

WC: Yes, it is possible that any of those could be working. It is also possible that our observations were due simply to chance. There are other studies that did not find any protective effect of multivitamin intake in cataract development. Ours is just one of a number of a studies which eventually will answer the question. It is unclear what specific components of multivitamins might be protective of cataracts. The other thing that should be stressed is this was an observational study; we didn't assign multivitamin intake and we didn't assign vitamin C or E supplementation for the participants. They chose to take these vitamins and people who choose to take various vitamins probably differ in a number of other ways that are also related to the risk of cataract development. Therefore, it is unclear whether any observed protective effect of multivitamins is due to the multivitamin itself, to some other behavior, or perhaps to some other nutritional factor associated with multivitamin intake. Randomized trial data, such as that being collected in the National Eye Institute-sponsored Age-Related Eye Disease study, as well as in the Physicians' Health Study and Women's Health Study being conducted here at the Brigham and Women's Hospital, will be required to answer this important question regarding the potential benefit of vitamin supplementation in eye disease.

KH: *Was there a correlation at all between increased consumption of fruits and vegetables in this study or did you even look at that?*

WC: No, we didn't look at that.

KH: *Stepping back - what kind of lifestyle recommendations can you make for an individual to help prevent cataracts. Is there anything you can put your finger on that would be reasonable and safe?*

WC: I think there is fairly good evidence right now that cigarette smoking is probably involved with the development of cataract. There is also fairly good information suggesting ultraviolet light or excessive sunlight exposure can also increase the risk of developing cataracts.

KH: How about any dietary recommendation?

WC: I think any dietary recommendations for eye disease would be similar to the recommendations being made to protect against other diseases such as cancer and cardiovascular disease. That is, a diet rich in fruits and vegetables is the best thing going, although it remains unclear what exactly about fruits and vegetables is protective.

KH: Would you recommend your family member or parent take a multiple vitamin with some extra C, E and beta-carotene?

WC: I know there are a number of people who would go ahead and do that now. I personally wouldn't.

KH: If there was no harm, in your mind, why not take a multivitamin?

WC: I can think of a couple of reasons for not making broad recommendations at this time. For some, the use of vitamin supplements would be viewed as an excuse for not changing other behaviors which are demonstrated to be associated with various pathologies. I think, for example, it would be a shame if an individual decided not to give up smoking because they were taking multivitamins, which may or may not be protective against a number of diseases linked to smoking. Additionally, I believe we spend about $4 billion a year in this country on supplements. If they are ineffective, that money certainly could be used for better purposes. Finally, there are issues concerning potential toxicity of megadoses that need to be explored. ◆

Cerebral Palsy and Magnesium

Judith K. Grether , Ph.D.
California Birth Defects Monitoring Program
1900 Powell St., Suite 1050
Emeryville, CA 94608-1811 U.S.A.
(510) 653-3303 ext. 347/ (510) 653-1678 (FAX)

"Can Magnesium Sulfate Reduce the Risk of Cerebral Palsy in Very Low Birthweight Infants?",
Pediatrics, February 1995;95(2):263-269. #21802

Kirk Hamilton: Could you please start out by telling us your educational background and then your present position?

Judith Grether: I have a Ph.D. in sociology from the University of Oregon. I started working in maternal and child health in the State Health Department in 1977. That is when I discovered epidemiology. I was then working with a sudden infant death syndrome program administered by the State Health Department. In 1982, when the Birth Defects Monitoring Program started, I took a position with this program, largely because I knew it would allow me to work as an epidemiologist and work with other epidemiologists.

KH: How did you get involved with birth defects and, specifically, cerebral palsy?

JG: We consider cerebral palsy a birth defect and started doing research on the assumption that a sizable proportion of cerebral palsy originates during prenatal development. Most people think of birth defects as structural abnormalities in various organs that develop during the first trimester or the first 8 or 10 weeks of fetal development. We know that in most cases of cerebral palsy, the causal factors are operating later than 8 to 10 weeks in gestation.

KH: What evidence is there that cerebral palsy has a prenatal etiology? What made you suspicious?

JG: For a longtime, the assumption has been that most cerebral palsy, particularly in full term babies, really has to do with obstetrical events around the time of delivery and a lack of sufficient oxygen getting to the baby's brain during delivery. Some years ago, work in this country done by my colleague Dr. Karin Nelson at the National Institutes of Health and Dr. Jonas Ellenberg, a statistician who worked with her, analyzed extensive data sets that had been collected in the early 1960s when not very many low birthweight babies were surviving. Their research on term babies indicated many children who developed cerebral palsy had absolutely nothing unusual going on during their labor and delivery, and birth asphyxia could not possibly be the cause of their cerebral palsy. Their research also indicated that many labor and delivery complications were relatively common overall and were not more frequent in births of children with cerebral palsy compared to children without cerebral palsy. Only very extreme and prolonged difficulties were associated with increased risk of cerebral palsy. These were rare and were not present in the births of most children with cerebral palsy. In addition, they were able to identify a number of children with conditions that were known to develop earlier on in pregnancy. Some of these were malformations of the brain and other conditions of early gestation. So they came to the conclusion that less than 15% of the children in their data set had cerebral palsy that could possibly be attributed to what is classically thought of as birth asphyxia.

KH: Where did the magnesium thought come from?

JG: There is a growing body of animal studies on magnesium and brain injuries of various sorts. My colleague Dr. Nelson was aware of that data. In addition, some colleagues of ours in Boston, who have looked at brain hemorrhages in very low birthweight newborns, unexpectedly found in their data an association between magnesium and reduced risk of brain hemorrhages.

KH: Magnesium intake by the mother or just magnesium levels in the infant?

JG: Magnesium sulfate given intravenously to the mother as a tocolytic agent in an attempt to either slow down or stop the contractions of premature labor.

KH: Is that the definition of a tocolytic agent - to slow down the contractions in the premature labor?

JG: Or to stop contractions. Magnesium sulfate is given to moms for that purpose, and there are a number of other medications that also are used for that purpose. There is controversy among obstetricians about which of these medications, if any, are in fact effective in slowing down or stopping labor. Magnesium sulfate is also given to women who have what used to be called toxemia and now is called preeclampsia. In this situation, it is given to prevent the mother from having convulsions as a result of the preeclampsia progressing to what is called eclampsia.

KH: Is the theory, then, that somehow magnesium helps with oxygenation of the fetus during the last parts of pregnancy?

JG: There has been research in two directions. One is with the gray matter of the brain and the other is with the white matter. It is in the white matter where we see hemorrhages in very low birthweight babies. In both the white matter and gray matter, the assumption has been that in some way the magnesium blocks calcium from getting into the cell. Too much calcium, which is a consequence of various events associated with trauma, can cause a kind of permanent damage that we may be seeing in cerebral palsy.

KH: Can you give us an overview of your study and what you found?

JG: We had 42 children who weighed less than 1500 gm at birth and had survived to 3 years of age with moderate or severe congenital cerebral palsy. Those 42 children represent virtually every child with moderate or severe congenital cerebral palsy who were born during a 3-year period from 1983 to 1985 in 4 Bay Area counties and who were of that birthweight group. We randomly selected approximately 2 controls for every case from the population of very low birthweight babies who survived to age 3 and who did not have cerebral palsy. We collected extensive medical record data both from the mothers' and the babies' hospital records. We collected data on medications given to the mother, and among the 42 children with cerebral palsy, only 3 of the moms had been given magnesium sulfate. Twenty-seven of the mothers of the controls had been treated with magnesium sulfate. This was a difference of 7% among mothers of children with cerebral palsy and 36% in mothers of controls, which is a pretty dramatic difference, even though our numbers overall are small. It is about a 7-fold reduction in risk with magnesium, and you don't see that very often.

KH: *That is quite amazing considering it is just a therapy given during delivery, correct?*

JG: It is given prior to delivery and the length of time before varies among these women.

KH: *In other words, what mothers did during the 9 months of gestation wasn't really that important with regards to cerebral palsy?*

JG: We don't know the answer to that question, and the answer is probably complex. Our research indicates that a medication administered intravenously in the hospital prior to delivery may have dramatic effects for the babies.

KH: *That is pretty dramatic if magnesium sulfate therapy prior to delivery helped prevent such a tough problem.*

JG: Well, not only is it dramatic but wonderful! Magnesium sulfate is an existing medication that is used a lot in this country although not in other parts of the world. So the medical profession really knows what the mother can handle. We know how to monitor its use. We know what the side effects are. We know how to deal with them if they happen, and they are quite rare, but they can happen. It is not a new experimental drug.

KH: *It is also cheap.*

JG: It is very cheap. You know, there are a lot of unanswered questions. A big one of course is if we are right and there really is something going on here, what's the appropriate dosage to optimize the outcome for the fetus? And that may be somewhat different than the therapeutic doses that are being given to mothers at this point.

KH: *That's very, very exciting.*

JG: You know what has really been important to us? In the course of doing this work before we went to publication, we wanted to spread the word among our colleagues who may have data sets so that they could look to see if they would find anything. Several of them have seen similar patterns in their data. That is very reassuring. Because it was really, frankly, pretty scary to us. At the same time it was very exciting. But what if it is a fluke in our data set? We did everything we could to find an explanation other than magnesium sulfate for what we were seeing. In epidemiology we call it confounding. We looked at everything we could think of and we asked for help from colleagues to tell us what other things they could think of. We couldn't make this magnesium association go away. But, of course, we're still nervous because it is so important and has the possibility of raising too many hopes. We don't want those to be false hopes.

KH: *Is there a familial risk of cerebral palsy or does it come out of the blue?*

JG: There is no identified familial risk for most cerebral palsy, but premature babies are at especially high risk. If a woman is in preterm labor or is going to be delivering preterm for some other reason, the question is, "Should all women be given magnesium sulfate in that situation?"

KH: *What is the percentage of cerebral palsy babies that are premature versus full term?*

JG: In the era when we did our study, about 25% of our singletons were below 1500 grams. We suspect that if we were to do the same study right now, it would be somewhat higher because survivorship is higher in that group. More smaller babies are surviving.

KH: *So prematurity increases the risk of cerebral palsy?*

JG: Absolutely! The risk among preemies is about 48 per 1,000 preemies who survive to childhood. And that translates to about 1 in 20. And among full term babies, it is less than 1 per 1,000.

KH: *What other nutrients in your sphere, since you're at the California Birth Defects Monitoring Program, are of interest for prevention of birth defects?*

JG: As I mentioned to you before, Dr. Gary Shaw is doing research on folate and neural tube defects, and other structural malformations. ◆

Cholesterol and Vitamin C

Judith Hallfrisch, Ph.D.
Beltsville Human Nutrition Research Center
Building 307, Room 323
Beltsville, M.D. 20705 U.S.A.
(301) 504-8396 / (301) 504-9456 (FAX)

"High Plasma Vitamin C Associated With High Plasma HDL - HDL$_2$ Cholesterol",
<u>American Journal of Clinical Nutrition</u>, 1994;60:100-105. #20548

Kirk Hamilton: Share with me your educational and professional background.

Judith Hallfrisch: I have a Ph.D. in nutritional sciences from the University of Maryland. I was at the Department of Agriculture for 10 years. Then I was at the National Institute of Aging (NIA) for 7 years, and then I came back here to the Department of Agriculture as a research leader.

KH: What has been your main area of interest in the last several years?

JH: I started out in carbohydrate nutrition. I was interested in the negative effects of fructose and sucrose. Then when I went to NIA, I was the only nutritionist working on the Baltimore Longitudinal Study of Aging. So I got interested in nutrition and aging.

KH: How did you get interested in vitamin C and HDL cholesterol?

JH: There was some animal work that suggested if you give vitamin C, you increase HDL and lower LDL, and if you are vitamin C deficient, total cholesterol goes up and HDL goes down.

KH: Share with us your paper on plasma vitamin C and HDL cholesterol in the <u>American Journal of Clinical Nutrition</u>.

JH: My paper is not an intervention study. To give some background, you need to know about the Baltimore Longitudinal Study of Aging, which began in 1958. Its purpose was to study normal human aging. They didn't want to have the confounding effects of disease, poverty, drugs and other variables found in older patients in hospitals and nursing homes. The subjects were healthy, free living, well educated, upper middle class people. The study had only men in it until 1978 when women were added. The goal is to maintain a population of about a 1,000 people ranging in age from 20 to however long they live. I think they only had 1 centenarian, though. The subjects come to the gerontology research center in Baltimore every 2 years for an extensive battery of tests - psychological, physical fitness tests, body composition measurements, clinical blood parameters and cognitive function tests. Part of the study is to look at their nutritional intake, and that was the part that I was in charge of.

KH: Did you look at a subpopulation or all of the study participants?

JH: Every single part of the study is voluntary. I obtained plasma levels of vitamin C on about 800 people.

KH: Could you explain to me the difference between HDL and HDL$_2$?

JH: HDL$_2$ is just a subfraction of cholesterol of which there are something like 14 subfractions. HDL, or high density lipoprotein cholesterol, is the part that helps to remove the LDL, or low density lipoprotein cholesterol, from the blood. HDL cholesterol is considered the "good" cholesterol. LDL cholesterol is considered the "bad" cholesterol. There are some people who believe it is the HDL$_2$ fraction of the HDL that is the beneficial subfraction and that it is the HDL$_3$ fraction that goes up if you drink alcohol. There is some dispute about what subfraction of the cholesterol is the best and which one is the worst. Generally, people think the HDL$_2$ has the beneficial effect.

KH: What were your observations in your study with regards to vitamin C plasma levels?

JH: I divided them into quintiles of plasma vitamin C. The higher plasma vitamin C levels were significantly associated with higher levels of HDL.

KH: Is that higher within the normal range or above the normal range for plasma vitamin C?

JH: I would say the plasma levels of this entire population were pretty high. This same relationship or a similar relationship has been found in populations that have a low intake of vitamin C. In other words, if they are at the low end of the spectrum, you see a pretty significant increase in HDL and decrease in blood pressure and some other beneficial effects with highest plasma vitamin C. This is a very well-nourished group of people. In fact, their average consumption of vitamin C from just food, not counting supplements, was about 2½ times the RDA for vitamin C.

KH: Is there a theoretical explanation of the mechanism on how vitamin C might increase HDL directly?

JH: Some people believe it is vitamin C's antioxidant capacity that is working here as a preventor of LDL oxidation.

KH: It has nothing to do with actually increasing the HDL?

JH: In guinea pigs and rats unable to synthesize vitamin C, a classic finding of vitamin C deficiency is hypercholesterolemia. Cholesterol goes up, and it is the LDL fraction that goes up. In fact, HDL has been reported in a couple of studies to go down with vitamin C deficiency. This occurs because plasma vitamin C promotes the removal of oxidized LDL cholesterol. The exact mechanism by which vitamin C might increase HDL cholesterol is unknown, but

HDL cholesterol is also involved in the removal of LDL cholesterol.

KH: How much vitamin C in the total diet would you consider to be the low end for the optimal range after looking at all these dietary surveys?

JH: If you look at plasma levels versus intake, there is an increase with intake in the plasma level up to a certain point and then it levels off. There is a point that if you take more vitamin C, it won't increase your plasma level. This is assuming, but is not necessarily true, that the high plasma level is the optimal level. The point at which the curve no longer increases significantly as vitamin C intake goes up turned out to be 215 mg for women and 345 mg for men. These are based on 7-day diet records and not actually feeding people food in which the vitamin C is measured, therefore, the results are variable. Vitamin C is a very labile vitamin. If you pour a glass of orange juice and let it sit for a while, the vitamin C will disappear very quickly. So I would say these values are probably optimistic. Probably their intakes, if you actually measured the vitamin C they were consuming, wouldn't be this high. But intakes are well above the RDA, which is 60 mg for both men and women.

KH: Is that the major point?

JH: This population, without taking any supplements, was already, just from their food, taking in about 150 mg a day of vitamin C. So it is my personal opinion that 60 mg is not the optimal level and that is somewhere around 150 to 250 mg per day. For men the optimal level is probably higher than for women.

KH:Could you not theoretically saturate body compartments with a higher intake of vitamin C and prevent such conditions such as LDL oxidation?

JH: I don't know. Certainly, I have no evidence of that from my study. It should be emphasized that vitamin C is a vitamin that you can get plenty of from the diet. So I am not one who recommends megadosing on any kind of vitamin and especially for vitamin C. I don't think there is any need.

KH: I am a believer that in certain acute conditions, vitamin C is highly underutilized. My experience clinically has been tens of grams can do profound things in acute illness.

JH: That's a whole different thing. That is a pharmacological dose and I am not saying there aren't therapeutic uses for lots of vitamins because I believe there are. I am only talking here about a healthy, free-living population. I am not talking about people with disease because I think that, especially in the older age groups when you get up to 50, 60, 70, most everybody is taking chronic medication and the RDAs just don't have any meaning for them at all. They may need more of a variety of nutrients just based on the pharmaceuticals they are taking.

KH: The integration of nutrition into therapy and prevention of disease I believe is supported by the literature and will lead to true health care reform.

JH: Preventive care. That is what I'm for. Thank you very much for your interest in our work. ◆

Cholesterol, Lipids and Soy Protein

James W. Anderson, M.D.
University of Kentucky
Metabolic Research Group
VA Medical Center
2250 Leestown Road (111C)
Lexington, KY 40511-1093 U.S.A.
(606) 257-4058 / (606) 257-8410 (FAX)

"Meta-Analysis of the Effects of Soy Protein Intake on Serum Lipids",
New England Journal of Medicine, 1995;333:276-282. #22584

Kirk Hamilton: *Can you please share with me your educational background and current position?*

James Anderson: I am a graduate of West Virginia University and Northwestern Medical School. After completing training in internal medicine and endocrinology at the Mayo Clinic, I served in the U.S. Army for 3 years as a research physician. I then moved to Lexington, Kentucky, in 1973. I am currently professor of medicine in clinical nutrition at the University of Kentucky, chief of the Endocrine-Metabolic Section at the Veterans Affairs Medical Center in Lexington, director of the University of Kentucky Health Management Resources, acting division chief of Endocrine/Internal Medicine Department at the University of Kentucky, director of the Metabolic Research Group at the University of Kentucky, and founder and Director of the HCF Nutrition Research Foundation.

KH: *When did you get interested in soy proteins and their healthful properties, especially with regards to blood lipids?*

JA: About 4 years ago, I became interested in the possibility that soy proteins might sufficiently lower blood lipids.

KH: *What is so special or unique about soy protein as compared to animal protein, or even to the classic grain/bean type combination of vegetable protein?*

JA: Consuming soy protein selectively lowers serum cholesterol and LDL levels, without reducing HDL levels. This is unique because usually reductions in fat intake produce reductions in both LDL and HDL cholesterol.

KH: *What is a good cholesterol/HDL ratio?*

JA: A good cholesterol/HDL ratio is less than 4.

KH: *What is the difference between soy protein's effect on cholesterol in meat or poultry?*

JA: Whereas soy protein sufficiently lowers serum cholesterol values, regular intake of meat or poultry with their saturated fat, tends to raise blood cholesterol.

KH: *Is soy protein less oxidizable than animal protein and how does this effect vascular disease?*

JA: Because the proteins are digested/hydrolyzed in the small intestine and reconstituted in the liver and the muscle, the oxidizability of intake of protein does not have much effect on vascular disease.

KH: *What kind of dramatic results do you see with lipid levels on soy protein diets?*

JA: From the 38 clinical studies reviewed in our meta-analysis, soy protein intake was associated with a 9.3% reduction in serum cholesterol, a 12.9% reduction in LDL and a 10.5% reduction in triglycerides. The study indicates that consuming 17 to 20 grams of soy protein per day could have a meaningful effect on cholesterol levels.

KH: *If someone doesn't like tofu, how do you incorporate more soy protein into the diet? In what foods?*

JA: Individuals interested in adding soy protein to their diets may do so by incorporating the use of soy flour in foods such as muffins, quick bread, pancakes or waffles (about 1/4 or 1/3 of all purpose flour can be reconstituted with soy flour); using unflavored soy beverage (also known as soy milk) for baking, with cereals and puddings, or for drinking; using textured soy protein in chili, sloppy joes, spaghetti sauce, tacos or a substitute in any recipe where ground beef or turkey is used; using isolated soy protein in different beverages, casseroles, soups and baked goods (Power Bars and sports drinks often include this form of soy protein). Also, you can include soy protein beans in vegetable, soup and chili recipes. They are prepared similar to any bean or lentil. Even people who don't care about tofu can add it to their diets in a way that is appealing. One way is to blend tofu to make puddings, dips or dressings, or adding to tomato sauce when making lasagne.

KH: *Where can interested health professionals or the lay public get recipes or resources regarding soy protein or the role of high fiber, high complex carbohydrates diets in disease treatment and prevention?*

JA: The HCF Nutrition Research Foundation (P.O. Box 22124, Lexington, KY 40522) may be contacted at (800) 727-4423 for a variety of periodicals and resources that include information and recipes about diet, fiber and healthy life-style/living resources.

KH: *Does soy milk have the same isoflavonoids and phytoestrogens as the soy powders in tofu?*

JA: Soy milk has the same isoflavonoid estrogen effects as soy powders and tofu.

KH: *How do you incorporate soy flour into the diet?*

JA: Soy flour can be incorporated into the diet by adding to it recipes calling for all purpose or wheat flour (substituting 1/4 or 1/3 with soy flour). Soy flour has a nutty flavor and adds a pleasant texture to baked products such as pies, donuts, cakes, rolls, muffins, breads and pancake mixes. You may also use soy flour to thicken gravies and cream sauces. Soy flour not only gives your baked goods extra protein, but also keeps them from becoming stale. Soy flour is free of gluten, which gives structure to yeast breads. Therefore, it cannot replace all the flour in a bread recipe. Soy flour creates baked goods that are somewhat dense and have a more moist quality. There are 2 kinds of soy flour on the market, full-fat (or natural) and defatted. Both add protein, however, defatted soy flour is more concentrated in protein than full-fat. Defatted has the oils removed during processing. All soy flour should be stored in the refrigerator or freezer.

KH: *Are there any adverse effects of consuming soy protein?*

JA: The adverse effects of consuming soy protein are minimal. Some of the less purified proteins such as textured vegetable protein may bind iron and decrease iron absorption in growing children.

KH: *How is consuming more soy and plant protein more environmentally conservative or efficient?*

JA: Soy protein requires much less energy, acreage and equalogic strand than does an equivalent amount of animal protein.

KH: *Do high complex carbohydrate diets raise or lower insulin levels?*

JA: Generous fiber intake lowers blood glucose levels, reduces insulin needs and improves blood glucose control. The HCF nutrition plan helps control diabetes with diet rather than medicine by using or eliminating the need for medicines or insulin.

KH: *What are the slow and what are the fast carbohydrates and their effects on our metabolism?*

JA: I am assuming that slow carbohydrates are complex carbohydrates, and fast are the simple carbohydrates. Complex carbohydrates are those produced in plants, which are insoluble, nonsweet forms of carbohydrate in which plants store energy. They are normally found in grains, nuts, legumes, root vegetables and potatoes. Fruits have much less of these complex carbohydrates. Simple carbohydrates are what we typically think of as "table sugar" such as candies and other sweets. Carbohydrates are hydrolyzed and absorbed in the body, in the small intestine, where pancreatic amylases and intestinal disaccharidases complete the job on most carbohydrates present. It does not take long for digestion and absorption of carbohydrates. Absorption rates depend on the type of food, what other foods are eaten at the same time, and the individual. The simple carbohydrates do digest more rapidly and into the blood stream, resulting in an increase in blood sugar at a quicker rate.

KH: *Are you from the "no fat" camp or are there good fats like monounsaturated fats?*

JA: Being in the promadicate camp, I think people should use some fat in their diet. I recommend monounsaturated fats as extensively as possible when people are selecting fat to eat. ◆

Cholesterol Lowering and Pantethine

Francisco Coronel, M.D.
Nephrology Service
San Carlos University Hospital
28040 Madrid, Spain
39 1 330 3492 / 39 1 330 3182 (FAX)

"Lipid Lowering Treatment With Pantethine in Renal Transplant Patients,"
<u>Nephrologia</u>, 1995;15(1):68-73. #22741

Kirk Hamilton: *Could you please share with me your educational background and current position?*

Francisco Coronel: I received my M.D. in medicine at the Complutense University of Madrid, Spain in 1969, and I did my specialty in nephrology at the University Hospital San Carlos of Madrid. In 1987 I received my Ph.D. degree with the thesis entitled "New Perspectives in The Treatment of Terminal Diabetic Nephropathy." I have presented approximately 155 communications in national and international meetings, and I have published about 65 papers in the nephrology field. I am in charge of the Peritoneal Unit of the Nephrology Department in the University Hospital San Carlos, Madrid, and I am an associate professor of medicine in the Complutense University of Madrid.

KH: *Why is there a problem with lipid lowering drugs in renal transplant patients?*

FC: Most of the lipid lowering drugs have many secondary effects if a certain degree of renal failure exists. This is not unusual in many renal transplant recipients with functioning grafts. On the other hand, some of these drugs can interfere with lipid metabolism.

KH: *When did you get interested in the role of pantethine and the lowering of lipids?*

FC: I used pantethine in renal hyperlipidemic patients with good results. Pantethine is a physiological substance, being the biologically active form of pantothenic acid, and for this reason I thought that it could be used in transplant recipients.

KH: *Can you describe the results of your study with regards to all the lipid parameters?*

FC: The administration of pantethine to renal transplant patients with hyperlipidemia achieved a significant decrease in total cholesterol, triglycerides, low density lipoprotein cholesterol, very low density lipoprotein cholesterol, and the cholesterol/HDL ratio at 2, 4 and 6 months of treatment.

KH: *How did pantethine affect HDL cholesterol levels?*

FC: High density lipoprotein cholesterol levels increased at 6 months, but without statistical significance.

KH: *Were there any toxicities noted with pantethine?*

FC: No changes were seen in renal function nor were there any other biochemical changes in the parameters studied. Two patients complained of gastric discomfort. Pantethine did not interfere with immunosuppressive therapy.

KH: *Do you think that pantethine may be used in nonrenal transplant patients for lipid lowering?*

FC: It has been efficiently tested in hyperlipidemia associated with different clinical conditions. In 1991, we published our experience with pantethine and hyperlipidemic diabetic patients treated with hemodialysis and peritoneal dialysis in <u>The American Journal of Nephrology</u>. I do not see why this substance cannot be used in nonrenal transplant patients, but as far as I know, it has not been tested in those cases.

KH: *How does pantethine work to lower cholesterol?*

FC: The action of pantethine on cholesterol metabolism could be related to its capacity to increase the availability of CoA with the subsequent enhancement of the Krebs Cycle and reduce the utilization of acetate for cholesterol synthesis.

KH: *At what doses should pantethine be used to lower cholesterol?*

FC: In our study, pantethine was given at 300 mg, 3 times daily. ◆

Cholesterol Oxidation and Olive Oil

Francesco Visioli, M.D.
Chair of Experimental Pharmacology
Institute of Pharmacological Sciences
School of Pharmacy, University of Milan
Via Balzaretti, 9
20133 Milan, Italy
39 2 20488309 / 39 2 29404961 (FAX)

"Low Density Lipoprotein Oxidation is Inhibited *In Vitro* by Olive Oil Constituents,"
<u>Arteriosclerosis</u>, 1995;117:25-32. #23014

Kirk Hamilton: Could you please share with me your educational background and current position?

Francesco Visioli: I received my Ph.D. in pharmaceutical chemistry from the University of Milan. After a postdoctoral fellowship at the Louisiana State University Neuroscience Center in New Orleans, I came back to Milan to work at the Institute of Pharmacological Sciences and obtained a Doctorate of Research in biotechnology. I am currently waiting for a permanent position.

KH: What got you interested in the role of olive oil and its effect on lipid peroxidation of LDL cholesterol?

FV: Actually, the whole lipidic portion of LDL undergoes oxidation, surface phospholipids being the first component to be oxidized, and cholesterol and cholesterol esters, in the core of the LDL particle, being the last ones. To answer your question, the notion that olive oil is more resistant to oxidation than other fats (e.g. butter and other vegetable oils) although it contains relatively little amounts of tocopherols, prompted us to investigate the antioxidant properties of some minor components, such as oleuropein (see Visioli and Galli, <u>Life Sciences</u>, 1994;55:1965-1971) and hydroxytyrosol, that are correlated with the stability of olive oil.

KH: What are the components in olive oil that may affect LDL cholesterol oxidation?

FV: Extra virgin olive oil contains various so-called minor components, which are responsible for its flavor, aroma, and taste and are also correlated with its stability. Most of them are phenolic in nature and have complex structures that are still under investigation. Oleuropein, the bitter component in olives, is particularly abundant in olive oil and can be hydrolyzed to yield simpler molecules such as tyrosyl, hydroxytyrosol, oleuropein aglycone, and others. All these components add up to approximately 500 to 800 mg/kg of oil, depending on the manufacturing process, the cultivar and the storage.

KH: What are other properties of olive oil that may be of benefit in cardiovascular protection?

FV: The lower incidence of coronary heart disease associated with olive oil consumption is mostly due to its high content of monounsaturated fatty acids (MUFAs) (approximately 70% oleic acid) and polyunsaturated fatty acids (specifically linoleic acid whose proportion, again, varies according to the brand of olive oil). MUFAs intake has been shown to lower LDL but not HDL, so the beneficial

effect of the Mediterranean diet has been so far attributed to its particular fat composition. Our study suggests that other components of the Mediterranean diet, such as olive oil-derived antioxidants, might in part be responsible for the low incidence of coronary heart disease by preventing LDL from being oxidized and, therefore, becoming atherogenic.

KH: Does extra virgin olive oil have more of these phenolic compounds that have antioxidant properties than a more refined olive oil?

FV: Indeed. Extra virgin olive oil contains most of the phenolic fraction, and refined olive oils, such as ones that are just labeled "olive oil," are virtually devoid of these compounds. Moreover, the amount of phenols in extra virgin olive oil varies according to the cultivar, the manufacturing process (olive oils are not <u>extracted</u>, they are obtained by physical pressure of the olive paste), the degree of ripeness of the olives and the storage of the oil. The phenolic composition is currently employed as a marker of the quality and freshness of the olive oil and can actually reveal the area of origin of each batch of olive oil (extra virgin, that is).

KH: Do other polyunsaturated fatty acids have these constituents removed from them or do they not naturally contain them?

FV: Most vegetable oils, such as canola, sunflower or peanut oils, are higher in polyunsaturated fatty acids, (i.e. linoleic acid) than olive oil, but contain virtually no antioxidants, except for tocopherols that are sometimes removed to "clear" vegetable oils from an unpleasant reddish color. For this reason, vegetable oils, which it should be remembered are extracted from seeds rather than being separated from the whole fruit as is olive oil, are less resistant to oxidation and usually go rancid much faster. It seems like the polyphenolic fraction is peculiar of extra virgin olive oil, as you can tell from its peculiar sharp, fruity aroma and pungent taste.

KH: Can your research be of any use to a physician, and how should we direct the general public with regards to olive oil's use?

FV: Physicians in the Mediterranean area often prescribe a higher olive oil-containing diet to people with high blood cholesterol levels because of its beneficial effects as described above. Following these studies, however, a high quality, antioxidant-rich extra virgin olive oil should be suggested, as the increased antioxidant intake could prevent the formation of atherogenic oxidized LDL. These results should also be a suggestion for olive oil producers (now expanding in the United States) to strive for the best quality of olive oil. The only drawback of extra virgin olive oil consumption is its high price and its pungent and sharp taste (the more antioxidants the oil contains the sharper the taste) which some people don't like. It should also be kept in mind that olive oil, although at its best when eaten raw, is very resistent to high temperatures because of its antioxidant content and can replace other vegetable oils normally used for cooking. Again, its bitter taste can add an undesired taste to the dish.

KH: *Natural antioxidants are becoming increasingly popular. Can olives and olive oil be considered a source of such compounds?*

FV: Olive oil itself is probably too expensive to be considered a source of natural antioxidants. However, we have recently demonstrated (Visioli et al, Experientia, 1995;1:32-34) that a by-product of olive oil production, the so-called waste waters, are rich in natural antioxidants that are currently disposed of which could be recovered and probably be of some use to preservative chemists. ◆

Chronic Disease and The Vegetarian Diet

Richard W. Hubbard, Ph.D., C.N.S.
Associate Professor of Pathology, Biochemistry and Nutrition
Schools of Medicine and Public Health
Loma Linda University
P.O. Box 596
Loma Linda, CA 92354 U.S.A.
(909) 824-4400 / (909) 824-4832 (Fax)

"The Potential of Diet to Alter Disease Process,"
Nutrition Research, 1994;14(12):1853-1895. #22584

Kirk Hamilton: Can you please share with me your educational background and current position?

Richard W. Hubbard: I hold both an M.S. and Ph.D. in biochemistry from Purdue University. Nutritional biochemistry has been a central theme in my work during my years at Purdue, the University of Michigan, Stanford Research Institute (under contract to NASA) and here at Loma Linda University where I have appointments in pathology, biochemistry and nutrition.

KH: What are the 3 major risk factors of chronic disease with regards to the Western diet?

RH: 1) Animal protein consumption, because it causes hypersecretion of insulin. 2) Animal fat, because it contains an excess of saturated fats compared to its unsaturated content and because of its cholesterol content. 3) The absence of fiber.

KH: With dietary change can we reduce, by more than 50%, the major degenerative diseases such as cancer, cardiovascular diseases, diabetes, arthritis and bone loss?

RH: Certainly in the Western world, and we can also include stroke, hypertension and renal disease.

KH: You have been a protein or amino acid specialist for years. What is wrong with the type of or the way we eat protein in the Western diet?

RH: Animal protein diets contain twice the protein content that we need. Also, all animal protein, except for egg whites, contains too much of the essential amino acids, particularly the branched chain amino acids. This causes hypersecretion of insulin, which can be reduced by 50% by dietary plant protein.

KH: Does plant protein versus animal protein have a different effect on insulin levels?

RH: Yes. Plant protein causes a much lower secretion of insulin than does animal protein. Also, glucagon secretion is increased by plant protein. Therefore, there is a reversal of the insulin/glucagon ratio found in subjects on the U.S. Western diet.

KH: How does plant versus animal protein affect cardiovascular disease?

RH: Isolating dietary animal protein away from its lipid content (substituting plant fat for animal fat in the diet with animal protein) allows us to show the way that plant protein lowers insulin levels which, in turn, lowers lipogenesis, translating to cholesterol and triglyceride level reduction.

KH: Is there too much protein in the American diet? If so, what harm can excess animal protein have with regards to heart disease and bone loss?

RH: The excess of animal protein in the diet is absorbed as amino acids, which must be excreted in the urine by the kidneys, which receive a direct blood supply from the heart. Of course, the more animal protein, the more consistent is the high insulin level problem. This high animal protein binds to dietary calcium and causes rapid excretion of calcium, meaning we cannot achieve calcium balance without an excess of calcium in the range of 1500 to 1800 mg per day. A plant diet can achieve calcium balance on 400 to 500 mg of calcium per day.

KH: What benefit can vegetable protein have on cardiovascular disease and bone loss?

RH: Plant protein lowers insulin and raises glucagon secretion following a meal. This lowers lipid levels. It also raises metabolic rate which appears to elevate thyroid stimulating hormone levels coming from the pituitary to the thyroid gland. This causes a lowering of body weight which in turn stimulates cholesterol reduction. Bone loss is greatly diminished and calcium balance is achieved at lower calcium intake levels.

KH: Where is the evidence, if any, that protein in cow's milk inhibits the absorption of calcium?

RH: The references 165 to 173 in my article covered this. Heaney, R. P., et al, Journal of Laboratory and Clinical Medicine, 1978;92:953-964 and Zemel, M. B., American Journal of Clinical Nutrition, 1988;48:880-993 are the most conclusive. Please remember that beef, pork, turkey, chicken, egg yolks and even fish protein also provide the same kind of protein as do the caseins from cow's milk.

KH: What types of fat are beneficial and what types are harmful (saturated, polyunsaturated, monounsaturated and/or trans fatty acids)?

RH: Ideally, you need about 25% saturated, 50%

polyunsaturated and 25% monounsaturated. Some monounsaturated substitution for part of the polyunsaturated would also suffice. However, monounsaturated fatty acids cannot substitute for all of the polyunsaturated fatty acids. *Trans* fatty acids may very well be the cause for the very serious reduction in the levels of delta-6-desaturase which, is causing a major essential fatty acid deficiency in the Western world.

KH: What role do nuts and seeds play in a diet that is to prevent degenerative disease?

RH: They serve as sources of a variety of minerals including calcium and magnesium. They include a variety of anticancer compounds and certainly a variety of fatty acids that are mostly unsaturated fatty acids. Also, as the advertisements always say, they are cholesterol free. They are all an excellent source of plant protein. Almonds are especially noted for their protein and calcium content. Walnuts are an excellent source of alpha-linolenic acid, which is the first fatty acid in the omega-3 fatty acid metabolic chain.

KH: Is it hard for vegetarians to get enough protein? How do we mix amino acids to get an appropriate amino acid mixture?

RH: Most vegetarians get more than enough protein to meet their dietary needs. Also, remember that vegetarians eat more and weight less because of their higher metabolic rate. Fortunately, the amino acids in plant protein come in the right amounts to meet our normal needs. The reduced essential amino acids in plant protein meet our needs and reduce our degenerative diseases over what is found in animal protein.

KH: Is there a different hormonal response in consuming simple carbohydrates (added sugars, fruit, etc.) versus complex carbohydrates (beans, whole grains, potatoes, etc.)?

RH: I am going to answer this on the basis of the higher fiber content of complex carbohydrates. The simple sugars start a preinsulin series of reactions in the gut that do not occur by comparison with the complex carbohydrates until further down the intestinal tract and even then at lower rates of glucose absorption.

KH: Can a whole food diet benefit arthritis?

RH: The rheumatoid arthritic patient consuming the vegetarian diet, on the average, greatly benefits by reducing the dietary intake of animal protein. Sometimes even part of the grain proteins must be reduced, but the dietary effect on arthritis is dramatically improved for these protein reactive people.

KH: Do you believe in the Paleolithic Diet concept - that we were essentially foragers consuming large amounts of leafy plant food, some berries, fruit and to a lesser degree nuts and seeds with an occasional gorging on some type of meat? If so, standing agriculture and the availability of whole grains is a relatively new phenomenon in our dietary and physiologic evolution, is it not?

RH: A general plant diet supplemented on rare occasions by meat would cause a rather severe disturbance in the gastrointestinal tract where all of the plant adapted microflora would not be able to assist in the digestion of the meat. In general, I believe that we had tillers of the soil and/or herdsmen and hunters who had meat to eat on a regular basis.

KH: Are there any advantages to the consumption of soy protein?

RH: Soy protein is more able by itself, compared to other plant proteins, to cause maximum growth compared to animal protein. However, if any 2 plant proteins are eaten at each meal or within 1 day, growth will be at a higher rate than with animal protein in growing children.

KH: What role does exercise play in the prevention of chronic disease?

RH: Exercise makes many of our receptors more sensitive. Insulin receptors as an example are much more sensitive after exercise than before. Also, exercise stimulates the release of growth hormone. Exercise increases the appetite. A variety of hormones, including the sex hormones in the male are stimulated by exercise. Exercise improves circulation and enhances oxidative processes versus storage as fat. ◆

Chronic Obstructive Pulmonary Disease (COPD)
Magnesium and Beta-Agonists

Morton Skorodin, M.D.
11A Veterans Affairs Medical Center
Honor Heights Drive
Muskogee, OK 74401 U.S.A.
(918) 683-3261 / (918) 683-3261, Ext. 309 (FAX)

"Magnesium Sulfate in Exacerbations of Chronic Obstructive Pulmonary Disease,"
Archives of Internal Medicine, March 13, 1995;155:496-500. #21987

Kirk Hamilton: *Could you please start off by sharing with me your educational background and present position?*

Morton Skorodin: I was born in Chicago, and I got most of my early education there including medical school at Northwestern University. Subsequently I did an internship, and then I was in the Indian Health Service for several years. I did some of an internal medicine residency in California. Then I came to Hines VA Hospital outside of Chicago to have my pulmonary fellowship training, and I stayed there for 15 years on staff. I have just recently moved to Oklahoma.

KH: *How did you get interested in the role of magnesium and chronic obstructive pulmonary disease?*

MS: By becoming aware of work that was done in asthma using magnesium. In 1989, I noted that The Journal of the American Medical Association had an article by Skobeloff and colleagues that showed that magnesium sulfate was useful in the treatment of acute asthma in the emergency room setting. So I thought the next logical step for our elderly patients with emphysema (seen commonly at the VA hospitals) might be magnesium sulfate when they had their acute spells.

KH: *How does magnesium theoretically work on a chemical basis?*

MS: Nobody knows for sure. It has been known since 1912 that magnesium can relax bronchial smooth muscle. The reports on this were sparse until the 1980s really. As far as its mechanism of action, we know it has a direct relaxing effect on bronchial smooth muscle. It might work by antagonizing the effects of calcium, much as the famous calcium channel blocker drugs do. It may work by augmenting beta-agonist function. Beta-agonists are problematic in their use in asthma and perhaps also in chronic obstructive pulmonary disease. As you have published in your newsletter, we are quite concerned about toxicity from beta-agonist drugs. It also may work by paralyzing the nerve endings of the cholinergic system. In other words, part of the autonomic nervous system may be paralyzed by magnesium, and this may keep the bronchial muscles from contracting. But we don't know this for sure. None of these mechanisms are definitely proven with regard to their effects on obstructive lung disease whether it be emphysema or asthma.

KH: *Tell me a little bit about your study - the basics of it and the results.*

MS: We used magnesium sulfate after using a standard beta-agonist treatment. We gave intravenous magnesium sulfate at 1.2 grams over 20 minutes, a fairly low dose. We noted that the patients had improvement in their index of bronchodilation, which we call peak expiratory flow. Magnesium sulfate is a safe drug to use unless, for instance, you gave that same dose in 5 seconds. That could be quite hazardous. There have been case reports of serious problems when given that rapidly. But in general, it is quite safe.

KH: *Now why did you choose a 1.2 gm versus the frequently used 2 gm initial loading dose?*

MS: A recent review of the world literature on magnesium's use in cardiac and pulmonary diseases showed the dosage given to be quite variable. We copied the work by Skobeloff and Spivey as mentioned above with asthma treatment in the emergency room, except we did it with emphysema. There were other minor differences in our protocol, but the dose was the same.

KH: *And your results in this study?*

MS: We did show that there was improvement in peak flow with magnesium. In other words, the index of bronchodilation was improved. There was a trend toward less need for hospitalization in the magnesium treated dose, but this was not statistically significant.

KH: *The one thing that comes to mind after having quite a lot of individual experience with intravenous magnesium in our clinic over the last 12 years is that you get an initial effect, but it doesn't hold unless you keep them on I.V. magnesium at a slow drip, and that seems to me to be the problem. If you could maintain the intravenous magnesium, I am sure that you would see a more sustained bronchodilating effect and I would be willing to bet a significant reduction in hospital admissions and stays.*

MS: That is one of the many problems with magnesium research. You have hit upon it there. We go from one extreme to the other. We go from the acute use intravenously to the studies that look at what whole populations are doing in terms of their dietary intake. I would like to point out to you a study by a researcher named Britton from Great Britain.

KH: *Isn't that the gentleman who found that increased dietary intake of magnesium led to a reduction in wheezing?*

MS: You are familiar with the study entitled "Dietary Magnesium, Lung Function, Wheezing and Airway Hyperreactivity: A Random Adult Population Sample," published in The Lancet last year. I met Dr. Britton at a meeting last May and it is quite interesting. Respiratory function was grossly linked to the dietary intake of magnesium. He has studied several thousand people, in a cross sectional study in his area of Great Britain. He postulated, or he inferred, from his study that we probably need a higher recommended daily allowance than is currently the case. I believe that he felt that it should be about 400 mg a day and that usually people would get 200 to 350 mg a day. So we go from one extreme to the other. What about the in between state? Very little work has been done on the patient that is subacutely ill.

KH: Did these patients get admitted?

MS: In our study, the decision to admit was strictly on clinical grounds. So some did and some didn't, and there was a trend toward fewer patients who got the magnesium requiring admission.

KH: What would be interesting to me is if the people who received the magnesium could be put on a low maintenance magnesium drip to see if this would result in a shorter hospital stay. Or would they get stabilized more quickly?

MS: That sort of study should be done. To my knowledge nothing like that has been done. One group took people who had asthma so severe that they required mechanical ventilation. They were given magnesium. There was improvement in their respiratory parameters. If I remember correctly, one patient was able to be taken off the respirator as a direct result of the magnesium. But there are very few studies like that. What needs to be done are subacute studies giving them low dose magnesium over 24 to 48 hrs or even a longer period intravenously. When we give magnesium orally there is a limit to what the gut will absorb. Magnesium can have a pretty dramatic laxative effect.

KH: What type of magnesium do you give orally if you do give it?

MS: Magnesium oxide is what we have been using....

KH: And the dosage of that?

MS: Four hundred milligrams of magnesium oxide 2 or 3 times a day. But it is my understanding that most magnesium products are well absorbed, and there is not too much variability in the bioavailability. You know, another problem with magnesium is the variability of results in the published studies. I have reviewed all the studies on myocardial infarction and all the studies on asthma. I cannot explain why, but sometimes it works and sometimes it doesn't.

KH: We use intravenous magnesium quite a bit in our patients. In our asthmatic patients, more than 50% of the time you see acutely that relaxation, that easing of breathing. But the frustrating thing is that it is hard to hold that benefit. I have always wondered how great it would be to be able to have a slower drip in a hospital for these people because I know it probably would continue that effect to a certain degree.

MS: Well one wonders that. That is one possibility. Other possibilities are the use of nebulized magnesium sulfate.

KH: There was one article a long time ago.

MS: I'm aware of 2 articles. One was with magnesium chloride and one was magnesium sulfate. And the magnesium sulfate was done in children with status asthmaticus. The magnesium chloride was 100 mg inhaled and there was no benefit. That was in adult patients. The other study was with children with magnesium sulfate inhaled and that was a much larger dose of 750 mg, and they showed improvement in the peak expiratory flow and in their total clinical situation.

KH: Our I.V. nurse, Ray Balestero, and I did an experiment. We put magnesium sulphate into a nebulizer and I inhaled it. I did it because I was curious to see if it would give the same relaxation effect as I.V. magnesium. The hope was that this would be a way to have a sustained bronchodilating effect in patients who initially had received I.V. magnesium. I can't remember specifically the dose, but I think it was between 1 to 2 grams. All I got was a sore throat though!

MS: If you give an asthmatic something that is hyperosmolar or hypoosmolar, you can make them wheeze. Then too, the magnesium sulfate can be irritating. I would like to try to use magnesium chloride because chloride is the more frequent anion in the body than the sulfate. For instance, just give magnesium chloride (the pure powder with no preservative) and mix that in with water (not normal saline, but water), and see if in a higher dose it would be helpful. But that also hasn't been done. I don't have current plans to do that. What we're doing now is we are giving higher dose magnesium sulfate with an anticholinergic drug versus a beta-agonist drug for emergency treatment of COPD, and we have already enrolled 2 patients in that study.

KH: Excellent! I would like to talk about beta-agonists for a while.

MS: One of my major concerns, and one that peaked my interest in magnesium's use in obstructive lung disease, is about the toxicity from beta-agonist drugs.

KH: Please tell me about that. My understanding was that if they are used just on demand, there is probably not a big problem. If they are used at a regular oral dosage for chronic treatment, then you might get a rebound effect. What's your opinion?

MS: I did write a paper on this subject. I had a debate in print with somebody who was in favor of beta-agonists. What I think happens is that you develop tolerance to the beta-agonists. We have our own endogenous catecholamines that act as beta-agonists, and then once we get used to an excess, we can't respond normally to our own. This might actually cause worse bronchoconstriction. It is like cocaine for the bronchial tubes. This is my fear about beta-agonists. I have had several patients that I have taken off beta-agonists who have had dramatic remissions (at least one was a complete remission) with cessation of use of beta-agonists. One man was taking prednisone for 28 years. When I got him off the beta-agonists, I got him off the prednisone. ♦

Circadian Rhythm, Adrenoleukodystrophy (ALD) and Methyl Vitamin B12

Akemi Tomoda, M.D.
Department of Child Development
Kumamoto University School of Medicine
1-1-1 Honjo
Kumamoto 860, Japan
81 96 373 5197 / 81 96 373 5200 (FAX)

"Circadian Rhythm Abnormalities in Adrenoleukodystrophy and Methyl B12 Treatment,"
Brain and Development, 1995;17:428-431. #24043

Kirk Hamilton: *Dr. Tomoda, can you please share with me your educational background and current position?*

Akemi Tomoda: I received my M.D. degree from Kumamoto University School of Medicine. My medical internship was at Kumamoto University Hospital. I am currently an assistant professor of the Department of Child Development, Kumamoto University School of Medicine, Kumamoto, Japan and my major area of interest is pediatric neurology.

KH: *When did you get interested in the role of vitamin B12 and adrenoleukodystrophy?*

AT: From my clinical research thesis in 1993. This is where I studied about the biological rhythm disturbance in school refusal patients. My other work in this area is as follows:

"A School Refusal Case With Biological Rhythm Disturbance and Melatonin Therapy," Brain and Development, 1994;16:71-76.

"Single-Photon Emission Computed Tomography for Cerebral Blood Flow in School Phobias," Current Therapeutic Research, 1995;56:1088-1093.

"Disturbed Circadian Core Body Temperature Rhythm and Sleep Disturbance in School Refusal Children and Adolescents," Biological Psychiatry in Press, 1996.

"Progressive Myoclonus Epilepsy: Dentato-Rubro-Pallido-Luysian Atrophy (DRPLA) in Childhood," Brain & Development, 1991;13:266-269

"Two Patients With Distal Muscular Dystrophy and Autonomic Dysfunction," Brain and Development, 1994;16:65-70.

KH: *What is the difference between methyl vitamin B12, cobalamin or hydroxocobalamin? What is the rationale for methyl cobalamin's use in sleep-wake rhythm disturbances?*

AT: As I commented in our article, methyl B12 is speculated to have neuropharmacologic effects and normalizes aberrant circadian rhythms. As a mechanism of normalization, methyl B12 is considered to work as a coenzyme in tissue transmethylation and to function as a methyl donor, then the methyl base activates the serotonin, monoamine and melatonin synthesis systems.

KH: *Why did you choose a dose of 1500 mcg of vitamin B12 in the treatment of this condition?*

AT: We used 1500 mcg of methyl B12 during the treatment, because the maximum dose of methyl B12 available as an ethical drug is 1500 mcg. In Japan more than 1500 mcg of methyl B12 is not an officially approved medicine and can only be administered on a clinical trial basis.

KH: *What is the theoretic mechanism by how vitamin B12 or methyl B12 could help sleep rhythm disorders and the eventual production of serotonin and melatonin?*

AT: As a mechanism of normalization, methyl B12 is considered to work as a coenzyme in tissue transmethylation, and to function as a methyl donor, then the methyl base activates the serotonin, monoamine, and melatonin synthesis systems. In our article, in fact, the clinical improvement and the increase in melatonin secretion during the night after treatment in our patient also suggests that methyl B12 plays important roles in melatonin synthesis. Further studies are necessary on the role of methyl B12 in the improvement of rhythm disorders as well as its effects on the central nervous system.

KH: *How effective is the oral dose of 1500 mcg compared to the injection?*

AT: Unfortunately, we did not compare the effects of methyl B12 between oral and IV administration. In our article, however, the methyl B12 blood concentration was measured twice a month after the medication was started, and the patient's methyl B12 blood concentration was within a normal range before and after treatment.

KH: *Do you see methyl vitamin B12 as a way of stimulating melatonin synthesis just in general?*

AT: I assume so. I commented on how this might occur in previous answers.

KH: *Melatonin has strong antioxidant properties so is it possible that methyl vitamin B12 supplementation may enhance antioxidant status through melatonin?*

AT: I don't have any idea about the antioxidant effects of melatonin like N-acetylcysteine (NAC). So I cannot respond to this question at this time. ♦

Claudication (Intermittent) and Propionyl-L-Carnitine

Gregorio Brevetti, M.D.
Universita Degli Studi Di Napoli Federico II
Faculty of Medicine and Surgery
Clinical Medicine I
Via S. Pansini
5-80131 Napoli, Italy
39 81 7462229 (phone/FAX)
39 81 7462240 / 39 81 7462229 (FAX)
E-mail: Indolfi@ds.cised.unina.it

"Propionyl-L-Carnitine in Intermittent Claudication:
Double-Blind, Placebo-Controlled, Dose Titration, Multicenter Study,"
Journal of the American Journal of Cardiology, November 15, 1995;26(6):1411-1416. #23642

Kirk Hamilton: *Could you please share with me your educational background and current position?*

Gregorio Brevetti: I received my undergraduate training at the University of Naples, Italy. I subsequently trained in Cardiology at the Second School of Medicine of the University of Naples. I am presently head of the Angiology Unit at the Department of Medicine, University of Naples Federico II.

KH: *How did you get interested in the role of carnitine and intermittent claudication?*

GB: I first "encountered" carnitine in 1985, when I participated in a clinical trial investigating the effect of L-carnitine in patients with acute myocardial infarction. Reading the extensive literature on the role played by carnitine in energy metabolism, I became interested in the possibility that this substance could be used to improve phosphorylation efficiency in the ischemic skeletal muscle, and thus increase walking capacity in claudicant patients.

KH: *What is the theoretic mechanism by how carnitine may benefit this condition?*

GB: Carnitine allows the mitochondrial entry of free fatty acids for subsequent beta-oxidation. In addition, it is a physiological modulator of the mitochondrial pool of acetylCoA an end product inhibitor of pyruvate dehydrogenase. Therefore, adequate availability of carnitine is fundamental for energy production in the skeletal muscle. Patients with peripheral arterial disease have alterations in carnitine homeostasis that are related to the severity of functional impairment. In particular, patients affected by the most advanced form of intermittent claudication show a reduced availability of carnitine to meet the increased metabolic demand produced by walking (Circulation in press).

KH: *There are different forms of carnitine. Why did you choose propionyl-L-carnitine over plain L-carnitine or acetyl-carnitine?*

GB: Within the mitochondria, propionyl-L-carnitine is converted into free carnitine and propionylCoA. PropionylCoA is readily transformed into succinylCoA and then into succinate, an intermediate of the Krebs' cycle. Through this additional metabolic mechanism (anaplerosis), propionylCoA contributes to the beneficial action of carnitine in providing substrates for energy production to the ischemic muscle. In a double-blind study, propionyl-L-carnitine was more effective than an equimolar dose of L-carnitine in improving walking capacity of claudicant patients.

KH: *Could you please describe to us the results of your study?*

GB: Patients who receive propionyl-L-carnitine walked a longer distance than those who received the placebo. Slightly less than 67% of the patients can be expected to improve their maximal walking capacity by at least 30% if they receive 2 g/day of propionyl-L-carnitine.

KH: *Were there any side effects with the use of propionyl-L-carnitine at 1 to 2 gm per day?*

GB: Propionyl-L-carnitine is a naturally occurring compound and, thus, the number of side effects observed during the treatment was low (4%), similar to that in the placebo group (5%). Nausea and gastric pain were the most frequent effects in both groups.

KH: *Do you have any experience with the different forms of carnitine in acute myocardial infarction or other forms of myocardial ischemia such as angina pectoris?*

GB: My experience with carnitine in coronary artery disease is limited to the above mentioned trial on acute myocardial infarction. We found that patients treated with L-carnitine exhibited less fall in R wave voltage than placebo-treated patients. More recently, the CEDIM Study reported that long-term L-carnitine treatment attenuates left ventricular dilatation in the first year after myocardial infarction. ◆

Colonic Fermentation and The Medical Consequences

K.H. Soergel, M.D.
Medical College of Wisconsin
Division of Gastroenterology
Froedtert Memorial Lutheran Hospital
9200 West Wisconsin Avenue
Milwaukee, WI 53226 U.S.A.
(414) 259-3043 (of) / (414) 259-1533 (FAX)

"Colonic Fermentation: Metabolic and Clinical Implications",
Clinical Investigation, 1994;72:742-748. #21315

Kirk Hamilton: *What is your educational background?*

K.H. Soergel: I received my premedical and medical education in Germany. Essentially, all my postgraduate medical education was in the United States, with the exception of 6 months of immunology research in Erlangen, Germany.

KH: *What is your present position?*

KS: My present position is professor of medicine, gastroenterology and physiology at the Medical College of Wisconsin, and clinical professor of medicine at the University of Wisconsin. I am the director of the Gastroenterology Fellowship Program and coordinator of the Department of Medicine fellowship programs at the Medical College of Wisconsin, Milwaukee.

KH: *How did you get interested in colonic fermentation and its effect on gastrointestinal disorders?*

KS: My research mainly involved studies of absorption from the human intestine by the steady state perfusion method, using inert markers. More than 20 years ago, I attended a veterinary conference at Ames, Iowa, and heard about the importance of short chain fatty acids in ruminant nutrition. Because they derive about 80% of their energy from fermentation in the rumen, I was curious whether short chain fatty acids, which are formed by bacterial fermentation of fodder in the large forestomach, play a physiologic role in man. At that time, Oliver Wrong, a nephrologist in London, had measured short chain fatty acids in human stool and found they were the predominant solute in stool water. In other words, there are more short chain fatty acids there than any other solute, such as sodium, potassium or phosphate. In collaboration with the Department of Chemistry at Marquette University, we then worked out a simple method for measuring short chain fatty acids in biologic fluids. In a series of perfusion studies in human subjects, we found these acids to be readily absorbed from the jejunum, ileum and colon. Invariably, as they are absorbed, the fluid that's left behind in the lumen becomes alkaline. It turned out that bicarbonate is secreted into the lumen in exchange for short chain fatty acid anions. Then came Dr. Roediger, a surgeon in Adelaide, Australia, who found that these short chain fatty acids are the main metabolic fuel of the colonic epithelium. That is to say, these cells can only function and survive when they metabolize short chain fatty acids. About 400 to 500 mmol of short chain fatty acids are produced daily in the normal human colon by bacterial fermentation of 30 to 50 grams of nonabsorbed sugars, starch and fiber. Although butyrate is present in lower concentrations than acetate and propionate, it is preferentially oxidized by colonocytes. This is different from the metabolic requirements of the small bowel mucosa which depends on the availability of glutamine and glucose. We then applied this knowledge to diversion colitis. Nearly all patients who have their rectum and sigmoid disconnected from the rest of the colon develop inflammation in this diverted bowel segment. I speculated that this occurred because there were no short chain fatty acids present in the lumen for lack of a fermentation substrate. This inflammation completely disappeared when we instilled short chain fatty acids into the diverted segment of the distal large bowel. By that time, others, mainly Dr. Richard Breuer in Evanston, Illinois, wondered whether similar therapy might be helpful in ulcerative colitis. In the meantime, Roediger had found that in ulcerative colitis, the colonic epithelial cells have a greatly reduced ability to metabolize short chain fatty acids. The hypothesis was that ulcerative colitis and diversion colitis exhibit a defect in the availability or utilization of short chain fatty acids, respectively. There now is a group of about 150 to 200 investigators across the world who study some aspect of short chain fatty acids. Clearly, this is an emerging field of biomedical investigation. Another issue of major interest is that butyric acid has a differentiating effect on cancer cells in vitro. Butyric acid, added to standard cancer cell lines, causes these cells to acquire the characteristics of normal, nonmalignant cells. This obviously has tremendous potential implications and these issues have not yet been completely explored.

KH: *Have you utilized butyrate, either suppositories or enemas, in the treatment of either ulcerative colitis or any other inflammatory bowel condition?*

KS: Yes. There have been a number of pilot studies on the treatment of distal ulcerative colitis. You can only treat distal disease because enemas don't spread beyond the splenic flexure of the colon. These studies indicated that, indeed, short chain fatty acid enemas, similar to the ones we had used for diversion colitis, tend to heal ulcerative colitis. These were pilot studies, done in Italy, Germany and in the United States. Following this, there have been several randomized, placebo-controlled studies of this issue - the treatment of distal ulcerative colitis. None of these studies have been published yet. We just finished one and are in the process of analyzing the data. Let me add that in ulcerative colitis, it is not a question of low short chain fatty acid concentration in the colon. Rather it is decreased utilization of these short chain fatty acids by the colonocytes lining the colon.

KH: *How can you enhance that utilization?*

KS: The current treatment trials rely on a sort of mass effect to overcome a metabolic block. Another theory involves the bacterial reduction of sulfate in the colon. That happens in everybody, but to varying degrees. The products of bacterial sulfate reduction are highly toxic to the colonic epithelial cells. One hypothesis is that ulcerative colitis represents a type of autointoxication by compounds such as sodium NaSH (sodium hydrogen sulfite), which strongly interferes with the metabolism of colonic epithelial cells. There is preliminary evidence that ulcerative colitis patients have high levels of NaSH and other thiol compounds in their stool. It is possible that we're dealing with an excess of sulfate-reducing bacteria in ulcerative colitis. These are, at the moment, very interesting hypotheses, but none of them are proven.

KH: *Is there a way to dietarily enhance the levels of butyrate?*

KS: That is a very complex field because various carbohydrates fermented in the colon differ in the rate at which they are converted to, for instance, butyrate. In one study, colon cancer was induced in rats. When they were fed wheat bran, the tumor mass in the distal colon was greatly decreased. The reason is that wheat bran is slowly fermented, so the butyric acid is largely produced in the distal colon. On the other hand, if you use other fiber products such as psyllium, these are fermented and absorbed in the proximal colon and the cecum. Presumably, there isn't enough butyrate available in the more distal parts of the colon. Yes, there are ways of manipulating SCFA concentrations along the colon, but how effectively this can be done in man is, at the moment, highly speculative.

KH: *The actual treatment for colon cancer aside from resection is pretty poor, is it not?*

KS: I think, at the moment, the issue is early detection. If everybody had a colonoscopy at age 50 or 60, and had all their polyps removed, the mortality from colon cancer would decrease by about 70%. This is not a recommended health care policy for now.

KH: *I understand, but let's say you have polyps for example. Would that be a person that would want to enhance their butyrate production?*

KS: Again, this is all speculation. There is much geographic variation in the incidence of colon cancer. If one plots the incidence in various countries against the dietary fiber intake, then there is a strong inverse relationship. That is to say, the more fiber people eat, the less colon cancer. For instance, there is little colon cancer among the Bantu in Africa. Here, in the United States, with our highly-refined diet, low in bran and fiber, we have a fairly high incidence of colon cancer. The problem with these data is, generally speaking, the more fiber is consumed, the less fat and red meat is eaten. One can interpret the same data and say colon cancer is related to fat and meat consumption. It is nearly impossible to study this question in humans prospectively because one would have to get large groups of subjects to agree to drastic dietary manipulations over a period of 10 to 20 years. Butyrate cannot be taken by mouth because it is completely absorbed in the small bowel and never reaches the colon. Application by enema is not a very efficient way of doing things. One challenge to the pharmaceutical industry is to devise a retention enema - something that is easily tolerated and retained indefinitely. Another approach would be dietary supplements of resistant starch which reaches the colon intact.

KH: *I am interested in the role of carbohydrate malabsorption and diarrhea. We have kids who consume lots of fruit juices and things and they can get diarrhea. Can you explain that a little bit?*

KS: Basically, carbohydrate malabsorption causes diarrhea at a certain threshold value. In a normal adult, 25 to 50 gm of extra carbohydrate reaching the colon can be efficiently disposed of; the result is a lot of gas, but no diarrhea. Diarrhea coincides with the appearance of unfermented carbohydrate in the stool, which then acts as an osmotic cathartic. In other words, the mechanism underlying the diarrhea of carbohydrate malabsorption is that the limit to which the colon can ferment carbohydrate is exceeded.

KH: *Is it anaerobic bacteria that ferments, for example, antibiotic therapy?*

KS: That is the classical example. During antibiotic therapy, people quite often get diarrhea, not necessarily due to *Clostridium difficile*. True *C. difficile* colitis is actually quite rare. Many more people get simple diarrhea than colitis. It has repeatedly been shown that with the suppression of the colonic anaerobic flora by broad-spectrum antibiotics, the capacity to ferment carbohydrate is decreased. In this situation, the carbohydrate that normally reaches the colon, 40 to 50 gm a day, is no longer fermented completely. The intact carbohydrate is osmotically active and causes an osmotic-type diarrhea.

KH: *In your article, you say the obvious approach is to stop the antibiotic therapy when appropriate and then also the possibility of feeding enteric anaerobic bacteria that somehow pass intact from the mouth into the colon.*

KS: These are not commercially available, nor by prescription. Dr. Gorbach at Tufts, in Boston, reported that he has some strains of anaerobic bacteria which become established in the colon after feeding them to humans in a lyophilized form. I haven't heard much about that since. Commercially available lactobacillus preparations, including those in yogurt, are not active in the colon. So, there are possibilities, but they have not yet been realized.

KH: *There has been a great addition of corn syrup and fructose to the American diet. Could that be a part of the problem of some functional bowel disorders?*

KS: Absolutely. The main sweetening agent in soda pop is high-fructose corn syrup, and people vary in their ability to absorb free fructose. It is not a disease, but if you consume large amounts of soft drinks, apple juice or grape juice, you might get gas or diarrhea.

KH: *What about glutamine?*

KS: Glutamine is to the small bowel what butyrate is to the large bowel.

KH: *Have you done any studies or followed the glutamine therapy?*

KS: The issue arises in patients who are unable to eat and receive total parenteral nutrition. The lining of the small bowel becomes atrophic because it is not used and because there is no glutamine to enter the mucosal cells during absorption. When feeding by mouth is resumed, these patients get diarrhea for a few days until the mucosa has recovered. The problem is that glutamine, a nonessential amino acid, is not present in TPN solutions. The reason is its very poor solubility and stability. One can add glutamine in the form of a stable dipeptide to the TPN solution. This maneuver succeeded, both in rats and in humans, in preventing this starvation atrophy. That is, starvation as far as the small bowel is concerned. However, this is not a critical clinical problem.

KH: *What are 2 or 3 dietary recommendations that would be of benefit for good health of the gastrointestinal tract?*

KS: Eat wheat bran, not oat bran, because it is slowly fermented all along the colon.

KH: I guess I can interpret that to say unrefined?

KS: Unrefined, unprocessed wheat bran in a plastic bag. It is very cheap. Metamucil and other psyllium products are fermented rapidly in the cecum. They are more expensive and may be less effective.

KH: Any other dietary recommendations do you see that would help just in general? You talked about corn sweeteners. We eat a fair amount of those.

KS: I wouldn't worry about them unless one develops diarrhea that could not be explained by anything else. There is nothing wrong with fructose, and it may cause less caries than sucrose.

KH: Or how about a lot of gas and flatulence?

KS: The other food item that commonly causes abdominal distress and diarrhea is sorbitol. This concerns many diabetics and people trying to lose weight. Sorbitol is frequently the sweetener present in dietetic food products such as sugarless gum, candy, chocolate and jam. Sorbitol is very poorly absorbed and can certainly cause diarrhea in the unsuspecting.

KH: Do you have any comment on the role of antioxidants in prevention of bowel cancer, taking into consideration the last study?

KS: No recommendation for the public because it remains a bit of wishful thinking. Clinical trials, to date, have been strikingly disappointing. I am sure you know the study from Finland.

KH: Right, the most recent one?

KS: Yes. One of the problems that people have is that if they did everything that has been suggested in the media, they couldn't eat anything resembling real food as we know it. There are too many messages out with too little clinical relevance to back them up. I think bran is good. Bran makes for better stools. It is good for simple constipation because it makes softer stools. It is good for nonspecific diarrhea because it makes watery stools a little firmer. Certainly, it also lowers cholesterol and there is some evidence that it decreases, over the long haul, diverticular disease, appendicitis and, possibly, colon cancer. So you can't loose. It is a perfectly harmless product and you might as well take it. ◆

Common Cold and Vitamin C

Harri Hemila, Ph.D.
University of Helsinki
Department of Public Health
P.O. Box 21 (Haartmaninkatu 3)
SF-00014, Finland
358 0 43 461 / 358 0 434 6456 (FAX)

"Vitamin C and the Common Cold: A Retrospective Analysis of Chalmers' Review,"
Journal of the American College of Nutrition, 1995;14(2):116-123. #22115

Kirk Hamilton: *Can you please share with us your educational background and present position?*

Harri Hemila: I am a biochemist and studied the molecular biology of *Bacillus subtilis* for my Ph.D. degree. I have had a long interest in vitamin C and changed my research topic after my Ph.D. For some years I have been working at the Department of Public Health as a research associate and concurrently have been studying epidemiology.

KH: *How did you get interested in vitamin C in health and disease prevention?*

HH: I first faced the unorthodox aspects of vitamin C in a television interview of Dr. Linus Pauling. The interview left me with a view that vitamin C may be more important than is generally accepted. I felt that either Pauling or his opponents had to be wrong. Now I believe Pauling was undeniably correct in the general conclusion that the physiologic effects of vitamin C are not limited to the prevention of scurvy, but he was over-optimistic of the eventual benefits of supplementation.

KH: *Why has there been so much controversy regarding vitamin C and the common cold? Is it a matter of bias or are people evaluating studies which have inadequate levels of vitamin C?*

HH: I believe there is no single and simple answer. It seems that many people believe that vitamin C has effects only on collagen metabolism in scurvy, without having studied what is known about vitamin C biochemistry. When a person believes that any effect on the common cold is simply absurd, he or she may unduly exaggerate the technical shortcomings in the studies with positive results. On the other hand, there is a huge amount of commercial exploitation in the field of vitamins with claims having no scientific basis even for an open-minded person, and such social background obviously arouses general skepticism in many people that are following the field from a distant perspective.

KH: *Is vitamin C beneficial in the common cold? If so, what are the reasonable dose ranges at which efficacy is present?*

HH: I think that a rational conclusion from the published studies is that vitamin C definitely has effects on common cold symptoms. However, there are no simple answers to the quantitative questions (i.e. what are the optimal doses and the maximal therapeutic effects?) as there have been great variations in observed results. On the average, studies with 2 gm to 6 gm of vitamin C have found greater benefit than studies with 1 gm, indicating that there may be a dose dependency even with doses above 1 gm per day. At best, large doses of vitamin C have decreased the duration of colds by half, whereas in some studies there has been essentially no benefit. Thus, it is not easy to derive any reasonable estimate of benefit. However, I think that the question of an exact estimate should not be the main question. We should not contemplate whether some estimated benefit is great enough to validate supplementation for all persons. Instead, we should try to identify the characteristics of subgroups in which the benefit is greatest and likewise the reverse insignificant. For example, Terence Anderson, et al, reported in 1972 that in subjects who had a low intake of fruit juices (less than 4 ounces per day), vitamin C supplementation decreased the total "number of days confined to the house" per subject by 48%, whereas the decrease was only 22% in those with a higher intake of fruit juices. Thus, the basic diet may be one of the factors modifying the effects of supplements.

KH: *Can you comment on the reported adverse health effects of taking vitamin C which includes vitamin C's reaction with iron that may generate free radicals promoting heart disease, cancer and other adverse sequelae; the destruction of vitamin B12 by vitamin C; the increased risk to oxalate kidney stones by vitamin C supplementation; the fact that vitamin C can be a pro-oxidant and increase the risk to certain free radical diseases; and the concern that vitamin C triggers a hemolytic anemia in those who are glucose-6-phosphate dehydrogenase deficient?*

HH: In 1987, Jerry Rivers reviewed 74 publications dealing with the proposed toxic effects of vitamin C and concluded that "large quantities of ascorbic acid will not result in calcium-oxalate stones, increased uric acid excretion, impaired vitamin B12 status, iron overload, systemic conditioning, or increased mutagenic activity in healthy individuals" (Annals of The New York Academy of Sciences, 498:445-54). There are small subgroups in which large doses can possibly be harmful such as subjects with iron overload and subjects with glucose-6-phosphate dehydrogenase deficiency, but mostly the claims of toxicity have been pure speculation. For example, none of the common cold studies using rather large vitamin C doses (1-6 gm per day) found any obvious harmful effects from supplementation.

KH: *In what discipline do you see vitamin C's value to be the most significant with regards to the literature - cardiovascular disease, cancer, infection control or as a prevention of eye disorders?*

HH: I believe it is not yet the right time to compare the possible effects of vitamin C on different diseases. We simply need large-scale intervention studies to better estimate the various effects of supplementation.

KH: What doses of antioxidants, and specifically vitamins E, C and beta-carotene, do you consume on a daily basis if you do so?

HH: Usually, I take about a gram of vitamin C per day but much more when I catch a cold, and about 400 mg of vitamin E per week. There are no good data to infer the best doses for the general population. I think that the recommended level of vitamin C at 60 mg per day is too low, even for normally healthy people. ◆

Constipation and Cow's Milk

Antonio Carroccio, M.D./G. Iacono, M.D

Via Coffaro No. 25 Palermo
91024, Italy
39 91 6552995 / 39 91 6552936 (FAX)

"Chronic Constipation as a Symptom of Cow's Milk Allergy",
The Journal of Pediatrics, January 1995;126:34-39. #21598

Kirk Hamilton: Can you please share with me your educational backgrounds and current positions?

G. Iacono: I graduated at the University of Palermo in 1971, later specializing in pediatrics in 1974 and in gastroenterology in 1986. I am a senior consultant of the II Division of Pediatrics at the Ospedale Di Cristina in Palermo; I have been carrying out clinical research in the Sector of Pediatric Gastroenterology for 10 years in collaboration with colleagues of the department of internal medicine of the University Hospital of Palermo.

Antinio Carroccio: I graduated at the University of Palermo in 1984 and specialized in gastroenterology in 1988. After graduation I worked in the INSERM Laboratories in Marsielles, where I became familiar with a number of research methodologies, especially in the sector of pancreatic disease. I also started to collaborate with Dr. Iacono. Our clinical research has mainly investigated food allergies, celiac disease and gastroesophageal reflux.

KH: How prevalent is cow's milk allergy in infants with regards to constipation?

GI: *Cow's milk protein allergy (CMPA) in all its numerous clinical manifestations is one of the most frequent diseases we encounter in our every day experience. Approximately 50% of the infants hospitalized in my department for gastroenterological problems are suffering from food allergy.* The considerable number of patients presenting with CMPA has allowed us to observe a wide, and often unusual, range of clinical manifestations. Among these we have recorded a fairly high frequency of constipation, which we have demonstrated as being directly correlated with cow's milk status.

KH: How does cow's milk cause constipation?

GI: The constipation, pathogenetically speaking, probably stems from anal and perianal inflammatory lesions. These micro-cutaneous lesions (erythema, bleeding, cleavages, ulcerations) cause pain, which intensifies during the passing of stools and eventually inhibits their evacuation.

KH: Do these patients have increased intestinal permeability?

AC: Patients with CMPA generally develop damage of the intestinal mucosa, leading to altered intestinal permeability. However, the constipated patients we studied did not undergo intestinal permeability testing.

KH: Did you evaluate the intestinal flora of these patients?

AC: We didn't consider studying intestinal bacterial flora in our patients; however, the simple culture we performed did not show the presence of pathogenic germs such as salmonella, shigella, etc.

KH: Can other foods cause constipation?

GI: The problem with food allergy is obviously not limited to cow's milk protein. *Almost all the most frequent manifestations observed in patients with CMPA can also be found in the case of allergy to other food antigens.* Among the foods most frequently involved in causing food allergy in our experience are eggs, tomatoes, fish and citrus fruit. These foods also play an etiopathogenetic role in cases of proctitis we have described. Furthermore, it is interesting to note that in patients with constipation secondary to CMPA, there is an aggravation of the clinical picture when the above foods are also eaten. Thus, we normally exclude these foods from the diet, in addition to cow's milk and its derivatives.

KH: What alternatives to cow's milk do you recommend for infants and young children?

AC: Our usual practice is advising a source of protein alternative to cow's milk protein depends chiefly on the age of the infant and their general condition. In unweaned infants, aged under 6 months, and in patients with a more severe picture of malnutrition, we normally suggest a semi-elemental formula with hydrolyzed proteins. These formulas guarantee a lower risk of further sensitization and offer a valid energy supply. In older infants, in those usually suffering from constipation and proctitis, we would prefer to advise a soy protein formula; although this can quite often cause food allergy. In our experience, it has the advantage of being considerably less expensive and has a much more pleasing taste than the semi-elemental formulas. Finally, there are also a number of natural foods which can be used, such as ass's milk, where available; we have successfully given ass's milk to patients as alternative sources with excellent results from the point of view of immunologic tolerance and nutrition. We must also say that ass's milk is a complete food, with a composition and, therefore, digestibility almost identical to that of human milk and should be considered as the first therapeutic approach to be suggested in cases of CMPA.

KH: Are there any tests beneficial in diagnosis of cow's milk protein allergy?

GI: In many cases, a preliminary immunologic study (total IgE, RASTs, prick tests and IgG anti-beta-lactoglobulin assay) in a subject with a clinical presentation of suspected CMPA is useful to support the diagnosis of CMPA. However, to confirm the diagnosis of allergy to CMP, an elimination diet followed by cow's milk challenge is the best means of assessment. In addition, there still needs to be some light shed on the immunologic mechanisms which determine the various clinical pictures of CMPA. In fact, in our study on constipation, approximately 1/3 cases had no involvement of IgE or an increase in IgG anti-beta-lactoglobulin; and yet these infants benefited from a CM-free diet, with a clear relapse on each of the 3 challenges. The diagnosis must, therefore, always be essentially clinical, although where possible, facilitated by immunological data.

KH: *How important is the elimination diet in the assessment of cow's milk protein or CMPA?*

AC: The clinical evaluation of an infant must be complete. It is important to attempt an elimination diet in an infant with constipation and positive clinical history of food allergy, a clear family history of atopic disease, laboratory data indicating a hyperstimulation of the immune system or anal and perianal lesions as described above. However, it must be remembered that there can be many other causes of constipation in pediatric patients -- psychological causes, dietary problems (insufficient fiber intake) and organic problems associated with altered motility.

KH: *Is there much research on cow's milk allergy and constipation?*

GI: To our knowledge, there are no other studies in the literature which discuss the relationship between chronic idiopathic constipation and food allergy. In fact, in many reports on general and gastroenterological pediatrics, constipation is quoted as the possible symptoms of CMPA, but there have been no clinical studies to confirm this affirmation.

KH: *How does one clinically approach these young children with constipation?*

GI: The approach of the practitioner should vary according to the age of the patients. In infants, aged 2 to 3 years, there is a greater possibility of being faced with an allergic manifestation; therefore, in these cases, those aspects of clinical history, laboratory data and objective examination which may suggest CMPA should be assessed and an elimination diet advised. In school-aged children, it is less likely that the constipation is of an allergic pathogenesis and it is necessary to take into greater consideration psychogenic and interpersonal relationship problems. Furthermore, all organic causes of constipation must be considered and accurately excluded before labeling a case of chronic constipation with a different diagnosis. ◆

Coronary Bypass Surgery and Vitamin E

Don Mickle, M.D.
Toronto General Hospital
ES3-404, 200 Elizabeth Street
Toronto, Ontario M5G 2C4, Canada
(416) 340-3274 / (416) 340-4706 (FAX)

"Vitamin E For Coronary Bypass Operations: A Prospective, Double Blind Randomized Trial", Journal of Thoracic and Cardiovascular Surgery, 1994;108:302-10. #20760

Kirk Hamilton: Could you start off by sharing your educational background and your present position?

Don Mickle: I am a physician, a chemist, and a member of the Royal College of Physicians and Surgeons in Canada. My specialty is medical biochemistry. My current position is acting director of the Toronto Hospital Clinical Biochemistry Service Laboratory.

KH: Could tell us about your article entitled, "Vitamin E For Coronary Bypass Operations" in The Journal of Thoracic and Cardiovascular Surgery?

DM: We gave identical capsules, some of which contained corn oil and some which contained vitamin E that had the hydrogen labeled with deuterium. The reason for labeling the hydrogen in vitamin E was to allow for its identification in the heart tissue. You don't want to use radioisotopes because of the radioactivity. Deuterium is quite harmless - it is just heavy hydrogen. The dose of vitamin E used was 100, 300 and 900 mg.

KH: How did you get interested in the use of vitamin E for coronary bypass surgery?

DM: I had collaborated with Dr. Weisel, who is a cardiovascular surgeon at the Toronto hospital, for some years. I had done some research in water soluble analogs of vitamin E and had shown for the first time that it could prevent ischemia reperfusion injury very significantly. Because the water soluble forms were not FDA approved we thought we'd try plain vitamin E. There was no risk to these elective patients.

KH: Could tell us how much of a concern is ischemia reperfusion injury in bypass patients and what are the medical ways of dealing with it?

DM: Ischemia reperfusion injury occurs when blood flow to any organ decreases significantly and the tissue becomes ischemic. Then reperfusion, especially the initial reperfusion, appears to cause a lot of injury. This applies not only to the heart but to other organs including the brain.

KH: Is that because of free radicals being released?

DM: That's one component, but that is not the sole component. You lose a lot of energy. Your proteolytic enzymes could be released and damage the cell. Calcium can infuse into the cell. There are many other factors.

KH: Have there been any other agents tried besides vitamin E to help reduce the damage from ischemia reperfusion? Other natural

antioxidants or agents such as probucol?

DM: In this type of study - no. This study was done 3 or 4 years ago and it was difficult to publish because no one really wanted to accept the concept that vitamin E might be useful.

KH: Why did you not choose another antioxidant such as beta-carotene or vitamin C?

DM: I am not so totally sure that beta-carotene is an antioxidant. Vitamin C is very short lived and I was concerned that when interacting with iron vitamin C might act as a radical itself. Vitamin E is your natural antioxidant. It is probably your only lipid soluble antioxidant and that is why vitamin E was chosen.

KH: Why would you have more interest in a lipid soluble antioxidant?

DM: Because the earlier research showed that the lipid membranes had become injured by free radicals and the dominant injury appeared to be in the cell membrane, the external wall.

KH: Is this of the artery?

DM: No, of the heart cell. We had done some research here and fractionated the heart. It appeared that the external membrane, the sarcolemma, was the most susceptible organ. It's natural antioxidant is vitamin E.

KH: What dosages of vitamin E did you give in your study?

DM: We gave 900 mg., 14 days prior to surgery. None of the outpatients who were taking vitamin E were excluded. The patients received either plain corn oil or they were getting corn oil supplemented vitamin E. No one knew, neither the surgeon or anyone in the trauma hospital because the capsules were prepared in Ottawa.

KH: Were these actually coronary bypass patients?

DM: They were all elective patients who had angina and required coronary bypass surgery. They were a low risk group of patients because they had to wait a month or 2 for the surgery. So for 2 weeks prior to that, they took the vitamin E daily or the placebo capsules daily.

KH: Please share the results with regards to myocardial lactate production?

DM: Normally, the heart consumes lactate. The heart is a scavenger. It will take food from wherever it can get in the blood stream and lactate is a very convenient source because it bypasses glycolysis and can enter the TCA cycle. So the heart extracts lactate from the blood very avidly. There appears to be less injury because the tocopherol patients were extracting lactate while the controls were still releasing it suggesting that there was more of an injury in the control patients.

KH: *So when there is a damaged heart, there is more of a release of lactate versus consumption. Is that correct?*

DM: Yes, as a general rule. Also, the left ventricular stroke volume indices were higher in the vitamin E treated patients.

KH: *Were there any other positive findings from the vitamin E treated patients?*

DM: Yes. The creatinine kinase MB release after heart surgery was statistically less in the vitamin E treated patient which implied that they had suffered less ischemic heart damage. Now I would like to stress these are low risk patients. You wouldn't expect much damage. They all did well. But these metabolic measures of overall heart damage appeared to be much less with vitamin E. I believe if we get into the high risk patients and could give them vitamin E prior to surgery, then I think you would see a more profound effect. This was actually a perfect study in that no one in our hospital knew what we were doing or what we were giving the patient. It was absolutely blind.

KH: *If you're going to have heart surgery would you take vitamin E two weeks before hand?*

DM: Yes, I would take vitamin E prior to surgery. I presently take about 300 units every 2nd or 3rd day.

KH: *How long have you been interested in vitamin E?*

DM: I started in free radical research in about 1984 or 1985 and it is was just a natural evolution. I measured the damage and ones natural defense for it. It turned out in some of the lipid membranes to be vitamin E. We measured the amount of lipid peroxidation. So it was a natural logical development. ◆

Coronary Heart Disease and Antioxidants

Pauli V. Luoma, M.D.
Regional Institute of Occupational Health
Aapistie 1
FIN-90220 Oulu, Finland
358 81 537 5681 / 358 81 537 6000 (FAX)

"High Serum Alpha-Tocopherol, Albumin, Selenium and Cholesterol, and Low Mortality From Coronary Heart Disease in Northern Finland",
Journal of Internal Medicine 1995;237:49-54. #21749

Kirk Hamilton: Could you please share with me your present position?

Pauli Luoma: I am currently doing research in the Department of Public Health Science at the University of Oulu, Finland. I am an assistant professor of internal medicine at the University of Oulu and an assistant professor of clinical pharmacology at the University of Tampere, Finland.

KH: How did you get interested in the role of antioxidants and coronary heart disease?

PL: The mortality from coronary heart disease (CHD) in Finland is one of the highest in the world. I got interested in antioxidants and coronary heart disease in the early 1980s when the association of low serum selenium and high risk of CHD in Finland was reported. I have been interested in lipid and apolipoprotein risk factors and liver microsomes, cytochrome P-450, lipids and proteins. Serum selenium is related to liver cytochrome P-450, and hepatic microsomal induction (increase in cytochrome P-450) is associated with a beneficial, antiatherogenic change in the serum lipoprotein profile. Antioxidants protect microsomes, low density lipoproteins and whole organs against oxidative damage, and may prevent atherogenesis and retard the manifestation of CHD.

KH: Was there any surprise to this study, in particular higher levels of cholesterol in the group that had the lower incidence of coronary heart disease?

PL: It is of particular interest to study reasons for a low CHD mortality in this country, well known for its high CHD mortality. The explanation for the association of high cholesterol and low CHD mortality might be found in some factor in genotype, diet, lifestyle or environment. The men of Sami origin (ethnic minority) living in northernmost Finland show a high frequency of apolipoprotein phenotype E4/4 and e4 allele which may in part explain the high concentration of serum cholesterol observed in the low mortality area. However, a major factor in the low CHD mortality in the north may be an adequate antioxidant status preventing the atherogenic modification of LDL also in people with a high serum cholesterol level.

KH: How would antioxidants protect against CHD?

PL: The antioxidants prevent the oxidative modification of LDL that has been suggested to have a major role in the development and progression of atherosclerosis and coronary heart disease.

KH: Why does reindeer meat have higher amounts of the antioxidants selenium and vitamin E? Are there other foods that are higher in these antioxidants that the Sami consume?

PL: Vitamin E and selenium in reindeer meat are derived from the natural sources. Reindeer researchers report that particularly lichens and mushrooms are rich in selenium. The consumption of margarine, plus vegetable oils and cereals, which are important sources of vitamin E, is higher in the Sami area than the neighboring regions to the south. Serum selenium is related to the consumption of fish, which is an important constituent of the diet in the north.

KH: You talk a lot about antioxidants, but how about the effect of omega-3 fatty acids in not only the fish but also in the Northern Reindeer fat even though the total fat is less?

PL: There are some differences in the consumption of food items between the two areas which may have significance. The consumption of reindeer meat and margarine plus vegetable oils is higher and that of milk lower in the low mortality area than the reference area. The intake of fat and saturated fats is lower in the low mortality area than the reference area. Reindeer meat has relatively high contents of unsaturated oleic acid. It has one double bond and is much more resistant to oxidation than linoleic acid which contains two double bonds. An increase in the consumption of oleic acid may beneficially reduce the atherogenicity of the diet. There are differences in the consumption of saturated and unsaturated fats between the two areas but we do not have data on omega-3 fatty acids.

KH: Do you consume basic antioxidants in supplemental form (C,E or beta-carotene) as part of a preventive approach to CAD?

PL: Not regularly. A Mediterranean type of diet is a good goal. Further studies are needed for a general recommendation to use antioxidants in the prevention of cardiovascular diseases. ◆

Coronary Risk Factor Intervention
Aerobic Versus Strength Training

Ben Hurley , Ph.D.
University of Maryland
Professor of Exercise Physiology
Director, Exercise Science Laboratory
Department of Kinesiology
College of Health and Human Performance
College Park, Maryland 20742 U.S.A.
(301) 405-2486 / (301) 314-9167 (FAX)

"Aerobic or Strength Training For Coronary Risk Factor Intervention?",
Annals of Medicine, 1994;26:153-154. #20476

Kirk Hamilton: When did you get interested in the subject of lowering cardiovascular risk by either strength or aerobic training?

Ben Hurley: It started when I was doing a postdoctorate fellowship at Washington University School of Medicine in St. Louis. We were recruiting some world class strength athletes and one of the things I noticed was some of the people in the masters competition (older than 45 years of age) - seemed to look younger than some marathon runners we were also testing. So that sort of intrigued me to examine the research literature on the health related effects of strength training compared to aerobic exercise training. After finding very little information in the literature, we decide to launch our own investigation. It started off as a subjective observation based on physical appearance and ended up as a research project in which we studied some people in both groups -both the marathon runners and some competitive power lifters.

KH: What is the role physical inactivity plays in heart disease?

BH: Until recently, it was believed that physical inactivity was only a minor risk factor and it was only secondary to the other risk factors, i.e. inactive people were thought to be at high risk only because they were more likely to be obese, smoke cigarettes, have high blood pressure and high cholesterol. A number of epidemiological studies since then clearly show that the independent effect of just physical inactivity, i.e. independent of the other risk factors - has a similar likelihood or relative risk as the 3 major risk factors - cigarette smoking, hypertension and high blood cholesterol. In fact, there are more people across the country that have physical inactivity as a risk factor than all the other 3 major risk factors combined.

KH: Is the public message that physical inactivity could be of greater risk when taken in total than the other 3 risk factors?

BH: Right. But what has not been known is what type of training modality is best. We have known that physical inactivity is a risk, but if you're going to try to reverse that and cause people who were previously inactive to become active, what do you tell them to do? That is the question that we have tried to address.

KH: Let's say a gentleman patient of our clinic comes in who is normal weight, but he has cardiovascular disease. Am I going to

encourage him to go out and walk, do circuit training, power lifting or encourage him to become a marathoner?

BH: Based on the data available right now, we have to go with aerobic exercise training. However, there is so much more information on aerobic exercise training than there is on strength training. Until 1980 there was little or no research on the potential health effects of strength training. Whereas, by the 1980s, there were hundreds maybe thousands of papers already published about the effects of aerobic exercise training on risk factors to heart disease and other health parameters. There is certainly more evidence available from good quality studies showing lipid profiles, for example, seem to be more favorably altered with aerobic training than with strength training. There are many studies showing no changes in lipid profiles with strength training. Some risk factors such as abnormal glucose metabolism seem to be affected similarly whether you use strength training or aerobic training. But if you look at all the risk factors that are important for heart disease, and you put them together in some kind of an overall risk profile index, there is probably more data available right now showing aerobic exercise training would be the training of choice when used as a risk factor intervention technique.

KH: Could I tell someone walking for 10 minutes, 4 times a day, is as good as going out and doing 40 minutes straight?

BH: The answer is yes as long as the intensity is the same, but practically speaking, how many people are willing to exercise 4 different times a day at a sufficient intensity?

KH: Does the aerobic exercise have to be greater than 60% or 70% of your maximum heart rate or can a person work in his garden vigorously for a half hour or 20 minutes?

BH: This has been a controversial issue because there is evidence that low to moderate activity is associated with a substantial improvement in longevity. However, there is no question that the intensity needs to be up there somewhere around the 60% minimum threshold to get optimal changes in cardiovascular function and that is much better than doing gardening or any other kind of activity that doesn't sustain this level of intensity. But there is confusion about the difference between improving cardiovascular function versus increasing longevity. Nevertheless, research clearly shows that as far as improving the cardiovascular system to the optimal level, that the alternative you are talking about is not as effective.

KH: *If someone did circuit training - light weights, frequent reps and moved from station to station versus heavy lifting, resting several minutes in between - is there data on this particular comparison?*

BH: We addressed this questions in one of our studies.

KH: *And, what did you find with regards to blood pressure, blood fats and glucose?*

BH: We had people go through circuit weight training and had their target heart rate sustained at least as high, and in most cases even higher, than the same people would when they go out to run. There were no rest periods. They moved quickly from station to station to sustained this high heart rate. Even at the end of 16 weeks of doing that, there was no significant increase in their maximal ability to utilize oxygen (VO$_2$ max), which is an index of the functional capacity of the cardiovascular system. To answer your question, there were no changes in blood pressure or any other indicators of cardiovascular function during exercise, despite some improvement in blood fats and glucose metabolism.

KH: *And if they would have done jogging?*

BH: We found that the amount of oxygen utilized would be substantially greater if they jogged at the same heart rate. Thus, the exercise intensity at the same energy cost as circuit weight training amounted to a slow to moderate walk.

KH: *So the pulse rate didn't make that much difference?*

BH: The pulse rate was even higher on the circuit weight training than it was walking on the treadmill. But with each heart rate there was less oxygen utilized by the muscle (i.e., a lower oxygen pulse). So oxygen pulse is lower when you do circuit weight training than it is when you do the same intensity of exercise using the large muscle groups, such as walking or jogging. We found a catecholamine response which caused the heart to beat faster, but it wasn't followed by a concomitant increase in oxygen consumption. So that explains why you cannot get a cardiovascular training effect from circuit weight training like you can from aerobic exercise.

KH: *Well, that blows my theory. I have always felt that while I am doing circuit training if I keep my heart rate up and if I move from station to station, that I was having the same cardiovascular benefit.*

BH: No, in fact, even when our subjects exercised to complete exhaustion through circuit weight training, there was no significant change in their maximum oxygen consumption (Vo$_2$max) and there was no change in any of their hemodynamics during submaximal exercise at the intensity they would normally use while jogging.

KH: *It appears you are sayig that aerobic training is still what we have the most data on and it is definitely the thing producing the most cardiovascular benefit, even though activity in general, long-term studies show, decreases mortality. Strength training has a lot less data, but definitely does have some positive benefit. Is it equal to aerobic exercise on its effect on lipids, blood pressure and glucose metabolism?*

BH: If you take all the literature available, there is more data showing aerobic exercise training is effective for improving lipid profiles than there is strength training. Secondly, with blood pressure, there is more consistent evidence that aerobic exercise training will favorably alter blood pressure than there is for strength training.

However, there is the impression among a lot of people, including many physicians, that because strength training elevates blood pressure acutely, it has a long-term adverse effect on resting blood pressure. That is just not true. In fact, there are isolated studies showing a reduction in resting blood pressure and other studies showing no effect on resting blood pressure. But there are no well-controlled published studies showing blood pressure increases at rest as a result of strength training. The effect on blood glucose metabolism is the most consistent of anything we have ever studied with strength training or aerobic exercise training. We have repeatedly found in about 5 separate and independent studies that both aerobic and strength training improve glucose metabolism by reducing the amount of insulin necessary to metabolize the same amount of glucose. The term used to define this is insulin sensitivity. Strength training increases insulin sensitivity and is just as effective as aerobic exercise training.

KH: *Can you give me a short definition of strength training?*

BH: Yes, it is exercising against resistance to strengthen skeletal muscle.

KH: *Strength training is definitely better than nothing as far as improving cardiovascular benefit?*

BH: Yes, it probably is. In almost every one of our 15 or so longitudinal studies, the mean value for V0$_2$max is a little bit higher after strength training than it is before training and it usually increases anywhere from 3% to 6%. If you have the same people exercise for the same length of time and everything else is equal with aerobic training, you will see a 15% to 25% increase in VO$_2$max.

KH: *Would you say the ideal workout is doing aerobics in combination with some kind of strength training?*

BH: You have to define the objective that you want to get out of it before you can answer that question. If all you're concerned about is cardiovascular fitness, I don't think you need to do any strength training. If all you're concerned about is strength and muscle enlargement, I don't think you need to do aerobic training. However, if you want to improve your total health and fitness and time is not a factor, then both training modalities should be recommended.

KH: *Well you are a 70-year-old person who is trying to keep his balance and coordination intact and not break bones?*

BH: In that case, if you have to choose one or the other, and you only have time to do one, strength training may be the training of choice.

KH: *As you get older?*

BH: Yes. Again, if the person is willing to spend the time to do both in an optimal way, then certainly both would be recommended. But the evidence coming out recently shows remarkable changes for older people with strength training.

KH: *What is the minimum time frame for aerobics that you would recommend on a 4-day-a-week basis if somebody is doing it to get significant benefit? Twenty minutes?*

BH: Twenty to 30 minutes has been shown to be optimal. That doesn't mean you can't get some benefit if you do it less than that. There are plenty of studies showing even 10 minutes will produce changes. But as far as optimal changes, it looks like 20 to 30 minutes is around the minimum threshold for optimal benefits. ◆

Depression, Aerobic Training and Physical Disabilities

Catherine P. Coyle, Ph.D.
Myra Santiago, Ph.D.
College of Health, Physical Education, Recreation & Dance
316 Seltzer Hall (062-62)
Philadelphia, PA 19122 U.S.A.
(215) 204-8706 / (215) 204-1455 (FAX)

"Aerobic Exercise Training and Depressive Symptomatology in Adults With Physical Disabilities," Archives of Physical Medicine and Rehabilitation, 1995;76:647-652. #22928

Kirk Hamilton: *Drs. Coyle and Santiago, could you please share with me your educational backgrounds and current positions?*

Catherine Coyle: I obtained my Ph.D. in educational psychology from Temple University and I am an assistant professor of the Therapeutic Recreation Curriculum at Temple University.

Myra Santiago: I received my Ph.D. from the University of Minnesota and I am an associate professor in the Physical Education Department and Biokinetics Research Laboratory at Temple University.

KH: *How long have you been studying the role of exercise and depression?*

MS: I have been interested in exercise physiology since the onset of graduate work in 1981.

CC: I have been interested in depressive symptomatology among adults with disabilities since 1986. Dr. Santiago and I joined forces at Temple University through a grant which the Therapeutic Recreation Curriculum received from The National Institute on Disabilities and Rehabilitation Research, U.S. Department of Education. The portion of the grant involving aerobic exercise began in the spring of 1990 and was concluded in the summer of 1991.

KH: *What are the physiologic mechanisms by how exercise may reduce depression?*

CC & MS: There are various hypotheses that have been described about the possible mediating mechanisms for a physiologic effect of aerobic exercise and depression. These hypotheses can be summarized in the 4 areas: (1) Physiologic feedback messages from an improved cardiorespiratory fitness; (2) Increased levels of endogenous opiates (i.e.; endorphins); (3) Changes in monoamine neurotransmitter secretions (i.e.; norepinephrine, dopamine and serotonin); and (4) Tranquilizing effects of increases in core temperatures.

KH: *What roles do endorphins play if any?*

CC & MS: The endorphin hypothesis has been very popular, but has recently been questioned due to the fact that many of the exercise studies measured blood serum level changes of this variable during exercise versus its levels in the central nervous system. Furthermore, current consensus is that the overall mechanism of changes in depression with aerobic exercise are likely to involve a combination of both physiological/biochemical and behavioral/ psychological adaptations to exercise. Results from our study provide support for this combined hypothesis in individuals with physical disabilities.

KH: *What are the results of your study with regards to exercise training and depressive symptoms in individuals with physical disabilities?*

CC & MS: Our research examined the ability of aerobic exercise to improve the physical and mental health of adults with physical disabilities. We tested 19 adults with a variety of physical disabilities ranging from stroke to spinal cord injury. The exercise program was done either in the individuals' homes or in a community based aerobic class. Results from our study indicated that exercise dramatically improved the fitness level and decreased the reported amount of depressive symptoms. Aerobic exercise improved fitness levels (VO_{2peak}) in the exercise group by 23% and decreased depressive symptoms by 59% after 13 weeks of aerobic exercise. In contrast, individuals who chose not to participate in the exercise program showed marked losses in fitness (19%) and increases in the reporting of depressive symptoms (6%) after 24 weeks of physical inactivity.

KH: *Could exercise programs be utilized as adjunctive treatments for depression in other individuals who do not have physical disabilities, and what impact do you see with regards to exercise as a whole on society if done on a much larger scale with specific emphasis on behavior?*

CC & MS: It is possible. Some research has shown that aerobic exercise is a beneficial adjunctive treatment for individuals with clinical depression, while other researchers have shown that aerobic exercise can be helpful in reducing the risk of depression in the general population. Aerobic exercise has also been well documented to improve mood levels in many individuals. Our study results confirm the possible mental health promoting effects of aerobic exercise in individuals with physical disabilities who, by the nature of their primary disability, are at risk for increased physical and/or mental problems. ◆

Depression and Exercise

Thomas L. Schwenk, M.D.
University of Michigan Medical Center
Department of Family Practice
1018 Fuller Street, Box 0708
Ann Arbor, MI 48109-0708 U.S.A.
(313) 998-7128 / (313) 998-7335 (FAX)

"Using Exercise to Ward Off Depression",
The Physician and Sports Medicine, September 1995;23(9):44-56. #23164

Kirk Hamilton: Could you please share with me your educational background and current position?

Thomas Schwenk: I am currently professor and chair of the Department of Family Practice at the University of Michigan. I received my medical training at the University of Michigan Medical School, then pursued a family practice residency and fellowship at the University of Utah. I returned to the University of Michigan in 1984 and completed my primary care sports medicine training during a sabbatical in Australia in 1993. I recently passed the examination for a certification of Added Qualification in Sports Medicine From the American Board of Family Practice. During my career, I have also been involved in research on psychiatric problems in primary care, particularly depression.

KH: When did you get interested in the role of exercise and depression?

TS: My 2 major career interests, sports medicine and depression, seemed to come together naturally in this regard. I have also found exercise to be very important to me personally as a stress reducer and as a buffer against the inevitable stresses of work and family life.

KH: What evidence to date is there that exercise can affect depression?

TS: Morgan, et al, administered the Zung Self-Rating Depression Scale to 101 healthy male college professors before and after participating in a 6-week exercise program. He found that only the 11 professors who were assessed as depressed by the pre-exercise scores significantly decreased their post-exercise scores. In another study, 15 moderately-depressed patients experienced a significant decrease in their Beck Depression Scale Scores after undergoing 10 weeks of aerobic exercise as compared to 2 weeks of stretching without aerobic activity. This decrease was even more marked at a 6 month-follow-up for those who continued to exercise. Some studies investigated whether exercise helps only depressed people. North, et al, conducted a meta-analysis and found that exercise significantly reduces depression ratings in those who were depressed, in those "feeling down" and in those who were apparently healthy. In a study by Roth and Holmes, researchers found among college students who were exposed to high life stress, those who had a low physical fitness level (as assessed by a submaximal cycle ergometer) subsequently developed more problems with health and scored higher on the Beck Depression Inventory. With regard to the long-term effects, it was found that regular exercise lead to a decrease in anxiety and depression in 5,000 college students in a mental health course. These students continued to show benefits for up to 7 years after leaving the course if they continued to participate in some form of exercise.

KH: What are the assumed physiologic effects that help the exercising depressed individual?

TS: Many mechanisms have been proposed on how exercise exerts its effect both psychologically and biological mechanisms have been proposed. Among the biological mechanisms, the most well known one concerns the effect of endogenous endorphins. The brain and other structures produce various endorphins that have a morphine-like action and can reduce the sensation of pain and produce a state of euphoria. Markoff, et al, found that this hypothesis can be both supported and rejected depending on the specific investigation one chooses to cite. The more well accepted hypothesis suggests that the improved effect associated with exercise can be obtained through the alterations of the major brain monoamines (i.e. dopamine, serotonin and norepinephrine). Depression is associated with impaired transmission at certain central aminogenic synapses, due to defects in production, transfer, reuptake or breakdown of those amines. By improving this transmission, the depression may be alleviated. Evidence for this hypothesis comes from studies which reveal that major urinary metabolites of serotonin, dopamine and norepinephrine are reduced in depressed patients. This presumably reflects a decreased rate of amine release at central synapses and presumably a decreased level of function of these synapses. Animal studies have shown that exercise may enhance transmission in neurons that contain norepinephrine or dopamine. Studies involving humans have found that depressed patients increase their secretion of amine metabolites when they engage in exercise. An additional proposed mechanism, for which there is little support currently, is the thermogenic hypothesis in which the elevation in body temperature that accompanies exercise could lead to antidepressant effects.

KH: What are the beneficial psychological aspects of exercise?

TS: The distraction hypothesis is an example of a psychological mechanism. It may be that distraction from stressful stimuli, as opposed to exercise per se, is responsible for the antidepressive effects. Two other psychological hypothesis deserve mentioning. The mastery hypothesis suggests that depression is a person's response to loss of control. Exercise therefore becomes a form of mastery or a way of regaining control of one's life. The social interaction hypothesis states that a substantial portion of the psychological benefits obtained from exercise stem from the social interaction that often accompanies participation in sports.

KH: *What type of exercise should be recommended for depression?*

TS: Martinsen found that only those hospitalized patients diagnosed with major depression who had a greater than 15% increase in estimated maximal oxygen uptake experienced a significant decrease in their depression scores. However, in a more recent study, Martinsen found that patients who met the DSM-IIIR criteria for major depression, dysthymic disorder or a depressive disorder not otherwise specified had significant reductions in depression scores even if a significant increase in VO_2 max was not obtained. Sexton, et al conducted a similar study that compared joggers who showed at least a 15% gain in aerobic capacity to walkers who had no significant change in VO_2 max. There was no significant difference in the psychological benefits of exercise in these 2 groups. The lack of difference persisted at 6 month follow-up. These studies suggested that a primary care physician can prescribe rigorous exercise such as walking, for which compliance is likely to be much greater, and still expect to see psychological benefits. An exercise program that is fun, convenient and varied is associated with compliance. The program should not be perceived as a disruption of the patient's already hassled and unsatisfying life-style. *The program should be individualized so that the type of exercise that suits the patient's life-style and temperament can be used.* Greist, et al, used the following principals to minimize dropouts: *1. Make each run so gentle and comfortable that the patient will look forward to the next run. 2. Runners should finish with more energy than they had at the beginning. 3. Concerns about distance, pace and competition with others should be minimized.* There is no research-based guidance regarding the specific mode, frequency, intensity and duration that an exercise program should employ so as to maximize its psychological benefits. General guidelines provided by Hill suggest aerobic exercise 2 to 5 times per week with a duration of 30 to 40 minutes, including 10 minutes of warm-ups (including stretching) and cool down at each session. The exercise should be performed at 60% to 70% of the maximal intensity. This program is compatible with the current ACSM recommendations for more general health benefits. Even though some studies demonstrate that anaerobic exercise is comparable to aerobic exercise in helping to alleviate depression, aerobic exercise should be recommended preferentially (if not contraindicated) so as to provide cardiovascular and other health benefits. In summary, a good rule to follow is to prescribe sufficient exercise to be challenging, but not so much as to be self-defeating. The threshold of self-defeat for depressed patients is probably lower than it is for non-depressed persons.

KH: *Do all depressed patients benefit from exercise?*

TS: Potentially all patients can benefit from exercise although the effect varies inversely with the severity of the depression. For patients with severe depression exercise is only an adjunct to more intense treatment with medication and counseling, whereas exercise may be the only needed intervention necessary in milder or intermittent forms of depression.

KH: *Is exercise as good in some cases as medication therapy or psychotherapy?*

TS: Greist randomly assigned 18 people to either running or 1 of 2 kinds of individual psychotherapy (10 session time-limited or time-unlimited). He found that running produced similar levels of improvement in depression scores as compared to both types of psychotherapy. In addition, he calculated the relative costs of treating depression with running to be approximately 1/5 that of psychotherapy. Harris concluded that depressed patients who experienced a combination of counseling and running significantly improved depression scores when compared to those who underwent counseling alone. North, et al, obtained similar results from a meta-analysis and concluded that exercise is as effective as psychotherapy but exercise plus psychotherapy is better than exercise only in mildly depressed patients. A study comparing exercise to antidepressant medication found that patients who exercised while also taking tricyclic antidepressants showed a larger decrease in depressive scores than those not exercising. In a subsequent study, Martinsen found that patients who received tricyclic antidepressants while exercising experienced larger reductions in depression scores than those who received antidepressants alone, although the difference was not statistically significant.

KH: *Are there any risk factors of exercise in depressed patients?*

TS: Even though exercise has many psychological benefits, negative consequences can result from excess. Athletes competing in endurance sports such as long distance running and swimming are commonly subject to periods of high intensity training in order to enhance performance levels. Overtraining or staleness is considered to be a general stress response to high volume, high intensity training with inadequate rest and recovery periods between training sessions. According to Kuipers and Kuizer, staleness may be encountered when the combined stresses from training, the environment, work and private circumstances exceed the individual's capacity to adapt. Symptoms of overtraining are similar to those of depression and include fatigue, loss of purpose, decreased energy levels, feelings of helplessness, hopelessness and incompetence, emotional lability, loss of libido, irritability, sleep problems, loss of appetite, weight problems and myalgia. Morgan, et al, found that approximately 80% of stale swimmers at a major university studied over a 10-year period were judged to have a diagnosable depressive disorder. Therefore, while exercise can help to alleviate depression, and inadequate exercise may be associated with depression, excessive exercise can lead to depression. Another risk is exercise addiction. Just as with other addictions, exercise addiction involves the same 3 classic characteristics - dependence, tolerance and withdrawal. Those who become dependent on the altered mood states associated with vigorous exercise may feel they must continually increase the exercise dose in order to achieve the desired effect. This results in developing an increasing amount of time exercising which can lead to compromising one's vocation, social, and family commitments. Morgan suggested that 3 signals indicate an addictive process: 1. The abuser devotes less attention to family and other close interpersonal relationships. 2. The abuser has less concern with external issues such as achievements at work since external rewards loose their importance as the exerciser begins to measure his or her self-worth by gains made in the training regimen. 3. The abuser starts to exhibit a pattern in which "feeling good" becomes more important than anything else. Endorphins may be involved in these changes in mood or affect but this has not been reliably proven.

KH: *What are physician responsibilities after an exercise prescription has been prescribed?*

TS: Educating the patient on the basis of exercise physiology can help to increase compliance. Also, physicians should be prepared to serve as role models for their patients by participating in an active life-style themselves, by encouraging exercise among their office staff, and by incorporating other related clinical preventive services in their practice. The physician should recognize the difference between an ideal exercise program and one with which the patient can comply. Benefits may be gained from even a minimal program. The key seems to be starting at low intensity, and gradually increasing the intensity consistent with the patient's progress. Of critical importance is designing a program that is likely to succeed, so the patient does not experience further failure and sense of loss. The physician must provide supervision, positive reinforcement, and feedback to keep the patient motivated, especially early in the process before the exercise becomes self-reinforcing. This should be done through frequent follow-up visits to maintain motivation as well as evaluate the therapy for desired effect. The severity of the depression can be followed with the Zung Depression Scale or other similar rating scales, providing feedback about improvement to both patient and physician.

KH: *Are there any type of antidepressant medications that exercise may interact with?*

TS: Many depressed patients being treated with exercise, especially those more severely depressed, will be taking antidepressants as well. Also, some patients who have already established an exercise program will subsequently develop depression. There are not good studies on the interactions between antidepressants and exercise. Common sense and an understanding of the mechanisms of action and side effects of the different classes of antidepressants suggests that the newer Selective Serotonin Reuptake Inhibitors (SSRIs) will rapidly become the agents of choice in this situation. The quinidine-like repolarization effects of tricyclics may be worrisome in athletes with increased heart rates, and their anticholinergic side effects will be annoying to many athletes. Monoamine oxidase inhibitors are difficult to manage due to dietary restrictions. The SSRIs including fluoxetin, sertaline and paroxetine, have rapidly become the most common first prescriptions by primary care physicians for depression and this preference need not be altered in patients who exercise.

KH: *Do you have any concluding comments?*

TS: Exercise has been shown not only to provide psychological gains to those with mild to moderate depression but to also serve as a preventive therapy for those not clinically depressed. The mechanisms by which these positive effects are achieved are unknown but the most likely mechanisms involve an improvement in the function of biogenic amine neurotransmitters. Exercise is most beneficial when combined with psychotherapy and/or medication. Physicians should prescribe exercise in an individualized manner, insuring that intensity and duration are not excessive. A continuum appears to exist in the relationship between exercise and mood state, with depressive symptomatology appearing at the extremes of too little and too much exercise, and optimal mood associated with a moderate exercise program. As with many aspects of a healthy life-style, moderation is the key to success. ◆

Depression, Caffeine and Sugar

Larry Christensen, Ph.D.
University of South Alabama
Department of Psychology
Life Sciences Building, Room B26
Mobile, AL 36688 U.S.A.
(334) 460-6321 / (334) 460-6320 (FAX)

"The Role of Caffeine and Sugar in Depression,"
The Nutrition Report, March 1991;9(3):17,24. #12081

Kirk Hamilton: Could you please share your educational background since college and your current position?

Larry Christensen: I received my Ph.D. from the University of Southern Mississippi. Then I went to Texas A&M and spent 25 years there. I worked my way up to a full professorship. This past year, I took a position as chair in the Department of Psychology at the University of South Alabama.

KH: When did you get interested in the roles of caffeine and sugar in depression?

LC: It was strictly a result of people "shoving books" about nutrition and behavioral disorders in my face. I read a couple of them. My ex-wife tried some of the things and they seemed to help her a little bit. There appeared to be something to what these people were saying. Many of them were saying things which I thought were all "smoke," but there appeared to be some "fire." I decided to make a commitment to take a look at it. That was back in 1980.

KH: In what area did you first focus on as far as nutrition goes?

LC: I focused on hypoglycemia because most of the books and writings at that time were talking about hypoglycemia. At that time, hypoglycemia was stated by some as the cause of the ills of the world. I didn't buy it, but that was the common denominator. I started looking at hypoglycemia and had about 23 people take oral glucose tolerance tests. Virtually none of them were shown to be hypoglycemic. However, when I put them on a diet I prepared, a few of them reported tremendous improvements. That is what kept me looking at the diet. I dropped the hypoglycemia immediately thereafter.

KH: What was your diet?

LC: It was a high protein, low carbohydrate diet, but I also eliminated caffeine. Then, over a period of years, I figured out what it was about the diet. Most people were talking about sucrose, which I focused on. Then, when I was doing my studies, I would give them the diet which would make them feel better, and then try and reintroduce the emotional distress by challenging them double-blind with sucrose or a placebo. In some of them, the distress would return and in some of them it wouldn't. There had to be something else about the diet. These people felt better, and some of them would feel worse by eating sucrose again. One of the subjects, after reintroducing the sucrose, didn't have any effect. I started interviewing her regarding her job. She worked at a restaurant where they constantly had coffee available. Other things seemed to point back to the caffeine. So I went and got a cup of coffee and had her drink it. Within an hour she started reporting that she was beginning to feel a little sad. I decided to look at caffeine in addition to sucrose. When I started looking at those two items, I found what would account for most of the people that were responsive to the diet. I continued to look at these two items and found that for sensitive people I can turn depression off and on.

KH: I would like to back track to the hypoglycemia concept. Granted, you didn't see blood sugar swings associated with the mood changes, but could it have been that to maintain the blood sugar there are other hormones "behind the scenes" that fluctuate sharply such as epinephrine or norepinephrine?

LC: Yes. There may be something to that. However, I saw no indication in the literature of that or of the other popular hypothesis that it is an alteration in insulin release. There is no consistent data that I can find to support that hypothesis. I also must say that I really haven't looked at it.

KH: You stated that when the study subjects consumed the caffeine they got depressed again?

LC: Yes, it would make them depressed. I wish I knew what in the caffeine made them depressed.

KH: Would it happen within minutes or would it take hours?

LC: Sometimes the effect of caffeine would take several days, and for some people it would be an immediate effect. Mostly, with caffeine, it would take 1 to 3 days for this effect to start showing up. With sucrose it could be within a matter of hours or it could take a couple of weeks.

KH: Now, is there not a connection between a high carbohydrate load and insulin release with increased tryptophan uptake?

LC: Yes, absolutely.

KH: Is there not, then, in some way a connection between carbohydrate consumption and serotonin release?

LC: This is a hypothesis by the Wurtmans at MIT which states as you eat carbohydrates, the carbohydrates stimulate insulin release. The insulin release then causes the peripheral cells to take up amino acids, and those amino acids are utilized by the peripheral cells. The one that is spared somewhat, though, is tryptophan because it binds to albumin. This increases the ratio of tryptophan to the other large neutral amino acids, meaning that more tryptophan crosses the blood brain barrier. Tryptophan is the precursor to serotonin. The Wurtmans have some data in rats showing nicely that if you give them a straight carbohydrate load, you get an increase in central serotonin. In humans, there is data indicating that you get only a little increase in the plasma amino acid ratio, but you can't test for brain serotonin levels. It is not enough to have much of an effect on central serotonin in humans.

KH: Clinically you observe, in many people, somnolence after a large meal, especially a carbohydrate-rich meal. Is there any explanation for sleepiness after the meal?

LC: There is some data on that in normal subjects, but it is not consistent across a lot of studies. I even did a study where I didn't get the sleepiness effect. So yes, it can occur, but it seems to occur in normal individuals when it does. Secondly, when it occurs it seems to be a very, very weak effect. It is not a strong robust effect by any means. That is my synthesis of that literature.

KH: You say caffeine has a depressive effect sometimes up to several days after ingestion and you're not sure why. When you talk about sugar, you are only talking about sucrose, correct?

LC: In the studies that I have done, I have not restricted natural sugars that are found in fruits, just added sugar.

KH: And what have you found with that?

LC: I found that sucrose can contribute to the fatigue and depression that some people experience.

KH: And is there any explanation?

LC: Explanation (laugh!)? I wish I had one. I don't know. I think it somehow has to be tied in with glucose. It's my speculation, I have no data whatsoever to back this up. My speculation is that somehow it is the sudden and massive release of glucose into the system. Now, does it have anything to do with the utilization of glucose because of a reduction in insulin receptor sites? That is a possibility. One of the things that you note is that as you consume a lot of glucose/sucrose and your blood sugar levels go up, the number of insulin receptor sites goes down. It is the body's way of regulating the utilization of things like glucose. Does that have any bearing on it? I don't know.

KH: Complex carbohydrates do not have the same effect, correct?

LC: They don't have the same effect.

KH: And what is your optimal antidepressive diet?

LC: It depends upon the sensitivity of the person. Some people are very sensitive to the sucrose and have to stay off it. Other people are very sensitive to the caffeine, and they have to stay off of it. The ones that are sensitive to the sucrose are probably not sensitive to the caffeine and vice versa. It is a matter of identifying the individual's sensitivity.

KH: How long do you have people stay off those two products? A week or two?

LC: I go two weeks. What I found is that if they do not benefit after two weeks, they're probably not going to benefit from it.

KH: Just from caffeine and sucrose? Would that include honey or maple syrup for example, and other added sugars?

LC: Probably so. One of the things that I find is that people who are sensitive to the added sugar can tolerate a little fructose, which is sugar also. I am focusing predominantly on sucrose, not fructose. Fructose is metabolized a little bit differently. It has to be converted to glucose in the liver so it is not going to create that immediate glucose infusion. Again, is that the reason? I don't know, but they can tolerate a little fructose. ◆

Diabetes Mellitus and Vitamin B6

Chandra Mohan, Ph.D
Calbiochem
19394 Pacific Center Court
San Diego, CA 92121 U.S.A.
(619) 450-5544 / (619) 453-3552 / (800) 776-0999 (FAX)

"Vitamin B6 Metabolism and Diabetes",
Biochemical and Metabolic Biology, 1994;52:10-17. #20478

Kirk Hamilton: *Please share your educational and professional background starting from college.*

Chandra Mohan: I received my Ph.D. in 1976 in biochemistry and physiology. Then I came to USC and worked as a post-doctoral fellow for 5 years. I was an assistant professor of pharmacology and nutrition for the next 10 years. Then I got a position in industry at Calbiochem. Right now, I am the supervisor and technical writer for the technical services department at Calbiochem.

KH: *Where did you get interested in the topic of vitamin B6 and diabetes?*

CM: Actually for the past 15 years or so I was mostly interested in diabetes. Diabetes is not just a simple matter of blood sugar going up and everything should be fine if you control the sugar. It is a very complicated disease and as the disease progresses, you get more and more complications. My basic interest was in the mechanism of insulin action and the metabolic effects of insulin. Dr. Rogers had done a lot of work on vitamin B6 metabolism and diabetes and on several occasions he visited our lab to work as a visiting scientist. We were collaborating on several projects. This was one of the projects we got interested in. I was interested in metabolism in general. Vitamin B6 in its active form, pyridoxal phosphate, controls and regulates the intermediate metabolism of insulin in several ways. That stimulated our interest in that particular project.

KH: *What are the specific ways that vitamin B6 is involved in either insulin's action or the enhancement or release of sugar?*

CM: Diabetes is a condition where the blood glucose level is high and the vitamin B6 level is low in the body. This is like a cause and effect relationship. If you have a low B6 level, then the insulin response is reduced and the circulating levels of insulin are lower. That leads to further increases in the blood glucose level. Also, if you have a major deficiency of vitamin B6 (not just skipping a day or two of B6 intake), storage of glycogen in the liver is impaired. This may lead to a hypoglycemic condition.

KH: *Are diabetics prone to vitamin B6 deficiency and can you define what deficiency means to you?*

CM: Deficiency is not a short-term deficiency - for example if you do not take the RDA amount of B6 will you be deficient? The answer is no. If you are below the minimum daily allowance (MDA) deficiency can set in over time. In prolonged uncontrolled diabetes with hyperglycemia people are more prone to B6 deficiency and this may eventually lead to complications.

KH: *So does the hyperglycemia cause you to either utilize more or spill more vitamin B6?*

CM: It causes one to spill more. Vitamin B6 is a water soluble vitamin. In diabetes, there is polyuria which leads to increased excretion of water soluble vitamins.

KH: *So, here is where I am a little confused. You say that vitamin B6 deficiency does not happen overnight?*

CM: That is correct.

KH: *Are you saying then that there is a whole lot of diabetics who are just not consuming any vitamin B6 at all?*

CM: No. What I am saying is you don't have to take supplements if your diet is well balanced and rich in sources of vitamin B6. But those who are deficient or their diet is very marginal - are more prone to develop deficiencies.

KH: *Are diabetics, in general, people who have marginal diets?*

CM: It depends on their income level and food selection. The poor who do not have enough variety of foods can get vitamin B6 deficient.

KH: *What is the best way to assess vitamin B6 status, either by an enzyme test or by blood levels?*

CM: Pyridoxal phosphate is the single best test to assess vitamin B6. The best assessment is made when both pyridoxal phosphate and pyridoxal are assessed rather than just the pyridoxal phosphate alone.

KH: *What impact does vitamin B6 deficiency have on diabetes when you're looking at - lets say - a national health survey. I mean, are there a lot of people, in your opinion, with vitamin B6 deficiency?*

CM: When a person is aware of his or her diabetes, I would suggest they eat a well-balanced meal as recommended by the American Diabetes Association's Guidelines - 20% of protein, about 50% to 55% carbohydrate, 30% fat, fiber from food sources and a variety of foods.

KH: *Do you happen to know the food sources that are rich in B6?*

CM: You can find B6 in meat products, poultry, a variety of grains, milk, green leafy vegetables - all of them provide enough B6.

KH: *Are there any studies that you know of where vitamin B6 is given and actually sugar or insulin requirements go down?*

CM: There have been some studies - only experimental - but not in clinical practice.

KH: *What if you just recommended to a diabetic patient to take a supplement as a precautionary measure - what dosage would you recommend they take in their multivitamin pill?*

CM: The RDA for vitamin B6 is about 2 mg per day. There is no need to go really too high because we really don't store any water soluble vitamins.

KH: *Is vitamin B6 deficiency a problem or not in diabetics in general?*

CM: Not widespread. Clearly, in this country, most of the population eats a well-balanced meal or at least healthy meals. This could be a problem in a small group of people.

KH: *Do you know if there are any other nutrients that work with vitamin B6 in diabetes mellitus?*

CM: Diabetics have low magnesium levels and I don't have the exact citation, but there are quite a few reports within the last 2 years which have shown a basic magnesium deficiency in diabetes.

KH: *Any other comments on vitamin B6 and diabetes that you would like to share?*

CM: In diabetes, there is a reduced level of B6 and an increased amount of blood glucose and uncontrolled hyperglycemia. Over a prolonged period of time, this can lead to damage of the eyes, kidneys, nervous and vascular systems, in general. But also reduced levels of vitamin B6 can cause problems with amino acid transport and maybe protein synthesis. Inefficient protein synthesis is one of the major problems in diabetics because you need insulin for protein synthesis. Low insulin levels and low amino acid transport would result in reduced protein synthesis. Also the diabetics have a high rate of protein breakdown because of the need of amino acids for the gluconeogenesis process. The tissues cannot detect the high glucose levels and uncontrolled glucose production occurs via gluconeogenesis - that is a breakdown of proteins and amino acids to produce glucose. We need at least 120 gm of glucose for the brain per day. If you have to estimate the amount of glucose needed (120 gms) and the amount of protein needed to produce 120 grams of glucose it comes close to about 200 gm of protein. The process is not all that efficient. Some amino acids are oxidized. Some of them are ketogenic amino acids and do not produce glucose.

KH: *Should diabetics take a vitamin B6 supplement in your opinion?*

CM: It is not something that everybody should get alarmed about. If you don't take vitamin B6 are you going to get diabetic complications? If you are a diabetic, consult your doctor, check your diet and if you have a marginal diet then supplements of vitamin B6 are appropriate. They are probably going to help. But the general population is not to be alarmed.

KH: *Do you have any upper limits for vitamin B6 as far as supplement intake in a diabetic?*

CM: It is a virtually nontoxic material. If somebody is taking 2 or 3 times the RDA level it is not going to cause complications. ◆

Diabetic Neuropathy, Vegetarian Diets and Vitamin B12

Milton Crane, M.D.
Weimar Institute
P.O. Box 486
Weimar, CA 95736 U.S.A
(800) 525-9192 / (916) 637-4111 / (916) 637-4443 (FAX)

"Regression of Diabetic Neuropathy With Total Vegetarian (Vegan) Diet," Journal of Nutritional Medicine, 1994;4:431-439, #21878. "Vitamin B12 Studies in Total Vegetarians," Journal of Nutrition, 1994;4:419-430. #21877

Kirk Hamilton: Can you please share with me your educational background and current position?

Milton Crane: I graduated from medical school in 1945. After an internship and residency in internal medicine I was involved in research and teaching in various fields of internal medicine, but particularly in cardiovascular subjects, hypertension, endocrinology and electrolyte metabolism at Loma Linda University for 30 years. Among other training, I spent 1 year at the University of Michigan on a fellowship in endocrinology. I am certified in internal medicine and I am a fellow of the American College of Physicians. In 1978, while at Loma Linda University, I began to apply a total vegetarian diet in the care of my patients. It became evident that a total vegetarian diet was a very effective modality to correct hypertension and alleviate Type-II diabetes. In 1982, I retired from Loma Linda University and became a professor emeritus of medicine and took the position of medical director and director of medical research at the Weimar Institute.

KH: How long have you been medically using the vegetarian diet?

MC: I advocated the lacto-ovo-vegetarian diet in my practice from 1946 until 1980. At that time I realized a more restrictive diet excluding milk, meat, eggs, refined foods such as sugars, refined cereals and free fats was very effective in alleviating hypertension, diabetes and coronary artery disease. I have been using this type of vegetarian diet ever since 1980.

KH: Could you define what vegetarian means?

MC: To me a vegetarian diet is simple. It does not include any food or drink that comes from animal, fish, meat, milk or eggs. We also go 1 step further and encourage our clients to eat whole plant foods. We believe that refined foods such as free fats (oil, shortening or margarine, etc.); free carbohydrates (sugar, syrups, starch, etc.); or refined cereals (white rice, white flour, etc.); or refined legumes (soy protein isolate or soy protein concentrate products) are detrimental to good health and should be kept out of the recipes and off the menus.

KH: What kind of dramatic health improvements have you seen?

MC: Eighty percent of the patients with systemic, distal diabetic neuropathy have relief of pain in 4 to 17 days, and the pain stays away so long as the patient adheres to the diet. One-third of the patient with Type-II diabetes and 10% of those with Type-I diabetes can be maintained with a fasting glucose level below 120 mg% with this program. Eighty percent of male hypertensives and 50% of

female hypertensives which are those with blood pressures of 160/90 or above can be maintained with normal blood pressure below 140/90 without medication after 1 month on the program. Clinical and laboratory regression of atherosclerosis occurs in 50% to 75% of patients with coronary artery disease or peripheral arterial artery disease. The addition of niacin, chromium and other modalities increase this percentage even more. Relief of pain of chronic degenerative arthritis of the knees, hips, and back, and remission of degenerative disk disease of the back occurs in more than half of the patients with this program. However, a "little oil" or a "little sugar" added to the diet prevents beneficial results. We see remission of rheumatoid arthritis, polymyalgia rheumatica and lupus erythematosus with prolonged adherence to the diet. With proper elimination of certain foods in addition to milk products and eggs, most people with allergies have marked relief of their allergic manifestations such as asthma, hay fever, and postnasal drip. In a few patients that we have seen with multiple sclerosis, the combination of the basic diet with elimination of certain food antigens and toxins, results in nearly complete remission of symptoms.

KH: What is the cause of diabetic neuropathy?

MC: The precise cause of diabetic neuropathy is not known. It is most likely related to a combination of factors related to faulty diet and inadequate exercise. It is thought that the changes within the nerve bundles as a result of faulty metabolism of carbohydrates results in tissue swelling and the production of pain. The 2 pathologic changes appear to be ischemia to the nerve, and/or an accumulation of certain metabolites of sugar within the cells that result from inadequate insulin.

KH: Can you describe the results of your study with neuropathy?

MC: Twenty-one sequential patients with definite, distal, diabetic, polyneuropathy were enrolled in a group session lasting 25 days in our live-in health education (NEWSTART) program. They were fed a low fat (10% to 15% of the calories), high complex carbohydrate, low simple sugar, high fiber, no cholesterol, total vegetarian (vegan-type) diet with meticulous exclusion of refined foods. They entered into the conditioning exercise program as they were able. The other main modalities consist of simply hydrotherapy treatments, adequate water, sunshine and rest. Alcohol, tobacco and coffee were excluded. They were counseled in stress management. Instructions included twice weekly physician visits, regular health lectures and cooking school demonstrations. It was observed that painful, tingling, burning, and/or stabbing pains disappeared in 17 out of 21 of the patients in 4 to 17 days. Two of the remaining 4 experienced partial relief. The numbness persisted, but sensation to touch was symptomatically improved. Follow-up for 12 to 48 months revealed that 16 of the 17 who could be followed continued to have the same relief of pain or were even further improved at home. All but 2 of them had remained on the diet quite well. During the 25-day period of the program, the 21 patients lost 0 to 21 pounds in weight, with an average of 10.8 pounds. Four of the 21 maintained fasting glucose levels below 120 mg% without insulin or oral agents. Their triglyceride and cholesterol levels had declined in 2 weeks by 25% and 13%, respectively.

KH: *How long did it take to start seeing results with this diet?*

MC: The earliest results were evident on the fourth day (average 10 days). The time of relief did not correlate with the duration (average 12 years) of the known diabetes, with the duration (average 4.1 years) of the painful symptoms of neuropathy, or with the age or sex of the patients.

KH: *What dietary or biochemical properties in the vegetarian diet allow for these effects?*

MC: The low-fat vegetarian foods furnish a good balance of omega-6 to omega-3 polyunsaturated fatty acids. Estimates are that about 1/2 of the fats in the diet were polyunsaturated fats. The use of whole plant food furnishes a more appropriate balance of naturally occurring vitamins, minerals and trace elements. The use of complex carbohydrates with restriction of simple carbohydrates, particularly refined carbohydrates, enabled the weakened pancreas to cope better with the load of carbohydrate at meal times. The plant foods furnish protein in amounts of approximately 40 to 50 gm per day. The avoidance of a high-protein diet contributed to the protection of the smaller blood vessel damage.

KH: *What role do essential fatty acids play in these changes? Is a no-fat diet the way to go? Or are omega-3 and monounsaturated fatty acids acceptable?*

MC: My opinion is that essential fatty acids play a very important role in these beneficial changes. We try to avoid fat in the "free" state. When it is taken in the form in which nature presents them, which is enclosed in cells in vegetable foods, grains, nuts or fruits, fats are wholesome and nutritious elements of foods. In general, low-fat plant foods contain approximately 1/2 or more of their fats as polyunsaturated fats and about 10% to 50% of these are omega-3 fatty acids. An example is soybeans (which are not low in fat). The green soybean contains approximately 50% of its total fats as omega-3 fatty acids and 9% as omega-6 fatty acids. Dry soybeans are the reverse - 50% occur as omega-6 fatty acids and 8% as omega-3 fatty acids. Sprouting the soybean results in a reversal of the fatty acid composition back to that of a green soybean. Less than 5% of total fat in meat, milk and eggs occurs as polyunsaturated fatty acids. Also, a key fatty acid is arachidonic acid, which is the precursor of the series-2 prostaglandins and thromboxanes. These series-2 prostaglandins and thromboxanes are vasoconstrictive. The omega-3 and omega-6 fatty acids, as they occur in the plant cell structures, provide linoleic, alpha-linolenic and gamma-linolenic fatty acids, which can be converted to other series of prostaglandins and thromboxane chemicals that have a vaso-relaxing effect.

What we advocate is a no "free-fat" diet and not a "no-fat" diet. Free fats induce an increased formation of endogenous cholesterol whether they are saturated or polyunsaturated. When fats are presented in the free state, they are subject to oxidation. Polyunsaturated fatty acids can be damaged by oxygen more than monounsaturated fatty acids because they have more double bonds.

Also, a high-fat diet of monounsaturated or polyunsaturated fatty acids can result in an excess of natural LDL within the wall of the artery. This excess LDL can become "modified-LDL" by oxidation, which is an initiating event in atherosclerosis.

KH: *Were vegetarians at risk for B12 deficiency in your study?*

MC: Our studies and others suggest that 60% of those who have been total vegetarians for a year or more have a value for vitamin B12 below 200 pg/ml. The remaining 40% have average B12 levels of 288 pg/ml, and an average mean corpuscular volume significantly larger than that of other individuals on total vegetarian diets who are eating foods which contain added vitamin B12. Our data suggests a safer level of vitamin B12 should be at least 350 pg/ml, which has been suggested by other studies following elevated serum methylmalonic acid levels. The only source of vitamin B12 is from friendly or harmful bacteria. It is not made by animals or plants. All total vegetarians (vegans) are at risk of becoming B12 deficient unless they allow germs to grow in their food or on their eating utensils on a routine basis. It may take a year or up to 10 years for evidence of vitamin B12 to become symptomatically evident. Vitamin B12 and folic acid, along with vitamin B6, are necessary for the change of homocysteine back to methionine. Thus, a deficiency of B6, B12 or folic acid can result in the accumulation of homocysteine and an increased risk to atherosclerosis. Omnivores are at risk from a lack of folic acid, while total vegetarians are at risk from a lack of B12. Either group can have elevated homocysteine levels, which increases atherosclerotic risk.

KH: *How do you get the best absorption from a vitamin B12 tablet? What is the best form?*

MC: Data indicates that vitamin B12 must be promptly combined in an acid pH in the stomach to a polypeptide in the food called an "R-binder." Next, in the duodenum, the intrinsic factor (made in the stomach) is exchanged for the R-binder hooked onto the vitamin B12. Thus, the R-binder and then intrinsic factor identify and guide the B12 so that it can be absorbed in the last portion of the small intestine. This appears to be necessary in order to select only the active B-12 from a maze of other corrinoids in the food which are not effective in the human, and which may be potentially competitive at the cell level. For this reason, a "hard" pill of vitamin B12 may not be readily absorbed. We recommend that the B12 pills be crushed or chewed unless it readily dissolves in the mouth. The small "B-12 DOT" marketed by Twin-Labs readily dissolves in the mouth.

KH: *Should vegetarians take vitamin B12 routinely? If not, what foods are good sources of B12?*

MC: My answer is a hearty, yes! There are no foods that are consistently eaten that contain vitamin B12 naturally or which have been supplemented by vitamin B12. The increasing concern over cleanliness in our society to avoid infectious diseases decrease the number of bacteria that would produce vitamin B12 in the foods. I believe strongly that it does not make sense to wait for vitamin B12 levels to go down before taking a supplement. When vitamin B12 is taken in adequate amounts orally, the intrinsic factor is the initial limiting factor and the intestinal wall is the second limiting factor. If excess B12 is absorbed, the excess is readily disposed of in the urine. Three sea vegetables, Arame, Wakame, and Kombu may be sources of vitamin B12 for the strict vegetarian, but studies indicate that this needs to be confirmed. The laboratory assay method must be one that avoids giving false high value for vitamin B12. Some assay methods include corrinoids in the assay which are not effective in the human body. ◆

Diarrhea, Malabsorption and Fruit Juice

J. Hans Hoekstra, M.D.
Department of Pediatrics
Bosch Medicentrum
P.O. Box 90123
5200 ME's-Hertogenbosch
The Netherlands
31 73 6862304 / 31 73 6862948 (FAX) / 31 73 6862443 (FAX)

"Fruit Juice Malabsorption: Not Only Fructose," Acta Pediatrica, 1995;84:1241-1244. #23680

Kirk Hamilton: *Can you please share with me your educational background and current position?*

Hans Hoekstra: I received my medical training at the University of Groningen in the Netherlands. After four years of training in pediatrics, I subsequently trained in pediatric gastroenterology and nutrition, at the Hospital of Ste. Justine, Montreal, Canada. I am presently head of the Department of Pediatrics, Bosch Medicentrum and am responsible for pediatric education and cooperation with the Amsterdam Medical Center.

KH: *What got you interested in evaluating fruit juice as something that could be potentially malabsorbed?*

HH: Of all the causes of chronic diarrhea in children, toddler's diarrhea, or chronic nonspecific diarrhea (CNSD), is the most frequent one in affluent societies. The child with CNSD does not normally suffer from its ailment, but the diarrhea may cause the parents to be extremely worried and frustrated. We have previously focused on the dietary aspects of this condition, in particular the high intake of fruit juices.

KH: *What did you find in your study regarding fruit juice malabsorption?*

HH: Malabsorption of free fructose, when ingested in excess over glucose, is considered a significant factor in apple juice induced diarrhea. Incomplete carbohydrate absorption was also found following the ingestion of grape juice and bilberry juice, although the last 2 contain equivalent concentrations of fructose and glucose. Surprisingly, the malabsorption was found to persist after a yeast treatment of the juices, which leads to major reductions in the fructose and glucose contents.

KH: *What are the components besides fructose that might be malabsorbed from the fruit juices?*

HH: We think that oligo-and polysaccharides in the juices are of importance. These substances are formed from the cell wall components of the plant, not only in the pressing step, but also by enzymes that are used in order to increase juice production.

KH: *What does increased breath hydrogen have to do with clinical symptoms if any?*

HH: This is a good question. Colonic fermentation of incompletely absorbed carbohydrate is mainly a beneficial process that gives nutrients for the organism as well as for the colonic

bacterial flora. Slowly fermented fibers are unlikely to produce clinical symptoms. On the contrary, the smaller carbohydrates are fermented very rapidly. Depending on the available quantities this may lead to symptoms secondary to rapid gas formation and increased colonic water overload.

KH: *How prevalent is fruit juice as a cause of nonspecific diarrhea in children?*

HH: The problem is mainly confined to the toddler age. The majority of children I see with this problem consume 400 mL or more of fruit juice, in particular apple juice. In another study (Archives of Diseases in Children, 1995;73:126-130), we showed the industrial processing of this juice is a very important factor as unprocessed ('cloudy') apple juice gave no symptoms, in contrast to clear juice.

KH: *What recommendations do you have for the introduction of fruit juice in young infants? Should they be diluted? Should they be avoid altogether?*

HH: Fruit juices are extremely popular with parents as well as children. There seems to be no reason to prohibit the consumption of moderate amounts. Parents should be aware of the importance of energy-dense foods at the toddler age and full-fat milk products should be advocated. Displacement of calories by the consumption of energy-rich drinks should be avoided. A diet that takes into account the importance of the 'four Fs' (fat, fiber, fluid intake and fruit juice) seems to be the best preventive measure with regards to CNSD. ◆

Ear Infections, Serous Otitis Media and Food Allergy

Talal Nsouli, M.D.
Watergate and Burke Allergy and Asthma Centers
Watergate Office Building
2600 Virginia Avenue N.W. #216
Washington, D.C. 20037, U.S.A.
(202) 342-1984 / (202) 342-1855 (FAX)

"Role of Food Allergy in Serous Otitis Media",
Annals of Allergy, September 1994;73:215-219. #20995

Kirk Hamilton: *What is your educational background?*

Talal Nsouli: I did my high school studies in Paris, France and then I moved to Brussels, Belgium, where I went to medical school. There, I received my M.D. with *Magna Cum Laude* distinction. I came to the United States and completed all my allergy and immunology training at Georgetown University School of Medicine in Washington, D.C. Later, I became part of the faculty as clinical assistant professor of pediatrics, allergy and clinical immunology at Georgetown University School of Medicine. I am currently a clinical research associate at the International Center For Interdisciplinary Studies of Immunology in Washington, D.C. I am also directing two centers, the Watergate Allergy and Asthma Center in Washington, D.C.; and I am the director of the Burke Allergy and Asthma Center in Burke, Virginia.

KH: *What is the medical necessity of the current situation with serous otitis media as far as the economics and the prevalence of the condition?*

TN: The main problem with this type of condition, in terms of the financial aspect, is that costs about $4 billion a year in surgical medical treatment. Due to the fact that there is a loss of productivity due to hearing loss from otitis media with effusion and otitis media, additional expenses include not only the medical and surgical treatments, but also specialized speech and developmental programs, costing another $30 billion a year in the United States.

KH: *Are you lumping together serous otitis media with frank otitis media?*

TN: Both could be connected and one might lead to the other. First of all, what happens initially is that the child gets an allergic reaction. This allergic reaction in the nose produces nasal congestion and then the congestion in the eustachian tube that goes from the nasopharyngeal area, which is the back of the nose to the middle ear. This tube, which connects these 2 structures, becomes extremely swollen and congested. When it becomes congested, negative pressure develops in the middle ear. This results in fluid accumulation in the middle ear. This fluid, in 50% of the cases, contains bacteria. This bacteria might proliferate and will give an acute or frank acute otitis media with pain, hearing loss, fever and discomfort in the child. Then the child requires antibiotics. Prior to this acute otitis media, is this fluid "behind the ear" that we define as otitis media with effusion, serous otitis media or, in England, it is called "glue ear." The reason for this name is because if you look at the fluid in the ear, it is so thick it looks like glue. Sometimes it is very difficult to get rid of this fluid because of its thickness. If we get a patient with an acute otitis media, a severe infection of the ear with pain, fever and discomfort, treatment with antibiotics, if the infection does not clear completely, might lead to otitis media with effusion - chronic fluid in the ear.

KH: *Can allergy, in the upper respiratory tree, increase the susceptibility to a viral or bacterial ear infection?*

TN: Yes, we published a study in the Annals of Allergy in January 1994 on allergy promoting sinusitis.

KH: *When did you get interested in food allergy as being a possible cause of ear infections and serous otitis media?*

TN: The reason why I became interested in otitis media in relationship to allergies in general is when I discovered there are more than 10 million children suffering from otitis media with effusion every year. I discovered that the No. 1 reason for visits to the pediatrician and ear, nose and throat specialists in the United States is for otitis media with effusion. We also discovered the No. 1 reason for pediatric surgery in the United States is ear tube placement for otitis media with effusion.

KH: *Why isn't it more prevalent that ENT specialists or allergist talk about food in relation to serous otitis media and then consequently acute otitis media - don't they tend to downplay the food connection?*

TN: That is correct. The dramatic numbers reported in our paper could be due to the fact that we are an allergy clinic. Maybe there is a certain bias for our belief and the number of patients that come to see us are self selected to be more allergic, even though we did not intend to select them for this reason. We only selected them for recurrent and repeated otitis media with effusion. The fact that we are an allergy center means we probably get more allergy people than we would see if we were not allergists. This means possibly an adjustment to the conclusion number -- 50% instead of 78% might be a real nonbiased noncontrolled type of scenario that you might be dealing with.

KH: *What is your definition of food allergy? You did skin prick testing, specific IgE tests and then you did food challenges.*

TN: I define food allergies as within the primary IgE mediated reactivity in order to be able to get objective data. The number appears to be high due to the fact that possibly some of these patients came to the clinic because they thought they had some parents that had some allergies or food allergies and they thought that the allergy clinic would help them at that time.

KH: *How many of these people had repeated antibiotic approaches?*

TN: The patients we screen are not regular patients with otitis media with effusion, these are refractory patients. They are recurrent, recalcitrant, challenging cases that no one has been able to help in any way and they landed in our clinic. This is a very important point of the paper.

KH: *Food elimination seems so simple that it still staggers my mind that ENT specialists and allergists aren't doing it routinely.*

TN: You're absolutely right. People we sent this paper to for publication initially sent it back to us because the reviewers checked their data base and there was no such connection found in the medical literature between food elimination and serous otitis media. So we called them and let them know that because of the specific reason, it is something new, it is a novel idea and this is why we came out and did this study. When they understood this, they looked at this paper.

KH: *Do you think that IgG$_4$ plays any role at all?*

TN: To tell you the truth, in 1989, we did a study at Georgetown University in our center directed by Dr. Joseph Bellanti and we came out with a paper on IgG$_4$ that could be related to food allergy. Then other papers came out saying there is no real correlation and some critical things due to the methodology of the different labs, which are not always reliable. Right now, my consensus on IgG$_4$ is it is something to look into. It could be a very valid criteria, but the book is not yet closed on this subject.

KH: *Let's say you're talking to a group of family practitioners or pediatricians, would you feel comfortable saying to this group that in individuals with recurrent infections it would be very reasonable to put them on an elimination diet for a month. Or what would you say would be a reasonable time frame?*

TN: We have to be careful. I don't feel very comfortable to blindly attack the patient and start to ask the patient not to eat this food and to avoid that food. Sometimes it could be the wrong food we are avoiding and these children very early in age need good nutrition. We don't want to have any hyponutrition due to some diets without a certain basis. With that said, we know that about 38% of the patients that we studied were allergic to cow's milk. I think cow's milk could be the one and the only one that should be tried blindly. You could probably take the child off milk for 6 to 8 weeks. Not only cow's milk but cheese, yogurt, ice cream and really the major dairy products, to see if the child will improve. If the child is going off cow's milk, he should be put on soy milk. If the child is even younger and the child is allergic to soy, put him on a nonallergic formula such as Nutramigen. The child, at that time, might receive a calcium substitute under the name of Neo-Calglucon at a dose of 2 teaspoons at bed time, depending on the age of the child.

KH: *Do you think even breast feeding mothers' - diet can have an effect?*

TN: Yes. A 1992 study by Dr. Asher showed that any food that the mother eats will go into the breast milk and to the baby with subsequent sensitization of the infant. Therefore, studies that were done by Asher, et al, showed that to prevent sensitization in the child, the mother should avoid, during the lactating period eggs, peanuts and eliminate completely cow's milk. Cutting down on cow's milk during lactation in a mother who is lactating will not any effect in any way her breast milk. I did some investigation and I spoke with Dr. Margit Hammosh, a specialist in breast feeding at Georgetown. She completely agreed with me that there is no relationship between the quality of milk coming in the breast and drinking milk in the mother. So to answer your question, yes, the mother during lactation should be careful.

KH: *Many times the treatment is to place the child on 3 to 6 months of antibiotics for serous otitis media. Aside from whether it helps the condition or not, do you see a harmful effect of the prevalent use of antibiotics in altering gut flora with subsequent changes in immune function or is that even something that you think about.*

TN: I don't have any concern, really, in using the antibiotics for serous otitis media for a short period of time. We like to use half the normal dose of the antibiotic and that should be used for about 2 to 4 weeks. This will be good enough to sterilize or clear the bacteria that could be in the fluid of the child with serous otitis media with effusion. The benefit of doing that, in my personal opinion outweighs the disadvantage.

KH: *My concern is that the chronic antibiotic therapy alters gut flora which can have an effect in and of itself and also it may allow for an imbalanced overgrowth of yeast in the intestinal tract. This may aggravate intestinal permeability allowing for more antigens to be absorbed with subsequent triggering of allergies and immune dysfunction that continue the problem of the serous otitis media with effusion or frank otitis media. Intestinal permeability may be altered by not only yeast but parasites and/or medications.*

TN: Unfortunately, we did not really look at this carefully. There are no double blind crossover studies dealing with the yeast question to prove it. It could be that there is some truth to it. I am not denying it nor confirming it. This is a topic that is open to debate! ◆

Enteritis (Radiation) and Lactobacillus

Eeva Salminen, M.D.
University Hospital, Turku, Finland
Department of Radiotherapy and Oncology
Turku 20520 Turku, Finland
358 21 2611611 / 358 21 2612809 (FAX)

"Adverse Effects of Pelvic Radiotherapy",
Fifth International Meeting on Progress on Radio-Oncology, May 1995;10-14:501-504. #23402

Kirk Hamilton: *Could you please share with me your educational background and current position?*

Eeva Salminen: I received my Doctor of Medicine degree in 1979 and specialization in radiotherapy and oncology in 1989. I completed my Doctor of Science in Medicine in 1991 and became a docent in clinical oncology and radiotherapy in 1993 at the University of Turku, Finland. Currently, I am also a specialist (consultant radiation oncologist) at the University Hospital in Turku, Finland.

KH: *When did you become interested in the role of Lactobacillus acidophilus in radiation enteritis?*

ES: My interest dates back to 1984 when I started working on radiotherapy side effects and potential ways of avoiding them.

KH: *Can you please share with me what happens to the gut during radiation enteritis and the subsequent symptoms?*

ES: Radiation therapy in the lower pelvic area causes irritation of the gut mucosa leading to intestinal inflammation, mucosal damage, and a permeability disorder. At the same time, disturbances of the normal intestinal microflora and gut motility take place. As a result, acute and long-term diarrhea and other side-effects such as intestinal fibrous strictures and fistulas may follow.

KH: *What were the results of your study with regards to supplementation of Lactobacillus in radiation enteritis?*

ES: Patients receiving *Lactobacillus* supplementation had significantly less diarrhea than the controls. More flatulence was observed after *Lactobacillus*. During follow-up less serious late effects were observed in the *Lactobacillus* group (see also ref. Salminen, E., Elomaa, I., Minkkinen, J., Vapatalo, H., Salminen, S., Preservation of intestinal integrity during radiotherapy using live **Lactobacillus acidophilus** cultures (Clinical Radiology, 1988;39:435-437).

KH: *Could you please go into detail about the doses of Lactobacillus acidophilus and the vehicle in which it was given?*

ES: We wanted to test a product that could potentially be a normal dietary adjuvant. Thus, the *Lactobacillus* was given in the form of yogurt with small amounts of lactulose, as the slowly absorbable carbohydrate substrate for the *Lactobacillus* in the intestine. The dose was 10^{10} colony forming units of viable *Lactobacillus acidophilus* (NFCO) 1748 daily. The patients consumed 150 ml of yogurt starting 5 days prior to radiotherapy, daily during the therapy and for 10 days after completing radiotherapy.

KH: *What are the mechanisms on how this Lactobacillus helps prevent radiation induced enteritis?*

ES: The main effect is the stabilizing effect on intestinal microflora and the prevention of excessive pathogen growth. Recent clinical studies have also indicated that some *Lactobacillus* strains may enhance the intestinal immune response and thus help in the prevention and the recovery of the damage in the gut.

KH: *Do you see other areas where Lactobacillus acidophilus could be used to either reinoculate intestinal flora or help prevent some of the adverse changes that occur during chronic illness in the gut mucosa?*

ES: Yes. There are now some carefully conducted double-blind and placebo-controlled studies indicating that specific *Lactobacillus* strains are useful in the treatment of acute infant diarrhea (bacterial and rotavirus). Adherent strains that are able to colonize the human intestinal tract may also be useful in antibiotic associated diarrhea and some forms of inflammatory bowel disease.

KH: *In your study did both groups eliminate whole grain cereals, raw vegetables, beans, peas, milk products with high lactose content and high fat foods?*

ES: Yes, they did. And the dietary counseling to do this was given to both groups.

KH: *Did this treatment extend the survival of cancer patients and if so what is the theoretic mechanism?*

ES: There was no statistically significant effects on survival. However, in the control patients there were deaths due to late adverse effects which are possibly related to the severity of acute effects. No such deaths were observed in the treatment group. This indicates that there is a need to further study *Lactobacillus* supplementation during pelvic radiotherapy. ◆

Exercise Performance and Caffeine

Terry E. Graham, Ph.D.
University of Guelph
School of Human Biology
Guelph, Ontario, N1G 2W1, Canada
(519) 824-4140 Ext. 3319 / (519) 567-1942 (FAX)

"Caffeine and Exercise: Metabolism and Performance",
Journal of Applied Physiology, 1994;19(1):111-138. #20801

Kirk Hamilton: Would you share with us your educational background and what your present position is?

Terry Graham: I did my graduate work at Queen's University in Kingston, Ontario in physiology and then did a post-doc in Copenhagen with Bengt Saltin. I then came to the University of Guelph where I've been in the Department of Human Biology ever since. I am currently a professor in this department where I am basically an exercise or metabolic physiologist.

KH: What does the word ergogenic means?

TG: Ergogenic means "work producing." Ergo is work and genic being producing. Technically, you could have either a negative or positive ergogenic aid - that is it either impedes your ability to work or promotes it. But by common acceptance, if an exercise physiologist says that this is an ergogenic aid, they mean it is a positive one that allows you to work longer or harder.

KH: How did you get interested in caffeine's effect on exercise?

TG: Well, I have always been an exercise physiologist - a muscle physiologist. But, actually, it was a bit of a serendipitous route that got me involved in caffeine. One of the areas of research I was working in was that of cold stress. In the 1980s, a number of investigators, some of them associated with the military, were very interested in trying to develop a cold pill that would stimulate metabolism and keep people or troops warm in a cold environment. They were using caffeine-like substances, which were prescription drugs. From these experiments, I began to wonder if caffeine could do the same sort of thing. Ken McNaughton, a graduate student of mine, and myself did a series of studies with people in a cold environment giving them caffeine either at rest or during exercise and found that caffeine did all the sorts of things in the body in terms of stimulating adrenaline or epinephrine, mobilizing fatty acids - all the things that should promote the muscle's ability to generate lots of heat but the muscle didn't do anything. So the caffeine was working as we thought it would in the body except for the fact that when the muscle was provided with these extra stimuli, it didn't respond. So at least, in our hands, caffeine was not a useful tool to be used in the cold stress. When I started to interpret our data, I believed there was so little work done with cold stress that I had to turn to the exercise literature. It became very apparent very quickly that there was tremendous controversy. Earlier work had suggested that caffeine definitely was an ergogenic aid, but subsequent work failed to corroborate this. As a result, a colleague of mine, Lawrence Spriet, and I decided to do a study which would prove once and for all that caffeine did not work in exercise. We have been studying it ever since.

KH: Because it did work?

TG: It worked tremendously!

KH: So why was there a discrepancy?

TG: I think there were several reasons for this. One of them was that a number of the studies had only indirectly measured some of the parameters, that is they had used qualitative measures for metabolism or performance and, as a result, their results were unclear. Secondly, a number of the studies were poorly controlled. They didn't control for whether the subjects were athletes, for dietary habits or whether or not they were caffeine users. Some of them compared decaffeinated coffee to coffee. Others compared a placebo to caffeine.

KH: Can you tell us the mechanism of action of caffeine with regards to being an ergogenic agent?

TG: The explanation you see quite often, both in the lay literature and also in published research, is that caffeine is stimulating the sympathetic nervous system to mobilize fatty acids which are then available to muscle. The muscle uses fatty acids preferentially, which spares the very limited muscle glycogen. Muscle glycogen is a useful fuel for endurance. We have been able to demonstrate this to some extent. However, we and others have demonstrated that even when that doesn't happen, caffeine still has a powerful effect on the muscle. So we believe, very strongly, that the first mentioned mechanism is working, but it is not the critical one. Caffeine is having a direct action on a variety of tissues of the body. A graduate student of mine, Mary Van Soeren, has recently done studies where she has been able to demonstrate that caffeine has a direct action on fat cells. Caffeine also has a direct action on the central nervous system and probably a direct action on other tissues of the body. What we're probably seeing is an integration of a number of these actions, which combine to cause the skeletal muscle in the human to be able to work harder or longer.

KH: What is the effective dose to get a response?

TG: We did a study in which we tried to establish the lowest effective dose and found that even the lowest dose that we used, which was 3 mg of caffeine per kilo of body weight was effective. Keep in mind that we only use pure caffeine, not coffee.

KH: Which is this amount, in terms of cups of coffee, for the individual?

TG: That's the question that is always asked and for some reason, we're not quite sure how to answer that properly. But it would be about 1 to 1½ mugs of *strong coffee*.

KH: *That's the 3 mg of caffeine.*

TG: Yes. So that would be about 9 gallons of American coffee.

KH: *(Laugh!) - Well we (U.S.) have espresso shops now so we're getting there!*

TG: What I don't know is what occurs below the 3 mg level because we didn't go below that. We were sure that 3 mg would not be effective, however, it was quite effective. The bottom-line message is that even what you might call a moderate or a small dose is effective, at least in the way in which we administer it. I say that because we are giving capsules of caffeine, meaning even if that is equivalent to the mug or mug-and-a-half of coffee, you're taking in 1 swallow. So it is a real shot. You should also keep in mind that coffee has hundreds of chemicals and these may influence the actions of caffeine.

KH: *What type of exercise does caffeine benefit?*

TG: Originally, people thought it benefitted only long-term endurance exercise - exercise lasting 30 minutes to an hour or even 2 hours. It has quite a powerful impact at that level. But more recently, in the last 3 or 4 years, investigators in England and France as well as Michelle Jackman in our laboratory, have studied activities that are lasting 2 or 3 minutes or even less and are showing that caffeine can still have a positive effect.

KH: *Do you take the caffeine 2 minutes before the event, an hour before the event or during the event?*

TG: That has not been carefully studied. Traditionally, in our laboratory, we take the caffeine an hour before the exercise - the basis being that 1 hour after you ingest it, you are starting to experience the maximal caffeine concentrations in the blood. People have not actually done a systematic study where they vary when it is ingested or, as you suggest, even taking it during the exercise. I suspect that any of these would probably be effective.

KH: *I was just envisioning a marathoner instead of getting his little cup of water or Gatorade-type drink while running, he gets a little iced coffee.*

TG: That is not beyond the realm of possibility. Although it is speculation, I have heard narrators for the Boston marathon, among others, comment that it wouldn't be unthinkable that some of these concoctions that the top runners are taking are laced with caffeine. It is perfectly legal if you can use the terms of the International Olympic Committee (IOC).

KH: *I have read where the average urinary output, even when people ingest reasonable amounts of coffee, is usually always below their limit.*

TG: That's right. In our early experiments, we started off with very high doses up to 9 mg per kg of body weight, which is then 3 times this minimal effective dose that we now have. Even with this dose, we were hard pressed to get anybody over what could be termed the legal limit (12 ug/ml of caffeine in urine). I would now say anybody that gets caught with a caffeine level higher than that deserves to be penalized because they have overdosed themselves.

KH: *Can you overdose on caffeine? How does this affect your performance?*

TG: I can give you personal testimony to that effect having been a subject in some of the experiments where we used very high doses. I could never have believed it until I experienced it myself that it can really be mood altering. It obviously hits the central nervous system pretty hard. Anyone that has had a cup of coffee knows that. Usually, that simply increases your level of arousal, it increases your central nervous system activity level. But, in fact, when you get into the higher doses you have tremendous difficulty in attending to any mental tasks - something as simple as looking at the clock on the wall and trying to figure out what time it is.

KH: *Now we're getting back to the cup of coffee analogy. Do we have to consume 10 cups of coffee in 15 minutes to get this effect or...?*

TG: No. Normally we have our subjects go without any coffee, tea and caffeinated beverages for 2 days. In this particular experiment, we had them not withdraw at all and then gave them 9 mg/kg of caffeine which is equivalent to about 4 to 5 strong mugs of coffee. In those circumstances, there was tremendous mental confusion. Some of the subjects would use the term "a real buzz" and you had a great deal of muscle tremor. You could watch the person almost bouncing from the other side of the room and when they tried to exercise, and I was certainly one of them, my endurance was compromised considerably simply because I was so mentally confused I just couldn't handle it. My legs still felt fine but I had to quit. Afterwards there was a tremendous feeling of depression as you came down from that high. The other thing - you almost felt drunk. You know - giddy and "well I know I am being a little silly but who cares" sort of thing. It was really an unexpected experience.

KH: *You took it in tablet form obviously.*

TG: This was in tablets, yes.

KH: *Socializing and consuming caffeine beverages is getting to be quite a popular activity in atleast my area in Sacramento, California for late teens and adults in their early 20s. In your article you mention an estimate that maybe up to 800,000 Canadian kids possibly, if the percentages were correct, were dosing themselves with caffeine to enhance performance. I wonder if you can comment on that.*

TG: The Canadian Center For Drug-Free Sport did a survey of 16,000 Canadian youths aged 11 to 18 and came up with a rather surprising finding that approximately 1/4 of them had, in the last year, used caffeine for the purpose of increasing their exercise performance. That caffeine could have been in pill form or from a dietary source.

KH: *Your ending comment is that it could be a gateway drug.*

TG: That's right. That may seem a little dramatic, but I don't think it is. For example, if you have a 14-year-old competing in high school track-and-field event, he might be already saying, "I don't think I can win unless I go and have my cappuccino or my espresso." Then he finds out that didn't work quite as well as he'd had hoped, so he may have 2 next time. Then that doesn't quite work as well as he had hoped, so he goes to a drug store and, for a couple of dollars, buys these wake-up pills. Wake-up pills are pure caffeine and they are available to anybody. Once you start to make these conscious decisions in terms of ethics you're still at this point probably working within the legalities of the sports system. Now I am not saying that every child or every teenager that experiments with caffeine is going to move on to amphetamines and everything else. But once you start to say I don't think I can win unless I take this and then you find that didn't work so you move to the next step - I think there is certainly the strong possibility that some of these people will then move on to other drugs which are also established as ergogenic aids. I find this a great concern.

KH: I think you're right as well.

TG: We work with a physician who is interested in sports medicine. I remarked to him when I saw these results that I was sure they were just taking a coke or a cup of coffee. He said don't fool yourself. He grew up as an extremely good hockey player and was playing junior A hockey when he was a teenager which is a very high level of hockey in Canada and he said that he can distinctly remember on road trips, when the guys were tired, the coach coming in and going around the room and giving everyone 1 white tablet and saying swallow it. No body asked what it was and they just swallowed it. He said it was pure caffeine. That was back in the early 70s. So I would have to think when you get into serious track and field, bike riding, sprinting and some of these other things people are doing more than just having a cappuccino before they compete.

KH: It seems you either have to ban caffeine totally or have no limit?

TG: Well that's my attitude. Because when you have what is called a controlled drug such as caffeine where you can have a certain amount but not too much - looking at the concentration in the urine is not a good reflection of how much people took in an exercise situation. Because, you can imagine that if you're a marathon runner and I'm a 100 meter sprinter and we both take the same amount of caffeine and after our event we give a urine sample that you have had 2 or 3 hours to clear that drug into your urine and I being the sprinter have had perhaps 20 minutes. And you're dehydrated so the rate of production of urine is very different than mine and there is all sorts of factors that come into it.

KH: Did you find a tolerance to the caffeine?

TG: That's a tricky question. What we do find is those subjects that we get who are "caffeine naive," those who almost never ever have any caffeine in their diet - they are very sensitive to caffeine and they will respond very well to a small dose as you would expect. If we overdosed some people like we did as previously mentioned who did not withdraw from caffeine or whether they withdrew from caffeine for 2 or 4 days, followed by habituation, caffeine removal and then the consumption of different levels - we found the whole body level of performance and endurance was not effected by the withdrawal and that users and nonusers behaved the same way. But what we could see were subtle changes in terms of the concentrations of epinephrine and rate of caffeine excretion were some adaptations but it didn't manifest itself in terms of the overall performance of the individual. ◆

Fertility and Vitamin C

Martin Luck, Ph.D.
University of Nottingham
Department of Animal Physiology
& Environmental Science
Sutton Bonington Campus
Loughborough LE12 5RD, United Kingdom
44 1159 516309 / 44 1159 516302 (FAX)
email: SBZML @ SZN1 NOTT.AC.UK

"Ascorbic Acid and Fertility," Biology of Reproduction, 1995;52:262-266. #21764

Kirk Hamilton: *Could you please share with us your educational background and current position?*

Martin Luck: I graduated in 1974 in animal physiology at the University of Nottingham and subsequently gained MSc (steroid endocrinology) and Ph.D. (animal physiology) at the University of Leeds. After post-doctoral work at the University of Southampton, I moved to Hamburg. I worked in the newly-founded Institute of Hormone and Fertility Research. I established a research group there and spent 7 years studying cultured ovarian granulosa cells. I returned to the University of Nottingham in 1990, where I currently hold a lectureship in Animal Physiology.

KH: *Why did you get interested in the role of vitamin C and fertility?*

ML: A graduate student of mine found that follicular theca tissue enhanced oxytocin and progesterone secretion by cultured bovine granulosa cells. Paracrine control of the ovary was becoming trendy in 1986, so this was an exciting result. As a control, she tested other tissues and observed a strong stimulation with slices of adrenal medulla. We postulated that this was due to the catecholamines, so she next tested the effect of adrenaline on her cultures. I had read somewhere that catecholamines degrade quickly in culture but that this could be prevented using ascorbic acid as an antioxidant. So in went ascorbic acid, at an arbitrary concentration, along with the adrenaline. Fortunately, we followed the rules of the game and did a separate control for the ascorbate. We discovered a profound stimulation. We subsequently showed that granulosa cells responded in a dose- and time-dependent manner to ascorbate and that ascorbate synergizes with other stimulators (adrenaline, acetylcholine, etc.). About this time, Tony Flint showed that the amount of ascorbate in the sheep corpus luteum was far in excess of that needed for luteal oxytocin synthesis. Another line of inquiry converged. We showed that the inhibitors of collagen synthesis inhibited the spontaneous luteinization of cultured granulosa cells and that they interacted strongly with ascorbate. Collagen synthesis (proline hydroxylation) is well known to be ascorbate-dependent. So here was a second possible role for ascorbate in the ovary. With further research we discovered a 4:1 concentration ratio between the fluid and plasma concentrations of vitamin C, and both concentrations correlated very strongly with follicular volume.

KH: *Are low levels of vitamin C more of a problem in the reproduction process of males or females?*

ML: We are not really sure about the effect in either sex. Most evidence is anecdotal or circumstantial and greatly in need of further investigation. Some of the male data seems quite convincing and I am sure, with modern sperm analysis techniques, it would be easy to show some *in vitro* effects. A clear effect of scorbusis on male fertility *in vivo* is evidently more difficult to show, but needs to be attempted. In the female, apart from some intriguing early studies on guinea-pigs, adequate experimental work just has not been done. There is some good evidence that implantation and growth of the conceptus needs adequate vitamin C, presumably because of the intense tissue remodeling involved. Generally speaking, our knowledge of biochemical actions of ascorbate has far outstripped experimental work on its role in the reproductive system.

KH: *How are sperm affected by low vitamin C levels?*

ML: Vitamin C deficiency has been associated with low sperm counts, reduced motility, higher incidence of abnormal sperm and agglutination. Early studies reported an increase in cattle fertility following ascorbic acid administration.

KH: *How is vitamin C involved in ovarian function?*

ML: The ovary accumulates ascorbic acid, especially in the corpus luteum and certain parts of the follicle. There is a cyclical change in uptake, with an abrupt increase in retention at ovulation which can be detected in peripheral concentrations. There are several suggested functions: (a) facilitation of steroidogenesis, especially hydroxylation steps; (b) facilitation of local catecholamine and peptide hormone synthesis; (c) synergism with neurotransmitters regulating ovarian function; and (d) facilitation of collagen biosynthesis in the ovarian extracellular matrix during the tissue remodeling and growth which accompanies the ovulatory cycle. In my opinion, the collagen effect is likely to be quantitatively the most important. For example, consider that the follicle wall has a basement membrane made of collagen type IV which has to expand rapidly during follicular growth. This occurs with no increase in tension, so it must involve rapid tissue synthesis. Also consider that the early corpus luteum, which contains abundant collagen I and IV, is arguably the most rapidly growing non-pathological tissue in the adult body. Can these be limited by ascorbate availability? An early study in scorbutic guinea-pigs reported lesions characteristic of a breakdown in follicle wall structure.

KH: *How do vitamin C's antioxidant capabilities relate to its possible benefit in reproduction?*

ML: Protection against damage by free radicals is postulated as the mechanism of its beneficial effects on sperm and fertilization.

KH: *Can vitamin C supplementation enhance traditional ovulation induction techniques?*

ML: There has been no systematic study of this. One study reported an enhanced response to clomiphene treatment. Dietary supplementation during normal conception and pregnancy has been recommended, but actual evidence of the beneficial effects is hard to find.

KH: *Could vitamin C supplementation prevent birth defects?*

ML: Again, a single study supports this contention, but data is lacking. One of the sperm studies speculates that protecting sperm DNA from free-radical damage may reduce the incidence of fetal defects.

KH: *Are there any studies showing vitamin C supplementation improving the frequency of conception?*

ML: Not to my knowledge.

KH: *How important is vitamin C for healthy fertilization?*

ML: This is not known.

KH: *Would you like to see vitamin C supplementation trials, and if so, at what dosage and during what time period?*

ML: Not quite yet. I am, of course, very excited by the possibility that the follicular response to stimulation is ascorbate-limited. But I have to say that more, carefully controlled physiological studies are needed before clinical trials would be justified. The danger is that such trials would be working in the dark, mechanistically speaking, and would just add to the speculative literature. Many other studies on the medical benefits of vitamin C showed that its effects are confounded by lifestyle (diet, smoking, general health, other medications, drug induced, age, etc.). Furthermore, there has been a well-publicized trend in some quarters to promote the prophylactic value of massive oral doses of vitamin C. I have no idea whether these are of reproductive significance. In my opinion, clinical trials would need to start from a physiologically more rational basis. We need to be very sure about the particular physiological end point which we expect to be affected before attempting to look for benefits in relation to fertility and conception. We need to know, for example, whether couples seeking fertility treatment show any evidence of low ascorbate levels, whether sperm quality or the follicular response to IVF stimulation correlates with vitamin intake and what mechanisms of any such effects really are. On the other hand, if I was reading this as a patient at an infertility clinic, I would be substantially increasing my fruit intake!

KH: *What is the role of vitamin C in protecting the genetic material in the sperm or ovum?*

ML: If genetic material is susceptible to free-radical damage, vitamin C is a likely protectant.

KH: *Are there any other micronutrients that may be important in reproduction?*

ML: Many, without doubt. The interesting thing about ascorbic acid is that a person's inability to synthesize such a ubiquitously important co-factor is down to a single, well defined genetic defect which prevents gluconolactone oxidase production in the liver. Humankind has lived with this defect for millennia, but flourished as a species nonetheless, presumably by dietary compensation. Only in the second half of this century have we managed to induce fertility in couples with reproductive problems. In doing so, we must be maintaining problems in the population which are heritable and which would otherwise die out. That is not a criticism of reproductive medicine, nor meant to be in any way offensive to infertile couples. What it does mean is that we now have the chance to find out whether a tendency to low ascorbate, through whatever cause, is one such problem. At least if it is, it should be relatively easy to remedy. ◆

Food Advertisement and Children's Television

Krista Kotz, RD, MPH
Primary Care Program Manager
IDHW, Health Resources Section, 4th Floor
P.O. Box 83720
Boise, Idaho 83720-0036 U.S.A.
(208) 334-0669 / (208) 334-6581 (FAX)

"Food Advertisements During Children's Saturday Morning Television Programming: Are They Consistent With Dietary Recommendations?" <u>Journal of the American Dietetic Association,</u> April 14, 1994;94:1296-1300. #21597

Kirk Hamilton: *Can you please share with me your educational background and current position?*

Krista Kotz: I am a registered dietitian and hold a Masters of Public Health Nutrition. I am currently a doctoral candidate in public health nutrition with a minor in epidemiology. My current position is primary care program manager at the Idaho Department of Health and Welfare.

KH: *Why did you decide to look at food advertising on children's Saturday morning television?*

KK: The average child in the United States views more than 25 hours of television per week. This amounts to as much as 3 hours per week of food advertisements, the goal of which is to persuade the child to desire a particular food product. Therefore, we thought it would be useful to perform a current assessment of the types of food advertised and categorize the foods using food groups described in dietary recommendations.

KH: *What did you find in your study?*

KK: The most striking finding, though not terribly surprising, was that out of the 564 food advertisements viewed, absolutely none were for fruits or vegetables. Using the USDA's Food Guide Pyramid food groups, we found 43.6% of the food advertisements were for foods classified in the "fats, oils and sweets" food group, and 37.5% were for foods in the "bread, cereal, rice and pasta group (23% of these were for high-sugar breakfast cereals). About 11% of the advertisements were for fast-food restaurants. The remainder were for foods in the "milk, cheese and yogurt" or the "meat, poultry, fish, dry beans, eggs and nuts" food groups, or were advertisements for frozen combination meals.

KH: *Were there any "harmful" effects found in this study with regards to the health of children from a dietary prospective?*

KK: The purpose of this study did not include assessing the effects of advertisements. The *potentially* harmful effects would arise from the very unbalanced picture of diet portrayed to the American children through television advertisements. The diet depicted in Saturday morning television programming is the antithesis of what is recommended for healthful eating for children.

KH: *How powerful do you think television is in affecting children's food choices in a positive or negative direction?*

KK: Television is such an ubiquitous medium that it is difficult to distinguish its behavioral effects from confounding variables. Thus, it has not been possible to describe completely the connection between food advertisements viewed and dietary patterns. However, some studies have described a correlation between types of foods seen advertised and requests for these foods during grocery shopping. Another useful study showed that children who were shown advertisements for candy, embedded in cartoons, chose candy as a snack over fruit more often than children who were shown advertisements for fruit. As a parent of young children, I can't help but be influenced by the many requests I seem to get for a particular food item as it is being advertised to my children. I have also noted that it often works in a positive way as well; carrots seem to be a very attractive item while watching Bugs Bunny.

KH: *What message should be taken by parents from your study?*

KK: I think it is valuable for parents to understand what is being shown to children if they choose to allow their children to watch television. Parents' food choices have a large influence on the dietary patterns of children. By having lots of fresh fruits and vegetables on hand, and by enjoying them in front of the children, parents can do much to balance their child's view of what a healthful diet should include.

KH: *Do you think that this type of advertisement affects the health of these children in the future and the health of our country?*

KK: As were discussed, it is difficult to assess the direct effects of advertisements on food patterns. However, if children were to choose a diet similar to what is advertised on television, they would be more likely to suffer from one of the major chronic diseases in this country including coronary heart disease, stroke, atherosclerosis, diabetes and some forms of cancer.

KH: *Do you think this is a governmental issue or should parents just turn off the television?*

KK: The American Academy of Pediatrics contends that because young children are cognitively incapable of making informed decisions about products advertised, and advertisements aimed directly at them is inherently unfair. Therefore, the position of the Academy is that all television food advertisements aimed at children should be eliminated. This is probably unlikely given the political etiology of our country and the role that television plays in our culture. However, laws do exist to regulate the amount of total advertising per hour. In addition, one reasonable approach may be to put a small tax on the advertising budgets of food manufacturers and earmark these funds to develop public service announcements advertising fruits and/or vegetables, or other types of food absent from the current advertising menu. In the meantime, since parents are the main gatekeepers, less viewing may be the prudent choice for dietary as well as other reasons. ◆

Food Advertisements on Children's Television

Howard L. Taras, M.D.
University of California at San Diego
Community Pediatrics Division
9500 Gilman Drive, Dept. 0927
La Jolla, CA 92093-0927 U.S.A.
(619) 685-4825 / (619) 685-4828 (FAX)

"Advertised Foods on Children's Television",
Archives of Pediatric and Adolescent Medicine, June, 1995;149:649-652. #22563

Kirk Hamilton: *Can you please share with me your educational background and current position?*

Howard Taras: I am a practicing pediatrician with a special interest in "community pediatrics" and school health. I am currently an associate professor of pediatrics at the University of California, San Diego. I do research and develop programs that pertain to how children's health at home, in school and in day-care settings can be improved. Naturally, a sizeable portion of this work is in the field of prevention of disease

KH: *What inspired you to start looking at food advertising on children's television?*

HT: I recognized from previous research of my own and of others how much television children watch and that it may be associated with obesity. Televised advertisements for food are logically one of the reasons for this. However, there is no recent data describing what foods are being advertised on television during children's viewing hours.

KH: *How many commercials per hour do children watch on television?*

HT: On the average 21.3 commercials per hour.

KH: *How much of these commercials pertain to food?*

HT: Of these commercials 47.6% were food related.

KH: *What percentage of foods shown in the commercials were high in fat, sugar and/or salt?*

HT: Of the foods present in commercials, 91% were high in fat, salt or sugar. Only 9% do not have these "less than nutritious" characteristics.

KH: *Approximately how much television does the average child watch per day?*

HT: This varies from age group to age group. However, in my studies which looked at children between the ages of 3 and 5 years the hours watched were on the average of 21.4 hours per week.

KH: *What portion of children's food advertising is unhealthy?*

HT: Cereals were number "1". Candies and other snack foods were the second largest category of advertised foods. About 15% of food-related commercials were for restaurants - mostly fast-food.

KH: *What portion of children's food advertising is unhealthy?*

HT: None of the advertised foods should ever be restricted completely from any child's diet. Any food in a small enough portion to other foods is allowable. However, as 91% of the advertised foods were either high in salt, in sugar or in fat, all may be considered to be unhealthy if consumed in quantities or proportions that were that large.

KH: *What percentage of the cereals advertised were high in sugar?*

HT: Of the cereals advertised, 85% were high in sugar.

KH: *What percentage of the advertised beverages were sweetened?*

HT: Of the advertised beverages, a minority were carbonated (5.6%), 83.2% were beverages that were sweetened.

KH: *What percentage of sweets and candies were high in sugar? High in fat?*

HT: The majority of these foods were high and sugar and fat.

KH: *What would you tell parents about educating their children regarding food advertising on television and how do you teach children to discriminate between good and bad information?*

HT: Parents can educate their children about how to be more skeptical about what they see on television. Young children have the fewest "cognitive defenses" about what they see advertised on television. Many children younger than 8 years of age are unable to understand the selling intent of advertisements. Children as old as 10 years have the cognitive ability to see advertisements for what they are but don't necessarily use this ability. They must be prompted to do so. Therefore, for the older children, teaching "media literacy" (i.e.: the ability to question the desirability and validity of what is advertised) is a worthwhile effort. For all children young and old, parents should discuss their view of the nutritional content of foods. Also, parents can refuse to purchase those foods children request after seeing them advertised on television. Limiting the number of hours children watch television also limits the number of advertisements they are exposed to. Public television often has excellent children's programming without commercials.

KH: *Do you think that children's food advertising plays a significant role in the health of our children?*

HT: I think it plays some role and it is likely significant. Parents' dietary and exercise habits are also excellent indicators for what type of life-style children will have. Children model what their parents do (even though that may not seem to be the case for a few years around the time of adolescence).

KH: From your research on this subject what diet recommendations can you make for young children? Or said differently, what would you tell parents and children about why eating the foods advertised might not be good for the children?

HT: I think the famous "food pyramid" recently adopted by federal agencies to teach about nutrition is a very worthwhile tool for parents to use for their own diets and that of their children. After the age of 2, it is necessary to guard against excessive fat intake. The advertisements parents see on television, on buses, on bulletin boards, etc., are definitely factors that effect all of our diets. Parents should teach, preach and practice many of the "food pyramid" philosophies. Furthermore, they should lobby their school district and their school boards that govern those school districts. Schools are excellent places for children to learn what parents have difficulty teaching. Nutrition education should be pushed to become a mandatory course and there should be educational standards for students on this and other health education topics. *By standards,* I mean that at the end of certain stages of a child's public education, students should be expected to know a set of basic health material. This is done for reading and math and other subjects. Its absence for health is a major reason for the poor contribution that health education given during the school year has towards healthy life-styles thereafter. ◆

Food Intolerance, Intestinal Permeability and Gut Fermentation Syndrome

Keith Eaton, M.D.
Templars
Terrace Road South
Binfield
Berkshire RG12 5DU, United Kingdom
01344 53919 / 01344 306280 (FAX)

"Gut Permeability Measured by Polyethylene Glycol Absorption in Abnormal Gut Fermentation as Compared With Food Intolerance,"
Journal of the Royal Society of Medicine, 1995;88:63-66. #22682

Kirk Hamilton: Could you please share your educational background and current position?

Keith Eaton: I am a consultant allergist working at the Princess Margaret Hospital, Windsor, United Kingdom, and I am currently an assistant secretary of the British Society of Allergy and Environmental Medicine with the British Society of Nutritional Medicine. I have previously been an allergy consultant to Merck Pharmaceuticals and Tate and Lyle Research at the University of Reading. I have been involved in research of allergy, nutrition, toxicology and biochemistry since 1971. Of recent years, problems of abnormal gut fermentation have been my chief research interest.

KH: When did you get interested in assessing gut fermentation and the possibility of this causing adverse clinical symptoms?

KE: I first became interested in abnormal gut fermentation in the early 1980s when it was clear that it was a subject with a long anecdotal history and an extensive clinical background, but very poorly substantiated by any reproducible laboratory based studies or hard data.

KH: Could you please explain what abnormal gut fermentation syndrome is?

KE: Abnormal gut fermentation is a syndrome with a varying presentation. The majority of subjects have evidence of irritable bowel, catarrhal symptoms and mild cerebral dysfunction such as inability to concentrate, fatigue and "brain fog or fag." The individual patient may vary considerably, and other symptoms also may be involved. Currently, the digestive tract dysfunction appears to be the key area of research. We therefore prefer the term Dysfunctional Gut Syndrome (DGS).

KH: Can you explain how to assess gut fermentation?

KE: Currently, the best test is measurement of ethanol production on a fasting sugar challenge. The limit of normal is 22 micromoles per liter. The test becomes negative after treatment. However, some patients only show excess β-alanine excretion and there may be a significant cohort of patients who could be helped by appropriate management who do not show positives to either test.

KH: In your study you evaluated gut permeability in those who had food intolerance and those who had abnormal gut fermentation. Did they have different degrees of intestinal permeability or similar?

KE: We looked at 3 groups: normal subjects, patients with food intolerance, and those with dysfunctional gut syndrome. Both latter groups differed significantly from normal, but not from each other. Using polyethylene glycol (PEG), one cannot distinguish between the 2 groups.

KH: Do you believe there is evidence that increased intestinal permeability and the absorption of partially digested food particles can trigger immunologic reactions that may result in significant adverse symptoms?

KE: My first view is that there is anecdotal evidence that patients with these problems have increased gut permeability and now laboratory data that confirms this. Other work we are doing suggests a low level of stomach acid (known in allergy since the 1930s) and low levels of pancreatic enzymes. All these suggest an underfunctioning gut which will digest less efficiently and increase the probability of significant amounts of macromolecules in the bowel contents of the small intestine. Because of increased permeability the macromolecules are likely to be absorbed, and must by their nature, be immunologically active. If so, the relationship between DGS and food intolerance may well be a chicken and egg scenario, and the two may be related.

KH: Is it possible that in these conditions increased intestinal permeability can cause absorption of poorly digested food constituents that do not cause an immunologic reaction but a more metabolic reaction resulting in subsequent adverse symptoms?

KE: Yes.

KH: What is the clinical relevance of your work which shows that there is increased intestinal permeability in those who have abnormal gut fermentation and those who have food intolerance?

KE: There is an interdependence here. Some physicians treat the food intolerance first and some the DGS. I am not sure if it matters. Both approaches can obtain good results. However, in our study, ⅓ of patients with 1 diagnosis crossed over within 2 years and acquired the contradiagnosis. A sound clinical program is likely to address both factors, and give the best results.

KH: How quickly can gut permeability improve?

KE: This depends on the cause. Drugs like NSAIDS can produce very dramatic changes. However, the changes in intestinal permeability may be long term and take weeks or months to correct. I usually retest no more often than every 3 months in these patients.

KH: *I was under the assumption that "gut epithelium" turned over every 4-5 days. Three months for intestinal permeability to heal seems like a long time when the offending agents have been removed. Could you comment on this?*

KE: Your question assumes that "the offending agents" <u>have</u> been removed. Where is your evidence that we currently have enough knowledge to be able to do this? I suspect that at present our best endeavors may well be only addressing perhaps 10% of them. What we do thereby is to make a modest reduction in total load and as a result of nature being truly wonderful the result is that in spite of urban man's efforts in creating toxins many patients recovery processes are just enough to tip the balance in favor of healing. This would help to explain why the process is lengthy and why in some cases it is a failure. We can't yet be too smug about our achievements.

KH: *What nutrition and lifestyle factors can improve gut permeability?*

KE: A diet relatively low in fermentable, starchy and yeasty foods which tends to leave a diet high in unrefined starches and vegetables - we have to be careful about fruit. The diet may be higher in fats and protein than most nutritionists would advise for healthy individuals but is otherwise often better than the regime that they had before we started. Because of low nutritional status, we tend to add supplements of B vitamins and magnesium (the latter is probably suboptimal in terms of intake for most individuals). Because of the above, some patients also need to supplement with gamma-linolenic acid. Some workers use many more supplements. I find that one can often manage without, and the less one uses, the less burdensome it is for the patient.

KH: *What nutritional lifestyle factors can adversely affect gut permeability?*

KE: Consumption of refined sugars and a high intake of lectins may be the worst hazards.

KH: *Are there any other pathogens such as yeast, parasites or abnormal intestinal flora that could affect gut permeability?*

KE: Yes. However to my knowledge the work had not been done with most yeasts and parasites and we can only surmise that in view of the behavior of other gut pathogens the effects will be adverse. Certainly there is abundant evidence that bacterial gut pathogens increase permeability and I think there is evidence about some viruses. Certainly the latter, like parasites, have an adverse (disabling) effect on local gut immunity and this is likely to have a key effect in initiating dysfunctional gut syndrome and/or food intolerance. ◆

Headaches-Migraine and Magnesium Sulfate

Alexander Mauskop, M.D.
New York Headache Center
301 East 66th Street
New York, NY 10021 U.S.A.
(212) 794-3550 / (212) 650-9189 (FAX)

"Intravenous Magnesium Sulfate Relieves Migraine Attacks in Patients With Low Serum Ionized Magnesium Levels: A Pilot Study," Clinical Science, 1995;89:633-636. #23887

Kirk Hamilton: *Can you please share with me your educational background and current position?*

Alexander Mauskop: I am currently director of the New York Headache Center and director of the non-profit New York Headache Foundation. I am also an associate professor of clinical neurology in the State University of New York system.

KH: *When and why did you suspect that magnesium played a role in migraine attacks?*

AM: I was fortunate to meet Dr. Burton Altura, who was involved in magnesium research at the State University of New York. There have been many published reports of the possible role of magnesium in the development of migraine attacks. The previous studies have given inconclusive results. Dr. Altura has developed a very sensitive ion-selective electrode to measure serum ionized magnesium levels. Serum ionized magnesium levels appear to be a much more sensitive indicator of early magnesium deficiency than regular magnesium levels. Using this technique of measurement of ionized magnesium in the serum of patients with headaches, we established that up to 1/2 of patients with an acute migraine attack had low ionized magnesium levels.

KH: *Can you share with us about your study using intravenous magnesium sulfate in migraine headache sufferers?*

AM: Our follow-up study involved injecting patients, with an acute migraine attack, with magnesium sulfate. We used 1 gm of magnesium sulfate through a slow intravenous infusion. Approximately 50% of patients had low ionized magnesium levels, and of those 85% responded to infusions of magnesium sulfate. That is, their headache completely resolved within minutes of the infusion. On the other hand, patients who had normal ionized magnesium levels did not respond. Only 15% of those patients responded - that is their headache went away.

KH: *Were there any side effects to the intravenous magnesium therapy?*

AM: The only side effect of the infusion is a feeling of heat. One of the patients had a sensation of nausea and 2 patients felt light-headed when they sat up after the infusion.

KH: *Once again, Dr. Mauskop, what was the exact protocol for the magnesium therapy?*

AM: For the infusion, we used 1 gm of magnesium sulfate in a 10% solution administered over 5 minutes through an intravenous line. The patients remained in our clinic for 15 to 30 minutes after the infusion.

KH: *Would oral magnesium have a similar effect?*

AM: That is a logical question. Oral administration will not provide as quick a rise in magnesium levels as an intravenous infusion will. So the oral magnesium supplementation is not very good for an acute attack. But given prophylactically, oral supplements may relieve headaches in those people who are deficient. Unfortunately, most magnesium preparations on the market are very poorly absorbed through the stomach. That is why many patients take magnesium supplements without any obvious benefit. Some of these patients may not need magnesium (because as you remember, only about 50% of migraine suffers have low ionized magnesium levels). On the other hand, some people may have low levels of magnesium, but their oral supplement does not get absorbed. We often prefer a chelated form of magnesium that can be bought in health food stores and pharmacies.

KH: *Have you done any studies evaluating the use of oral magnesium prophylactically in migraine patients?*

AM: We do not have any clinical studies to prove that taking oral magnesium supplements prevents headaches. That is the next step. We do, though, have very solid evidence and good statistics on patients receiving intravenous infusions of magnesium sulfate. We also are working on trying to prevent not only headaches but also other symptoms of premenstrual syndrome (PMS) using magnesium supplements. That is another promising area that we are working on.

KH: *Does the intravenous magnesium therapy work on any other type of headache?*

AM: In patients who have tension headaches, the incidence of low ionized magnesium in those patients is only about 7% which suggests that migraine headaches may be a biologically different disorder than tension headaches.

KH: *How is magnesium theorized to work in preventing and treating migraine headaches?*

AM: A few words about the possible mechanism of action of magnesium. Magnesium regulates a very large number of various neurotransmitters and enzymes in the body including a very important one called NMDA. This receptor is intimately involved in pain transmission in the body. Magnesium ions sit inside this receptor and prevent calcium ions from entering the cell and causing the transmission of pain. So if you have a lot of magnesium in your cells it will be harder for the calcium to enter the cell. On the other hand, if your magnesium level is low an NMDA receptor may be easily opened for calcium flow. Magnesium also regulates the size of the blood vessels. If you deplete magnesium from the animal preparation the blood vessel in that preparation will go into spasm. If you add magnesium the blood vessel will relax. ◆

Hepatic Injury and Vitamin A

Y. Horsmans, M.D.
Universite Catholique De Louvain
University Clinics of St. Luc
Department of Internal Medicine
Avenue Hippocrate 10, B-1200
Bruxelles, Belgium
32 2 764 89 27 (FAX)

"Hepatic Injury and Vitamin A Ingestion",
American Journal of Medicine, April 1995;98:4224. #22235

Kirk Hamilton: Could you please share with me your educational background since college and your present position?

Y. Horsmans: I studied medicine at the Catholic University of Louvain, qualifying in 1985. I interned as a clinical assistant in Belgium and as a research fellow in INSERM U24, Clichy, France. In September of 1991, I joined the gastroenterology medical staff as a consultant in hepatology at St. Luc University Hospital (Catholic University of Louvain).

KH: How did you become concerned about the role of vitamin A in liver injury?

YH: During my training at St. Luc University Hospital, I met several patients with liver disease due to ingestion of large amounts of vitamin A, with some of these patients requiring liver transplantation.

KH: At what dosages have you seen vitamin A cause liver injury and over what time frame?

YH: Two kinds of liver disease may be observed after therapeutic vitamin A ingestion: cirrhosis and noncirrhotic portal hypertension. The mean total accumulative vitamin A intake is around 400×10^6 IU in cases of cirrhosis and 150×10^6 IU in cases of noncirrhotic portal hypertension. However, a wide variation can be observed. The lowest dose we observed which induced liver damage was 20×10^6 IU.

KH: Have the majority of these patients had irreversible liver dysfunction or reversible?

YH: The evolution of the majority of the patients with cirrhosis or noncirrhotic portal hypertension is characterized by deleterious evolution, even after vitamin A withdrawal. However, in some cases the evolution is more favorable and characterized by a normal expectation in life.

KH: What are the biochemical signs of liver injury that are characteristic of this condition?

YH: Biochemical signs include moderate elevation of serum transaminase levels and a slight anicteric cholestasis (elevation of serum γ-GT and alkaline phosphatase). An important elevation of serum immunoglobulin M is also observed. Biochemical signs of hepatocellular dysfunction are present in the cirrhotic stage.

KH: Did these individuals have prior injury to the liver or any type of dysfunction that may have made them more susceptible to vitamin A damage?

YH: No prior injury to the liver was present, and since most of the patients who take vitamin A are highly concerned by their health, it seems unlikely that another factor aside from vitamin A caused the damage seen in these patients.

KH: Can you give a safe dose range with regards to vitamin A intake in a healthy individual to avoid liver injury?

YH: The answer is very difficult because there is a wide interindividual variability. However, the total cumulative dose appears as a critical factor. A dose of more than 5,000 I.U./d is certainly not to be recommended.

KH: Are there any risk factors that you know of that may make individuals more susceptible to vitamin A damage to their liver?

YH: Until now there was no identifiable risk factor. However, it seems likely that an increased metabolism of vitamin A could favor the occurrence of liver damage. Thus, ethanol and drug inducers such as phenobarbital are not recommended for patients who consume great amounts of vitamin A. ◆

Hepatic Necrosis and Thioctic Acid

Burton M. Berkson, M.D., M.S., Ph.D.
P.O. Box 7538
Las Cruces, NM 88006 U.S.A.
(505) 678-2321

"Fungal Toxicology, Mushroom Poisoning, and Thioctic Acid",
New Mexico Supplement To The Western Journal of Medcine,
May 1995:162(5);2. #23950

Kirk Hamilton: *Can you please share with me your educational background and current position?*

Burton Berkson: I started my medical training in Chicago. My education took an unusual turn when I left medical school for a career in biology. I went on to receive a Ph.D. from the University of Illinois with a dissertation concerning fungal cytomorphology and cell biology. After that, I worked as a professor and researcher at Rutgers and the state universities of Illinois until I returned to medical school to earn an M.D. degree from the Autonomous Universities of Mexico. I spent my clinical medical school years in Cleveland and continued postgraduate training in internal medicine at Case Western Reserve Teaching Hospitals. I spent my second postgraduate residency year studying pathology. Because of my Ph.D. in mycology and my knowledge of unusual diseases, I had staff and consulting privileges at several hospitals. I also taught mycology and continued doing research in Ohio and was mycology research associate at the Cleveland Museum of Natural History. During that time, the FDA appointed me principal investigator and IND holder for thioctic acid due to my successful work in the treatment of acute hepatic necrosis. Following some work at the Max Plank Institute in Germany and publishing the results of some of my studies, a few American medical schools showed an interest in doing double-blind studies with thioctic acid. Dr. Fred Bartter of the National Institutes of Health, my mentor and research partner, believed that it would be unethical to withhold thioctic acid from a dying patient and the double-blind studies were never done. Without the studies, the American medical community lost interest in thioctic acid and our money for liver regeneration studies were lost as well. Today, I have small private corporation that contracts with the Department of Defense for medical services. I am also an adjunct professor at New Mexico State University and I am still a consultant on thioctic acid and mushroom poisoning with the Centers for Disease Control.

KH: *What is the basic physiology of thioctic acid and are there other names for thioctic acid?*

BB: Thioctic acid, also known as alpha-lipoic acid, is found to be active in various biochemical systems in mammals. Chemists and biologists have known of its involvement as a coenzyme in the tricarboxylic acid cycle for many years. As a coenzyme it is essential for and involved in, ATP production and cell efficiency. As an antioxidant, thioctic acid works alone and interacts with glutathione to protect the cell. I have found thioctic acid to be an antitoxin and research demonstrates that it has radioprotectant properties. Some European scientists have reported neuroregenerative effects with thioctic acid and I have personally observed liver regeneration using thioctic acid.

KH: *When did you become interested in thioctic acid and its role in clinical medicine?*

BB: I first used thioctic acid when I was a physician in training in Cleveland. I was asked to manage and take responsibility of the treatment of several patients suffering from severe hepatotoxic *Amanita* mushroom poisoning which resulted in acute hepatic necrosis. I was able to procure thioctic acid from Dr. Bartter at NIH and I treated the patients through IV administration.

Because mushroom toxins bind to the hepatocyte and destroy the RNA polymerase system within the first 12 hours after ingestion, I knew that thioctic acid must work on the cellular level rather than interfering with the *Amanita* toxin directly since no patients were treated prior to 19 hours post ingestion. Soon after receiving the IV thioctic acid, patients began to improve dramatically and all left the hospital after 2 weeks of treatment with normally functioning livers and without any signs of liver damage.

KH: *What is the role of thioctic acid in diabetic neuropathy?*

BB: In 1995, at the European Conference, several speakers described the reversal of diabetic neuropathies using thioctic acid. They concluded that this was probably due to the chemicals' hypoglycemic and antioxidant effects. In German studies, researchers showed that thioctic acid can actually regenerate nervous tissue and protect healthy neurons from the direct effect of high blood sugar.

KH: *What is the role of thioctic acid in liver failure or dysfunction?*

BB: As I mentioned earlier, I was involved with IV thioctic acid management of patients with acute hepatic necrosis. I have also had excellent results in the medical management of chronic cirrhosis, acute biliary cirrhosis and renal shutdown. The only adverse effect of high dose IV thioctic acid that was observed in these cases was hypoglycemia. Since all the patients were on glucose drips, hypoglycemia was easy to control.

KH: *Can you give a case report of how thioctic acid might be used in liver failure?*

BB: A young man arrived at a large medical center in Cleveland with acute and chronic liver disease. His SGPT was over 14,000 and he was a candidate for liver transplant. His physician called me for permission and consultation concerning the administration of IV thioctic acid. I sent the physician enough thioctic acid for 2 weeks and the patient recovered quickly and apparently regenerated a major portion of his liver with near normal hepatic function.

KH: *How would you compare thioctic acid with N-acetylcysteine as an agent used for hepatotoxic reactions?*

BB: N-acetylcysteine probably acts as donor molecule that indirectly increases glutathione levels. Thioctic acid would probably work as well or better than N-acetylcysteine since it increases glutathione levels in a more elegant manner for acetaminophen poisoning.

KH: *You have been doing work for many years with thioctic acid and it seems to be quite remarkable. Why did your colleagues not recognize this agent as a very important therapy to be used in these acute conditions?*

BB: There are probably several factors that have prevented widespread acceptance of thioctic acid therapy. Because thioctic acid is not patentable, it does not hold interest for pharmaceutical companies.   Another reason may be the discouragement of independent thought when it comes to patient treatment in America. Doctors who use non-traditional therapy risk losing board certification and encumbering lawsuits.

KH: *Could the use of thioctic acid with regards to the liver and the kidney help prevent the need for transplantation?*

BB: From my experience in administering IV thioctic acid to patients with acute hepatic necrosis and directly observing these recoveries, I would have to conclude yes.

KH: *Since you are on the editorial board of the New Mexico edition of the* Western Journal of Medicine *has it been easier to get your work known through traditional circles?*

BB: In 1995 I wrote an editorial on the politics and the use of thioctic acid (New Mexico Supplement To Western Journal of Medicine, May 1995:162(5):2).

KH: *If thioctic acid was fully utilized in medicine, to the degree that you have clinical experience with, what impact would it have on these different disease states?*

BB: From my personal experience, I believe thioctic acid reversed several types of acute and chronic liver disease.   Other studies show thioctic acid could also be used as an antioxidant, as a chronic disease protectant, as a radioprotectant, for organ regeneration, as an hypoglycemic agent in adult onset diabetes, and it may be able to reverse certain types of neoplastic disease. German research suggests that it increases active T-cell function.   It also appears to limit HIV viral replication *in vitro*.

KH: *Could thioctic acid have a beneficial effect in cardiovascular disease and/or cancer?*

BB: Research indicates that thioctic acid may be valuable in the treatment of cardiovascular disease and neoplastic disease. Russian researchers have studied thioctic acid in the treatment of heart disease. They found it as an excellent antioxidant by preventing damages to molecules that rid the body of excess cholesterol and it stimulates enzymes that breakdown lipids. The research also found that thioctic acid increased oxygen perfusion of the heart by 70%.

Thioctic acid may protect cells from neoplastic transformation by protecting the nuclear factors that are involved in preventing oncogene activation and it may also prevent free radical damage to genetic material.   In addition, it can protect the bone marrow and increase immune surveillance. ◆

Hip Fracture Risk Factors

Steven R. Cummings, M.D.
Prevention Sciences Group
74 New Montgomery Street, Suite 600
San Francisco, CA 94105 U.S.A.
(415) 597-9176 / (415) 597-9213 (FAX)

"Risk Factors For Hip Fracture in White Women",
The New England Journal of Medicine, March 25, 1995;12:767-773. #22016

Kirk Hamilton: Could you please share with me your educational background since college and your present position?

Steven R. Cummings: I received my M.D. and a fellowship in preventive medicine, general internal medicine and clinical epidemiology from the University of California at San Francisco. Presently, I am a professor of medicine in epidemiology at San Francisco.

KH: Why did you want to study hip fractures?

SC: Because 1 out of 6 white women will suffer a hip fracture that can sometimes cause death, commonly cause disability and account for perhaps $3 billion to $7 billion a year in medical expenses.

KH: What were the most significant risk factors you found in your study that increased the risk to hip fracture?

SC: Women whose mothers had a hip fracture were about twice as likely themselves to suffer a hip fracture in the future regardless of the degree of osteoporosis. Other risk factors included a past history of fracture frailty, (the inability to get up from a chair without assistance of another person), which carries a 2- to 3-fold increase in risk, and a past history of any kind of fracture. If you had a fracture in the past, you were at greater risk of hip fracture regardless of the level of your bone density. Next in importance was exercise. People who walked for exercise had a lower risk, and those who spent at least 4 hours a day up and around were at somewhat lower risk. These are important because they are simple things women can do on their own to minimize risk.

KH: What role did medications play in increasing risk?

SC: As other studies have found, those taking long acting sedative hypnotics had almost twice as great a risk of suffering a hip fracture. Those taking medications for seizures also had an increased risk though it was not because they had a hip fracture while seizing. It was for other reasons.

KH: How about impaired vision?

SC: People with impaired vision had a greater risk of hip fracture. But this is not the sort of vision testing one commonly does in the office. It is not just measurement of visual acuity. We measured depth perception. And we measured something called contrast sensitivity. Visual acuity testing, using the simple office tests, didn't have a relationship to hip fracture, but these more specialized tests did. So it indicates that some functions of vision that are lost with aging, especially in people with cataracts or glaucoma, really do increase the risk of hip fracture. But the doctors can't assess this risk just by a casual acuity test.

KH: How about the whole question of caffeine intake?

SC: Caffeine intake was a moderate to weak risk factor. The more caffeine someone took in, the greater the risk of hip fracture.

KH: Was there a threshold for a level?

SC: No. We didn't find a threshold suggesting that cutting down or cutting it out would be beneficial. But there is no safe magic number of cups of coffee.

KH: What would you like to see changed as far as preventive strategies for hip fractures?

SC: I don't know what women are doing around the country to prevent hip fractures. There have been no surveys of measures that people are taking already. However, in our data there are a lot of women (more than half the cohort are not walking for exercise) who could start walking, and that would be a big help. Those women who are inactive who sit and watch television should get up and do something else. That might go a ways to reducing risk. Ten percent of women in the country are using the long acting sedatives that increase hip fracture risk, and in addition about 10% of women are smoking. However, smoking doesn't appear in our list of official risk factors because women who smoked had several other risk factors that accounted for that increase. They were less likely to exercise. They were in poorer health. They had lost weight or hadn't gained the normal amount of weight with aging. For those reasons they were more likely to suffer hip fracture, and that 10% could do themselves a big favor by quitting.

KH: It sounds like a lot of these things are very, very basic and just require mass education.

SC: Yes. However, if a woman finds herself with several risk factors that she can't change, there are other things that she can do to reduce her risk, specifically things that increase bone density.

KH: Which include?

SC: Estrogen therapy, and in the course of the next year I expect that there will be new treatments approved, namely disphosphonate drugs, to increase bone density and prevent fractures.

KH: Isn't there some work regarding Japanese women who have less risk to hip fractures because they do more squatting and flexibility type things?

SC: There are some surveys suggesting that Japanese and Asian women have a somewhat lower risk of hip fracture. It is even lower in the native countries. Just why that is isn't clear.

KH: *What about the bone density as a risk factor?*

SC: The risk among women who already have some other risk factors depends a lot on the level of their bone density, which is something again that could be treated with estrogen or some other additional treatments that will be coming.

KH: *Can you tell me the technique for assessing bone density in your study?*

SC: There are several techniques for measuring bone density. At the beginning of our study we used a measurement of the heel, calcaneal bone density, which takes 10 or 15 minutes. This is very safe. Later on we measured bone density in the hip.

KH: *Using what technique?*

SC: That's using dual x-ray absorptiometry. And the first one was using single photon absorptiometry of the calcaneus. But we have previously shown that dual x-ray absorptiometry of the hip is a little better than calcaneal bone density in predicting hip fractures. So if a woman is concerned about her risk of hip fractures and wants to get more information than she has from this list of risk factors, I think she should have a measurement of bone density in the hip.

KH: *And you recommend the dual x-ray absorptiometry?*

SC: Yes, dual x-ray absorptiometry. ◆

Infertility and Dietary Aflatoxin

Dr. Isaiah N. Ibeh
University of Benin, Nigeria
Microbiology Department, Faculty of Science
Benin City, Nigeria

"Dietary Exposure to Aflatoxin in Human Infertility in Benin City, Nigeria",
International Journal of Infertility, 1994;39(3):208-214. #20837

Kirk Hamilton: *Tell me about your educational background.*

Isaiah Ibeh: I attended the School of Medical Laboratory Sciences, University of Benin Teaching Hospital, Benin City (1975-1980), University of Benin, Benin City (1986-1988;1989-1992). I hold the Associateship of the Institute of Medical Laboratory Sciences of Nigeria (AIMLT) in bacteriology, a Masters of Science (M.Sc) and a Doctor of Philosophy (Ph.D.) in microbiology (immunology and immunochemistry; food and industrial microbiology). In 1988, I successfully defended a thesis entitled, "Improved Method For Culturing Neisseria Meningitides in an Atmosphere of Carbon Dioxide" for the award of Special Fellowship (FIMLT) of the Institute of Medical Laboratory Sciences of Nigeria. I have also attended a short course on monoclonal antibody techniques at Royal Postgraduate Medical School, University of London, in 1986.

KH: *How did you get interested in environmental toxins, specifically aflatoxins and fertility problems?*

II: My father was a butcher. As an infant I observed, with keen interest, the techniques he applied in the preservation of fresh and dry meat and his frustrations with such methods, which sometimes failed, giving rise to meat spoilage. The Nigerian Civil War broke out in 1967, bringing with it hunger and starvation in the Biafran held territories. I saw people eat junk food and the out-break of marasmus and kwashiorkor. These experiences stimulated my interest in nutrition. I became vaguely aware that there may be a correlation between balanced/good nutrition and good health; that certain diseases could be prevented by controlling the quality of foodstuff consumed. These early observations set the line of research that would interest me in the future. Later, I found out that one of the problems affecting the food industry in Nigeria and, indeed, other developing African countries, is environmental toxin contamination of food. In this regard, mycotoxins captured my interest. Given the plethora of mycotoxins in existence, aflatoxin became more attractive for studies because of the tropical species and toxin production. If this toxin could occur in foodstuff at significant biological level, then it could have an impact on the good conditions in our country which favor easy proliferation of Aspergillus and the health of members of this community, given the mutagenic and carcinogenic potential of the toxin. I thought I should look at this issue from the angle of common diseases in this community which do not have clearly defined etiology. Such clinical conditions as liver cirrhosis, kwashiorkor and infertility problems readily came to mind. Then, I started the investigation with my research associates. We have published some of our findings, including those on the significance of aflatoxin and kwashiorkor and infertility.

KH: *How does aflatoxin exposure effect the male sperm and subsequent infertility?*

II: Exposure of male animals to low doses of dietary aflatoxin over a relatively short period may give rise to the development of sperm cells that are abnormal, in terms of structure, viability, motility and composition. The sperm cells become less viable, less motile; structural defects may include big or double heads, no tails, perforations of the cell membrane, leading to loss of cell inclusions. The deviation from normal sperm cells in terms of these criteria, indicates that the rate of fusion between male gametes (sperm cells) and female gametes (ovum) may be low. Although the mechanism by which aflatoxin impairs fertility is not completely understood, our findings suggest an interference of the level of development and maturation of the spermatogonia, lytic effect on preformed normal sperm cells which may lead to loss of cellular inclusion such as enzymes, hormonal insufficiency and fatigue which may lead to the inhibition of libido.

KH: *Have you done any research on how aflatoxin may effect the female ovum and fertility?*

II: I am working on the second phase of my study which includes the determination of the effects of aflatoxin on the female animal's reproductive system.

KH: *Do you know if antioxidants play any role in inhibiting the effect of environmental toxins, specifically aflatoxin on spermatozoal damage?*

II: I have not carried out specific studies on the effects of antioxidants on the toxicity of aflatoxin with respect to spermatozoal damage. However, I have an opinion. The activation of metabolism of aflatoxins involves a series of oxidative reactions, catalyzed by such enzymes as mixed function oxidases (MFOs). The susceptibility of an animal to aflatoxin is influenced by the rate of toxin metabolism and the type of intermediate products released. Fast metabolism of ingested aflatoxin to water soluble excretory products ensures quick elimination of toxin from the system, thus, providing immunity. If antioxidants enhance this process, then they would have contributed in inhibiting the effect of aflatoxin or other environmental toxins. Although the rate of metabolism of aflatoxin varies among animal species and is regulated by sex, age and nutrition, cellular metabolism in general, is influenced by vitamins. Some of the known antioxidants are vitamins, for example vitamin C. In this regard, I would say antioxidants could play a protective role in aflatoxin or toxin spermatozoal damage. It is also likely that toxin-induced membrane degeneration changes may be accompanied by the release of superoxides. The presence of antioxidants in such a situation will be combative to the deleterious effect of these oxides on cells and tissues.

KH: *Can you give an opinion on the overall role of environmental toxins on infertility problems?*

II: Because of structural differences in environmental toxins which may influence the modes of action, I think I should limit my opinion on the effect of toxins on infertility problems to aflatoxin. It is possible that aflatoxins constitute an etiology of infertility problems in man and other lower animals.

KH: Do antioxidant nutrients play a role in reducing the environmental toxins' effect on sperm?

II: Drawing from my answer to the previous question, I would say yes, there is a prospect that antioxidant nutrients could play a role in reducing the environmental toxins' effect on sperm. In addition, the literature has shown that vitamin A deficiency exacerbates the toxicity of aflatoxin in an exposed animal. Malnourished animals were also found to be more susceptible to the effects of aflatoxins. ◆

Lipids and Royal Jelly

Jozef Vittek, M.D., Ph.D.
Department of Medicine
Section of Endocrinology and Metabolism
New York Medical College
Valhalla, NY 10595 U.S.A.
(914) 285-8138 / (914) 285-8120 (FAX)

"Effect of Royal Jelly on Serum Lipids in Experimental Animals and Humans with Atherosclerosis," Experientia, 1995; 51:927-935. #23823.

Kirk Hamilton: *Can you please share with me your educational background and current position?*

Jozef Vittek: I received my doctoral degrees from the Komensky University, Bratislava, Slovakia. I am presently professor of medicine and dentistry at New York Medical College, Valhalla, New York. Among other interests, I did an extensive research with steroids as a member of the section of endocrinology and metabolism of the Department of Medicine for more than 25 years.

KH: What exactly is royal jelly and where does it come from?

JV: The royal jelly is a secretion from the hypopharyngeal and mandibular glands of the worker honey bee fed to the queen honey bee throughout their larval and entire adult life. Royal jelly consist of about 67% water, 12% protein, 12% carbohydrate, 5% fat, 1% minerals and about 2% other substances, i.e. vitamins, nucleic acids and probably other not yet analyzed chemical compounds.

KH: Why did you get interested in the role of royal jelly in atherosclerosis and serum lipids?

JV: As a student of medicine, I was also working at the Department of Biology as an instructor and research associate. At that time, we were doing some research with royal jelly for one of the pharmaceutical companies. Our results showed that royal jelly significantly decreased serum lipids and cholesterol in some individuals. In recent years, there were many reports in professional journals, as well as in the media, about the beneficial effects of various cholesterol-lowering products in the treatment of hyperlipidemia and atherosclerosis. Unfortunately, these cholesterol-lowering products have multiple side effects, so I reviewed the literature about the use of royal jelly for this purpose and published the results.

KH: Is there any evidence that royal jelly in human trials can lower serum lipids and of what type (HDL, LDL, total cholesterol, triglycerides, lipoprotein A, fibrinogen, etc.)?

JV: Meta-analysis of the controlled human trials showed that royal jelly significantly effects lipid metabolism in people by decreasing total serum lipids up to 15%, cholesterol by as much as 25% and normalizes HDL and LDL ratios by mainly increasing serum concentrations of HDL up to 35% only after short periods of treatment such as 15 days. In addition, royal jelly has an anti-thrombotic effect by decreasing the plasma concentrations of fibrinogen and causing significant vasodilation.

KH: How does one take royal jelly and in what dosage does it need to be taken to have these effects?

JV: There exist many preparations containing royal jelly in various forms. Royal jelly can be taking orally in the form of natural royal jelly mixed with honey or in the pharmaceutical preparations as pills, capsules, or as enteric coated tablets. (Enteric coating prevents disintegration of the royal jelly in the stomach and promotes dissolution of it in the intestine). Royal jelly can also be given by intramuscular injections. As shown by various studies, the usual oral form of royal jelly is 50-100 mg/day and an injectable form of 10-100 mg was sufficient to be effective when given for a short period of 10-20 days with the interruption of treatment for a week or two. However, if the royal jelly is taking by an ill patient it should be done under a physician's control with the appropriate laboratory testing.

KH: How do you know you're getting the appropriate substance?

JV: While there are many preparations containing royal jelly on the market, only very few are biologically effective. The most reliable are those preparations made by pharmaceutical companies. Hove, et al (J. Apic. Res. 1985;241:52-61) tested 15 commercial products of royal jelly and found that half of these products were either adulterated or did not contain any royal jelly. Storage of the royal jelly alone or in combination with honey or higher temperatures (as it is in the stores) may cause the destruction of royal jelly's biological effect up to complete inactivation.

KH: What is the theoretic mechanism by how royal jelly lowers serum lipids?

JV: Significant reduction of serum lipids and cholesterol by royal jelly suggests that royal jelly may act on the all important steps of cholesterol uptake, transport, biosynthesis, degradation and excretion. Royal jelly phytosterol, mainly beta sitosterol competes for sterol binding sites on enterocyte membranes, blocking the uptake of cholesterol in the gastrointestinal tract. Beta sitosterol may also prevent intracellular accumulation of cholesterol esters at the arteriole intima. Royal jelly also has an estrogenic effect and contains some estrogen. The estrogens may decrease the concentration of plasma cholesterol and LDL by suppression of HMG-CoA reductase and thus, hepatic cholesterol synthesis which activates the LDL receptors and promotes assimilation of lipoprotein from the plasma. In addition, unsaturated fatty acids, mainly 10 hydroxy-delta 2 decenoic acid has been shown to inhibit biosynthesis of lipids. Royal jelly also increases the utilization of oxygen and oxidative phosphorylation in the liver and inhibits ATPase activity, probably in part due to the increase of niacin in the liver. Thus, niacin content of royal jelly together with its increase in the liver may accelerate lipid catabolism in the liver and its excretion in the bile. However, the effect of royal jelly in the prevention of atherosclerosis is not only in the lowering of lipids and cholesterol, but also by its antibacterial (caused by royal jelly fatty acids and peptide Royalisin,) antiviral (caused by royal jelly glycoprotein which stimulates interferon production), antiproliferative (caused by Royal Jelly peptide ACE inhibitor and by estrogens) and antithrombotic (possibly caused by royal jelly fatty acids) properties. These effects of royal jelly may be responsible for the prevention, of the initiation and progression of atheromatic lesions. In addition, a vasodilation effect of royal jelly from the niacin acetylcholine and ACE inhibitor, present in royal jelly, may play a significant role in the control of high blood pressure and the prevention of atherosclerosis.

KH: Does royal jelly have any antioxidant properties that may also be beneficial in atherosclerosis prevention?

JV: I have no knowledge of this effect of royal jelly.

KH: What is the safety of royal jelly. Have there been any noted side effects?

JV: It is generally believed that royal jelly is nontoxic and safe to be eaten. The single ingestion of up to 15 gm had no adverse effect. Doses of 10 mg/kg in rats for 28 days had no adverse toxic effects. Doses of up to 100 mg/kg given to pregnant rats and mice have had no toxic effects on offspring. However, some pharmaceutical companies do not recommend its use in pregnant women and patients with some forms of cancer (inj. forms). In addition, allergy to royal jelly with anaphylactic reactions, as well as contact allergic skin reactions, have been reported.

KH: Is it a substance that is reasonable to take on a daily basis as a dietary adjunct to cardiovascular disease prevention?

JV: The long-term effect of royal jelly taken on a daily basis for cardiovascular disease prevention should be first evaluated before it is recommended, but it seems reasonable. ◆

Lung Cancer and Antioxidants

Kaarlo Jaakkola, M.D.
Kruunuhaka Medical Center
Phjoies Planadi 33 A
00100 Helsinki, Finland
358 0 626388 / 358 0 626312 (FAX)

"Treatment With Antioxidant and Other Nutrients in Combination With Chemotherapy and Irradiation in Patients With Small-Cell Lung Cancer",
Anticancer Research, 1992;12:599-606. #20848

Kirk Hamilton: *What is the rationale for the use of vitamins and minerals in theoretically reducing the side effects from chemotherapy and/or radiation therapy?*

Kaarlo Jaakkola: Chemotherapy and irradiation cause a cascade of free radical changes in the whole body. The effect of these kinds of treatments is partly based on ample changes in the free radical status. Vitamins and trace elements protect the antioxidant defense in normal cells. Because cancer cells do not have efficient antioxidative systems, vitamins and other antioxidants do not protect cancer cells. On the contrary, high concentrations of antioxidants can have similar effects to chemotherapy. This can be the reason that patients have less side effects and at the same time, a regression of the tumor.

KH: *Do you see a day when a vitamin and mineral supplement program, such as what you have done, is routinely given along with standard chemotherapy in the treatment of cancer?*

KJ: We are waiting eagerly for the day when these forms of therapy can be combined. More studies and international cooperation are needed, however.

KH: *With the use of antioxidant and multivitamin and mineral regimens, do you think this would reduce the risk to secondary cancers that sometimes occur from regular cancer treatments?*

KJ: When a broad spectrum of vitamins, trace elements and specific fatty acids are used in pharmacologic doses in combination with regular cancer treatment, our clinical results indicate that the risk for metastasization is reduced as well as the risk for secondary tumors.

KH: *Do you have any experience with antioxidants and other nutrients in the treatment of other types of cancers besides small-cell lung cancer?*

KJ: As previously mentioned, our clinics have experience with antioxidants and other nutrients in the treatment of several other types of cancer. Based on the theory that cancer, to a great extent, is a disease caused by free radical damage in an organ with decreased antioxidant defense, we have treated a huge number of different cancer forms. The results have been encouraging.

KH: *Do you have any particular nutrients which you think have a greater importance than others?*

KJ: The supportive treatment should be based on individual laboratory measurements and has to be individualized. With a treatment that has a broad spectrum, it is possible to obtain better results. Of main importance are those nutrients that can effectuate a chemotherapeutic or even a cancerosidic effect on tumor cells. Such elements are vitamins C and E, selenium in different medical forms, beta-carotene and pharmacological doses of vitamin A.

KH: *What was the rationale for vanadium, chromium and manganese in the nutritional supplements that you gave as far as their anticancer effects?*

KJ: Vanadium is important in the regulation of the ion pump. Most cancer patients have a deficiency in the function of sodium-potassium adenosidotriphosphatase. Vanadium plays an important role in the regulation of these enzymes. Many studies have demonstrated that daily intake of manganese and chromium in our country (Finland) is systematically too low. Chromium plays an important role in the regulation of sugar metabolism. Because cancer cells get their energy from glucose by an anaerobic metabolism, we think a normalization of the metabolic pathways are important. Manganese is important because it participates in the function of the prosthetic part of the MnSOD enzyme. The treatment is based on the individual whole blood determinations corrected with the hematocrit. This determination demonstrates the individual manganese status efficiently. In cancer patients there are frequently low manganese levels, which are furthermore an indication for manganese supplementation.

KH: *What was the breakdown of the types of fatty acids that you utilized (omega-6, omega-3, omega-9)?*

KJ: The treatment with different fatty acids in cancer patients is based on recent knowledge of the biochemistry of fatty acids. Before the treatment is started, the quantity as well as the percentage of different fatty acids are measured. Based on these measurements, a essential fatty acid (EFA) preparation is initiated. For example, if serum alpha-linolenic acid levels are low, or if omega-3 fatty acids (EPA, DHA, ETC) are decreased, the patient is given cod liver oil or similar products. Animal lecithins are additionally given to the patient. These products are important because a significant lipid peroxidation takes place in cancer patients. ◆

Mediterranean Diet and Health

W.C. Willett, M.D., Dr.P.H.
Harvard School of Public Health
Department of Nutrition
665 Huntington Avenue
Boston, MA 02115 U.S.A.
(617) 432-4111 / (617) 432-0464 (FAX)

"Mediterranean Diet Pyramid: A Cultural Model For Health Eating",
American Journal of Clinical Nutrition, 1995;61(suppl):1402S-6S. #22553

Kirk Hamilton: Could you please share with me your educational background and current position?

W.D. Willett: I trained as a physician and ended with a doctoral degree in epidemiology and joined the faculty at Harvard School of Public Health. I am presently a professor of nutrition and epidemiology and chairman of the Department of Nutrition.

KH: When did the Mediterranean Diet come on the scene as something that was of interest as far as health goes?

WW: The Mediterranean Diet has been on the scene for several decades. Much of the interest is owed to Dr. Ancel Keys, who first documented the very low rates of coronary heart disease in the Mediterranean countries compared to the Northern European countries and correlated the differences to diet. In particular, he noted that there was a much lower intake of saturated fats and higher intake of monounsaturated fat in the Mediterranean countries, while total fat was actually about the same in Greece as it was in the United States and other countries with high coronary heart disease incidence. It was really the type of fat that seemed to be the most different.

KH: In the traditional Mediterranean diet, we have a similar amount of total fat and they use, obviously, a lot of olive oil or oleic acid. What are the special properties of olive oil that make it of benefit?

WW: Since the Ancel Keys work, we have now come to understand some of the reasons why high olive oil consumption may be related to reduced coronary heart disease risk. It does several things. First of all, substituting olive oil for saturated fat substantially lowers the LDL or the bad cholesterol. But it doesn't lower the HDL or the "good" cholesterol, whereas substituting carbohydrate for saturated fat reduces both the good and the bad cholesterol. So, from metabolic studies, it looks like monounsaturated fats, which are very high in olive oil, are better than saturated fat or carbohydrate. Also, we have now learned more about the role of antioxidants in coronary heart disease. Monounsaturates produce LDL cholesterol that is resistant to oxidative damage and olive oil contains a lot of antioxidants. So you get a very favorable balance of resistance to oxidation and protection by antioxidants.

KH: When you talk about carbohydrates being substituted instead of the olive oil, you said that the carbohydrates lowered HDL cholesterol. Are you talking about simple carbohydrates, complex carbohydrates or carbohydrates in general?

WW: Whether they are simple or complex, they all lower HDL cholesterol.

KH: What is the role of milk products in the Mediterranean diet? I reviewed Ancel Keys' article and though they consume less amounts of milk, they did consume a lot of cheese. I was a little bit confused.

WW: Overall, dairy product consumption is moderate in the Mediterranean diet. It is lower than in many parts of the world, particularly much lower than in Finland where the coronary heart disease rates were the highest in Ancel Keys' study. It is probably not that the dairy products consumed are more in the form of cheese and yogurt that is beneficial, but rather the low to moderate consumption in general.

KH: What is the atherogenic property in milk products or do we know?

WW: We think it is mainly the high amount of saturated fat in milk products that is responsible for increased rates of heart attack. That has received the most attention. Also, that fat comes along without much antioxidant protection.

KH: What about the role of fruit in the Mediterranean diet?

WW: It looks like fruit and vegetables are a very key part of the Mediterranean diet. It is probably important to emphasize vegetables, because they are consumed in large amounts in the Mediterranean diet. From anyway we look, higher consumption of vegetables seems to be important. That may be in part because of their fiber, carotenoid and vitamin C content. Other substances contained in fruits and vegetables seem to have anticarcinogenic effects. So whether we consider cancer or heart disease, a high vegetable consumption seems to be good.

KH: Are grains consumed a lot in the Mediterranean diet? Is there a lot of pasta consumed or is pasta a side dish in the Mediterranean diet?

WW: The amount of pasta varies quite a bit around the Mediterranean diet. It is obviously higher in Italy than anywhere else. In Greece, which actually tended to have lower rates of heart disease than Italy in the Seven Countries Study, there was not much pasta consumption, but rather grains were consumed more as bread. The important thing about grain consumption is probably that it be consumed more as whole grain rather than in the refined form.

KH: Is there a concern that a high carbohydrate diet, even if it is complexed, can aggravate the insulin response and actually increase atherosclerotic risk?

WW: There is concern in the minds of many of us about the high carbohydrate diet, which is the opposite side of the coin of a low fat diet. There are metabolic changes that happen on a high carbohydrate diet that do not seem to be beneficial. One gets higher levels of blood glucose, higher insulin levels, higher blood levels of triglycerides and low HDL cholesterol, which all seem to be inter-related and lead in the wrong direction for reducing heart disease risk.

KH: *I know I seem to be repeating my question, but I am trying to get clear on types of carbohydrate - to me there is the "Western" carbohydrates which are refined white flour bread products versus a country that could be eating lentils, peas and beans. Do the complexed carbohydrate diet still cause those changes in insulin and such?*

WW: Even the relatively complex carbohydrate diets - of course almost nobody eats all their carbohydrates as lentils or legumes - seem to have some adverse metabolic effects. These are probably less if carbohydrates are less refined and more in the form of legumes. So I think that there is good reason to go for the less refined grains.

KH: *Does olive oil create a neutral hormonal response?*

WW: It seems to elevate insulin levels less. That may be one of the reasons why it is advantageous.

KH: *The diet that Ancel Keys talked about in the 1950s - has there not been a change in the Mediterranean consumption of foods and thereby an increased risk to heart disease in the last 40 years?*

WW: Yes. There has been a lot of change toward a more typical Western pattern.

KH: *What is the biggest difference between those 2 diets - the traditional Mediterranean diet and the newer Mediterranean diet?*

WW: Probably the biggest change has been a major increase in meat consumption which, obviously, contains lots of saturated fats and displaces other healthier parts of the diet.

KH: *What role does alcohol play in the Mediterranean diet?*

WW: Almost for sure, alcohol is partly responsible for the lower rates of coronary heart disease in some of these areas. There is overwhelming evidence that moderate levels of alcohol consumption reduce heart disease risk.

KH: *And what about physical activity?*

WW: Certainly, it has played a key role. In fact, I think being inactive is probably more important than the type of fat or the amount of fat that we consume.

KH: *Which brings us to the Mediterranean Diet Pyramid. We have the government's dietary pyramid and the one in this article the Mediterranean Diet Pyramid. What are the major differences?*

WW: There are some important differences. First, it is probably useful to indicate the similarities. Both emphasize high consumption of fruits and vegetables. There is great unanimity about that. The government pyramid talks about emphasizing carbohydrate but it doesn't emphasize so much whole grain forms of carbohydrate and the more we see the more that seems to be important. If you are going to consume carbohydrates, it does look like it is advantageous

to consume them in the whole grain form and not just for more fiber but also because micronutrients are lost when grains are refined. Some of the main differences are that the government pyramid is an expression of the general fat phobia and it doesn't distinguish between types of fat but just says reduce fat intake. But that flies in the face of an overwhelming body of evidence indicating that it is really the saturated and *trans* fats that are harmful and that other fats are either essential or at least neutral, particularly the polyunsaturated and the monounsaturated fat. So the type of fat really seems to be more important than the total amount of fat. The other major differences are in what is called the "Meat" group which is obviously a compromise with the meat industry. Meats are lumped along with legumes - and the government says it is healthy to have these 3 times a day.

KH: *Let's talk about **trans** fats for a moment. They are still very controversial. The harm of **trans** fats in your opinion?*

WW: They clearly appear to be bad. I don't think anyone at this point in time can look at the data objectively and deny that *trans* fats have adverse metabolic effects. There is an overwhelming body of literature behind that. They seem to be uniquely bad because they both raise LDL cholesterol, reduce HDL cholesterol, and also elevate lipoprotein (a). There is no other type of fat that has that combination of adverse effects. Some people say *trans* fats are only a small percentage of the diet, they are only on the average 2 or 3% of the American diet. But there is no other artificial chemical in our food supply that comes anywhere near that level, and we've worked out that this level of intake could account for about 7% of premature deaths due to heart disease which are about 30,000 deaths a year. Research by Scott Grundy, M.D., independent from ours, using a somewhat different computation than ours, came out with virtually identical results. He estimated 8% of premature deaths. We estimated 7%. That is not a trivial number of premature deaths per year, and they are quite unnecessary.

KH: *What are the major sources of **trans** fats?*

WW: Until not too long ago the major source was margarine, but the levels in some margarines have been reduced quite a bit. Yet, margarines really don't need to have any *trans* fats in them, but many still do. If we look in the grocery store, large amounts of those brick hard margarines are still being sold and thus many people consume margarines that are still very high in *trans* fats. Also, there are two other major sources now. Probably the most serious one is the fast food industry. They switched to using heavily hydrogenated fats around 1989. These fats contain up to about 25% to 35% *trans* fats and many people eat much of their food from fast food places. The other source is baked and prepared foods. One can consume a lot of *trans* fat that way.

KH: *This was a fabulous response! Now do you take antioxidants yourself? And what may I ask do you take and at what dosage?*

WW: First of all, I take a multiple vitamin which is in part to make sure I get enough folic acid. Secondly, I take 400 I.U. of vitamin E a day. Thirdly, I take 500 mg of vitamin C a day.

KH: *And you get your beta-carotene from fruits and vegetables?*

WW: Yes. I am able to enjoy them all the time. ◆

Mediterranean Diet and Public Health

Ancel Keys, Ph.D.
University of Minnesota
Division of Epidemiology
School of Public Health, Suite 300
1300 S. Second Street
Minneapolis, MN 55454-1015 U.S.A.
(612) 871-6396 / (612) 624-0315 (FAX)

"Mediterranean Diet and Public Health: Personal Reflections",
American Journal of Clinical Nutrition, 1995; 61(Suppl.):1321S-3S. 22547

Kirk Hamilton: Could you please share with me your educational background and current position?

AK: I am emeritus professor of epidemiology at the University of Minnesota, and my educational background was from the University of California where I have an M.A. and a Ph.D. in biology. I also received a Ph.D. from Kings College at Cambidge University in England.

KH: When did your interest in diet and heart disease begin?

AK: At the end of the war, I noticed that in the newspapers (I had been working for the War Department) lots of executives were "dropping dead" and I wondered how and why. Nobody else knew either. I said we needed to have a prospective study on executives. We had been noticing that in general, people who had coronary artery disease had high cholesterol values. We were finding that their cholesterol values were influenced by their diet. That was the beginning of an experiment on diet and cholesterol values. The second thing was that we were looking to see what the situation was in other countries. This led to the Seven Countries Study which began in 1957, and it is still continuing.

KH: Why did you get interested in the Mediterranean diet?

AK: Because as we were working on this question to some extent and when I was a visiting professor at Magdalen College, Oxford University, I had time off and we went down to Naples in 1952 to see whether it was true what the professors were saying that they had no coronary heart disease problem. When I got down there, I found that this was true. There was no coronary heart disease problem in general, except among the wealthy people going to private hospitals who consumed meat on a daily basis.

KH: What were the significant differences in the western diet versus that Mediterranean diet that you felt gave it its advantage?

AK: The first thing we noticed was that the people in that area in Italy consumed a diet that had much more green vegetables and fruit and much less dairy products and meat. The latter were only in small quantities.

KH: When you say much less dairy products, I do notice in the article that cheese was eaten a fair amount.

AK: Yes, but that was only a small part of the diet. The custom was to sprinkle a tablespoon of grated Parmesan cheese on pasta. Hard cheeses were eaten at the end of the meal on festive occasions.

KH: What types of fat are consumed in the Mediterranean diet?

AK: At that time, I was not aware of the importance of the different types of fat. Olive oil, though, was the only source of fat practically, but its consumption did vary. On the island of Crete, for example, it was in the order of 30% of the diet. In Italy, in our parts of Italy at least, it was somewhat less, but it was still very high.

KH: Is the Mediterranean diet today in 1995 the same as it was when you visited there in the 1950s?

AK: No. Unfortunately, it is changing. There is a lot more consumption of dairy products and meat. Their diet is converging to our type of diet in the United States.

KH: Did they eat a lot of desserts?

AK: No. In general, fruits were their desserts. Cakes were only for special occasions. For example, at Christmas time they had a special Christmas cake and at Easter a special Easter cake. But other than that, cakes were almost unknown.

KH: What are the major "villains" in the diet that we have acquired in comparison to the Mediterranean diet?

AK: Well, the saturated fat. That is the big difference.

KH: In the last part of your article you mentioned that if you wanted to promote good healthy eating, you have to start with children. Could you please explain that?

AK: With children for example, we would favor the use of 2% milk as we use ourselves, and we would discourage children from eating too much ice cream and things of that sort. Instead, encourage them to eat vegetables at dinner, especially green vegetables.

KH: Do we have to be as cholesterol conscious or should we spend more energy on just reducing our saturated fat?

AK: It is the saturated fat that is the big deal . . . cholesterol in the blood is bad, but cholesterol in the diet is not necessarily the major culprit that increases blood cholesterol. ◆

Menstrual Pain and Omega-3 Fatty Acids

Bente Deutch, Ph.D.
Nutrition and Home Economics
Arhus University
University Park
M50 DK-8000, Aarhus, Denmark
45 86 12 23 55 / 45 86 13 73 89 (FAX)

"Menstrual Pain in Danish Women,",
European Journal of Clinical Nutrition, 1995;49:508-516. #23498

Kirk Hamilton: *Could you please share with me your educational background and current position?*

Bente Deutch: I am biologist and received my Ph.D. from Aarhus University, Denmark. In the period after my Ph.D., I left the university and taught microbiology and chemistry to laboratory technicians and other individuals. About 10 years ago, I returned to the university as a teacher and later as a principal of the Institute of Nutrition and Home Economics. I soon became interested in human nutrition research.

KH: *How did you get interested in the role of omega-3 fatty acid intake and menstrual pain?*

BD: In the 1970's 2 Danish doctors Bang and Dyerberg studied the disease patterns in Greenland eskimos. They found a low prevalence of cardiovascular diseases, asthmatic bronchitis, diabetes, rheumatologic disorders and other inflammatory conditions. At the same time the eskimos had increased bleeding time and tendency, and therefore, a higher death rate due to brain hemorrhage. Their hypothesis to explain this pattern was based on a high intake of marine, long-chain omega-3 fatty acids among the eskimos. Omega-3 fatty acids are metabolized to a series of prostaglandins which generally give milder inflammatory and coagulatory responses than prostaglandins derived from the omega-6 family which are highly prevalent in the western diet. What inspired me was that none of these studies had been concerned with women and their biological functions and what might be influenced by this unusual diet. After all childbirth, abortion and menstruation are all involved with natural, spontaneous and self-limiting bleeding. Besides being involved in blood clotting, prostaglandins are also involved in vasodilation and constriction and smooth muscle contraction. It was natural to assume that menstrual symptoms could be influenced by them. I wrongly suspected that women with a high intake of omega-3 fatty acids would have more violent menstrual flow.

KH: *What is the mechanism of menstrual pain biochemically?*

BD: The biochemistry of menstrual pain is not known in detail. But uterine contraction in general is prostaglandin-mediated. This means that prostaglandin-synthetase inhibitors such as aspirin inhibit the contraction and thereby reduce the pain. The prostaglandins PGE_2 and $PGF_{2\alpha}$ are elevated in the blood and urine of dysmenorrheic women during painful menstruation.

KH: *How do fish or marine oils reduce some of this inflammatory cascade?*

BD: Fish oils contain a higher proportion of omega-3 fatty acids, and like omega-6 fatty acids they are metabolized to prostaglandins. But in general the prostaglandins formed from the omega-3 fatty acids such as PGD_3, PGE_3 and $PGF_{3\alpha}$ are less inflammatory than the prostaglandins formed from the omega-6 fatty acids, mainly those previously mentioned PGE_2 and $PGF_{2\alpha}$. Therefore in principal, by changing the diet towards a higher relative content of omega-3 fatty acids from fish oils, the bodily functions, such as menstruation, would be influenced by less aggressive prostaglandins resulting in less discomfort.

KH: *What is the amount of fish oil needed to be consumed on a monthly basis to help lower the risk of menstrual pain?*

BD: The studies showed that the total average intake of omega-3 fatty acids among women without pain was about 2 gm a day of which approximately .4 gm per day came from marine, long-chain fatty acids. This would be covered by monthly varied fish intake of 1.0-1.5 kg. So it is not very much. This is approximately 1 to 2 fish meals per week.

KH: *Could fish oil supplements be used to reduce menstrual pain in females?*

BD: In principal yes, but it needs to be tested clinically.

KH: *What is the role of high arachidonic acid containing foods such as meat, egg and dairy fat in aggravating menstrual pain?*

BD: I can only say that in this study the highest prevalence of menstrual pain was found among the vegetarians, thus dietary arachidonic acid itself was not seen to be aggravating. However, this is very difficult to explain because arachidonic acid of course is metabolized to the aggressive prostaglandin-series $PGF_{2\alpha}$, etc., when it is released from the phospholipids. But arachidonic acid was also formed from dietary linoleic acid which is much more abundant and ubiquitous in the vegetarian diet.

KH: *What is the role of omega-6 fatty acids that come from gamma-linolenic acid and the possibility of being beneficial in menstrual pain?*

BD: I have no personal experience with gamma-linolenic acid. I know of experimental evidence with gamma-linolenic acid which is very rare and not part of the natural diet. My answer, therefore, must be based upon the literature. Several authors suggest that gamma-linolenic acid favors the formation of prostaglandin E_1 which is another diversion from the formation of the aggressive PGE_2. It seems that gamma-linolenic acid works against PMS and menstrual pain in some cases.

KH: *Are there any other nutritional factors that you know of that can be used to reduce menstrual pain?*

BD: In the study 24 dietary nutrients were tested. None of these nutrients except omega-3 fatty acids and B_{12} showed any significant correlation with menstrual symptoms. We also saw no effect of vitamin and mineral supplements which were consumed by about 40% of the women. The effect of B_{12} is probably an indicator for fish intake and omega-3 fatty acid intake. However, it should be looked into and tested in an independent clinical trial. In fact of all of the nutrients, B_{12} showed the correlation with the highest significance. ◆

Mind - Body Connection and Health

C. David Jenkins, Ph.D.
University of North Carolina
Adjunct Professor of Psychiatry & Behavioral Sciences
School of Medicine
Chapel Hill, N.C. 27514 U.S.A.
(919) 962-8331

"The Mind and the Body",
World Health, March-April 1994;447(2):6-7. #20558

Kirk Hamilton: *Please share with us about your education background.*

David Jenkins: I received both a bachelors and masters degree from the University of Chicago, the latter in human development. After my masters and before I started on my doctoral degree I worked for the City of Chicago Health Department for 3 years as a psychologist and became involved with public health and prevention issues. While I was completing my Ph.D. in clinical psychology at the University of North Carolina, I started working at the Department of Epidemiology at the University of North Carolina School of Public Health. I learned epidemiology on the job and remained their 13 years becoming a professor there in 1970. I then moved to Boston University School of Medicine where I started the Department of Behavioral Epidemiology located within the larger Division of Psychiatry. In 1982, I came to the University of Texas Medical Branch at Galveston to be a professor of preventive medicine, psychiatry and behavioral sciences. Since then, I served a term as president of the American Psychosomatic Society and continue to be an executive editor of Behavioral Medicine.

KH: *Your article "Mind and Body" in World Health was excellent and was personally relevant to me. I enjoyed it. Can you weave a connection between psychology and how it eventually goes through our nervous, endocrine, and immune systems?*

DJ: As we experience things and see, think, and perceive, many emotions are generated. Messages arise both from cognition and from emotions. They go through the central nervous system and fan out to the peripheral nerves and then to the endocrine system. We now know the immune system is also strongly effected.

KH: *Are we able to actually measure an emotional event or a thought process through changes in our endocrine and immune systems?*

DJ: Yes we can. I have been working on a manuscript based on 100 nurses who went through a laboratory experience where their blood pressure and endocrine systems were monitored. Blood pressure and heart rate changed dramatically as the nurses performed different tasks and felt different emotions. The first challenge was a hand grip. Each person gripped the hand grip as hard as she could. This was measured and then released. Then she gripped again and held at 30% of maximum for 3 minutes. You would be surprised how much that hurts during the last minute. This drives the systolic and diastolic blood pressures up as well as the heart rate. We later had them do mental mathematics and that drove pressures up even higher than did the handgrip or other physical stressors. We also measured changes in stress hormones as well as self-reported feelings of anxiety and anger. *All of these interactions of mind and body can be quantified.*

KH: *In your article in World Health you present a model of ischemic heart disease and you talk about stress, hostility and type A behavior. Can you explain the difference between good stress that motivates us to go out and take action versus the stress that may create this relentless striving or whatever it is that causes damage to one's health?*

DJ: It has something to do with the intensity and duration of the stress. We know that people who are under intense stress for long periods of time will incur an increase in blood pressure - at least for that period of time. For example, the air traffic controllers we studied tended to get much higher blood pressures over time than men in other occupations. We think that is due to the fact that they are under this repeated stress. They never know quite when the other shoe is going to fall in terms of planes entering their space unannounced and the like. So there is a constant vigilance and this has been often associated with elevated blood pressure. There have been a number of studies showing, for example, that Type A people under stress generate more noradrenaline than Type B people under the same challenge.

KH: *Do these air traffic controllers get ill more often?.*

DJ: Yes. Our work says they do. They get more gastrointestinal disturbances. They get more hypertension particularly and a number of other disorders as well.

KH: *Is it a key factor that there is no break in the stress?*

DJ: It seems that way, and maybe also it is the way the individual handles stress. At the end of 3 years we had some people who had developed new hypertension and others who had remained normotensive. When we reviewed our records there was no difference in their work load. So it may be something to do with, the way they cope with it stress. The workers who claimed they had no anxiety, no work problems, and were happy with management developed sustained hypertension more often than those who recognized and talked about the problems and the negative emotional responses that they experienced.

KH: *Could you give a definition of the Type A behavior pattern? I think some people just assume that everybody who is a hard driver is Type A.*

DJ: Competitive aggressive, easily angered . . .

KH: *Always in a hurry and in a constant struggle against time and the environment?*

DJ: That is the classic definition. It is from Doctors Meyer Friedman and Ray Rosenman, the cardiologists who originally derived the concept.

KH: *It would seem like you could be working on a lot of things, but if you didn't internalize it and get frustrated with it, and constantly project this kind of relentless striving, so to speak, that would be okay?*

DJ: That's right. And, we have often found that people at higher executive levels are less Type A than some of the people that they supervise. So it is more a matter of how you climb up the ladder than just being at the top.

KH: *You discuss the role of hostility in ischemic heart disease. I wonder if you could elaborate on that?*

DJ: Science has fads and fashions. There was the decade of the Type A which probably was the 70s. The 1980s has been the decade of hostility, and Type A became kind of "old hat". I think hostility is certainly a valid risk factor, both for ischemic heart disease (coronary disease) and for other causes of death. Some people claim that the only thing about type A that is noxious is the hostile portion. I think that is not correct because there are some studies that have looked at separate components of Type A and even controlling for hostility - - the competitiveness, hurry and other job related Type A features still have a correlation with disease.

KH: *I have a grin on my face because as I read your article and talk to you I see myself. Fortunately I am not a hostile person but I am a driver and usually in a hurry! Can you give our readership some practical steps on how to live in this fast-paced world of communication, intensity and work and still develop a healthy response to it?*

DJ: Well there are a lot of stress management books available, and they say it better than I can, but I can reiterate some of their points. *Part of it goes with reperceiving yourself and the world you operate in. And, a lot of us Type As like to think that the world will collapse if we don't keep holding it up by ourselves.* And we are really not that important. A lot of us feel that we have to prove our worth everyday. We tend to feel worthless in the evening if we haven't reasserted our worthwhileness by productivity during the day. A person doesn't have to be productive every day to be a worthwhile person. A person doesn't have to correct all the ills in the world to be a worthwhile person. Another thing is that many Type As are looking for new challenges, but I am trying to control my own Type A behavior and look away from challenges, and not fall for the bait of hurrying or trying to do all these different things. I am spacing out my schedule. Some of us have more control over that than others. Dr. Bob Eliot has done much cardiovascular research. He talks about "the hot reactor", the person who has a big physiologic reaction to every frustration. *He says there are only two rules to control stress: 1. Don't sweat the little stuff. 2. It is all little stuff.*

KH: *Well this is a very appropriate interview for me - let me tell you. Because I came in here today stressed. I have too many things to do and not enough time to do them. Obviously that's just my own choosing.*

DJ: We have talked about some of the psychological things you can do to relieve stress. There are physical things you can do too. One of these is Dr. Herb Benson's relaxation response. There are various types of meditation practices, yoga practices that really change physiological function and they might very well change immune function as well.

KH: *Well for me - a "lazy man's" meditation is exercise. After about 10 or 15 minutes, if I am vigorous about it, I start to focus on one or no thoughts. All the other ones get pushed out. My cluttered mind before my workout is clear afterwards and much more peaceful.*

DJ: Well I think that is a Type A way of reaction. Someone gave me a relaxation tape to listen to and comment on. It was about 30 minute long. After about 10 minutes or so I got so itchy that I wanted to put it on fast forward. I knew that something was wrong at that point. I personally will get more relaxation out of vigorous exercise, than I would from sitting and meditating. So I'm in your corner.

KH: *In the era of health care reform -- and I mean true health care reform, not just juggling dollars around -- How does awareness of the mind-body interaction play a role? -- Where would you like to see it as an emphasized entity?*

DJ: *I think the bottom line is that we have to take individual responsibility for our own health and that includes our behavior* - such behavior as getting immunized, eating a good diet, getting exercise and keeping our weight under control, avoiding tobacco and health-damaging behavior. In addition, we need a positive frame of mind and way we think about the world. In short, the way we take care of ourselves, and the way we deal with stress. Somebody -- and I wish I knew the originator of this -- said: *Your health is too important to leave in the hands of a doctor. You have to be responsible for yourself.* Of course, you need a doctor as a consultant at certain times. The idea is to know when to go and when not to go. But if we take much more responsibility for our own health and practice a lot of these things mentioned in the "Mind - Body" article as well as other parts of your PEARLS and newsletter, I think we'll reduce the number of trips to the doctor and cut health care costs. There are 3 ways to cut health care costs: 1. Reduce the cost of each unit of service. This means cutting doctor's incomes and hospital's incomes. 2. Secondly, is to reduce the number of units of service that are rendered per patient. Basically that means rationing. 3. *The third is reducing the need for service by having more people stay healthy more of the time. Unfortunately, very little is being said about that in this health care debate.* ◆

Morbidity in the Elderly and Glutathione

Mara Julius, Sc.D.

Department of Epidemiology
School of Public Health
University of Michigan
109 Observatory St.
Ann Arbor, MI 48109-2029 U.S.A.
(313) 764-5435 / (313) 764-3192 (FAX)
(313) 668-7248 (PHONE/FAX)

"Glutathione and Morbidity in a Community-Based Sample of Elderly,"
The Journal of Clinical Epidemiology, 1994;47(9):1021-1026. #21961

Kirk Hamilton: Could you please share with me your educational background and current position?

Mara Julius: My graduate training was in physiological psychology and philosophy at the University of Zagreb, Zagreb, Croatia. With a Ford Fellowship for foreign scholars, I did postgraduate work in social psychology at the department of psychology, and in survey research methods at the Institute for Social Research, University of Michigan, Ann Arbor, Michigan. My doctoral thesis was in psychosocial epidemiology and my masters thesis in social psychology. I have been doing research in psychosocial epidemiology at the Department of Epidemiology, School of Public Health, University of Michigan since 1970. I went into early retirement because I wanted to devote more time to glutathione research. My current emeritus status combines the University of Michigan resources with personal freedom to choose what I like to do most.

KH: When did you get interested in glutathione's role in the elderly?

MJ: In the early 1980's, I started to conduct epidemiologic studies of aging populations, which included aspects of both psychosocial and physical health. I was not satisfied with the existing measures and their ability to predict aging. Therefore, I started searching the literature for a more basic biological system which, if measured, could give a better diagnostic tool for predicting health/disease, longevity/death in aging populations. Given at that time (1980s), the technological advances of the second scientific revolution (e.g., electrospectrography, computers), I was sure that in the fields of molecular biology and biochemistry there were scientists identifying at a cellular/molecular level some of the essential biological systems for survival. For almost 2 years, I could not find any such work. I was about to give up when serendipitously, I found an abstract describing Dr. Calvin A. Lang's work on the role of glutathione in aging in healthy elderly women in Louisville, between the ages of 60 to 102 years. The abstract was literally forgotten on a poster panel after presentation at an annual gerontological meeting in 1984. Just by reading the abstract convinced me that this was the biological parameter I was searching for in the past several years. I immediately contacted Dr. Lang and we have been collaborating ever since. My study of "Southfield Elderly," reported in the Journal of Clinical Epidemiology, 1994, is a joint effort between Dr. Lang and my research teams. Dr. Lang is professor of biochemistry and director of a research on aging program at the Department of Biochemistry, University of Louisville Medical School in Kentucky.

At the time we met, he had more than 3 decades of glutathione research on animal models (mosquito, mouse, rat) and humans. The other two scientists instrumental in our collaboration, are Lang's long standing associates and former graduate students, Dr. Betty Jane Mills, associate professor of biochemistry at the University of Louisville, and Dr. John P. Richie Jr. who is presently research scientist at the American Health Foundation in Valhalla, New York. Even though we are at different institutions, our strong interest in the role of glutathione in aging, health and disease, plus the modern means of communication, makes for continuous collaboration among us. Informally, we call ourselves "The Glutathione Research Group."

KH: Do we make our own glutathione?

MJ: Yes, we do. Practically all living cells have glutathione and cannot live without it. That suggests strongly that glutathione was one of the early entries into the compendium of living matter.

KH: What is glutathione made from?

MJ: It is a tripeptide composed of glutamic acid, cysteine and glycine. The description of biological aging, that the cell loses the ability to replicate/regenerate, and the immune system decline coincides with the major functions of glutathione in the body, protecting cells against the destructive effects of reactive oxygen intermediates and free radicals; detoxifying external substances such as drugs and environmental pollutants; maintaining cell membrane stability; regulating protein and DNA biosynthesis and cell growth; enhancing immunologic function through it's effects on lymphocytes. These widespread functions suggest that the level of glutathione has major health effects on the molecular, cellular and organ levels of the individual. Lang's initial work using animal models of the mosquito, mouse and rat, suggests that glutathione declines with old age and parallels the survival curves. Correction of glutathione deficiency can enhance longevity in the mosquito by 40%. In his studies of healthy men and women in Louisville, glutathione levels were significantly lower in the elderly (60 to 79 years) when compared to mature (40 to 59 years) subjects. However, levels in the very old (80-99 years) were similar to those of the mature group. This curvilinear pattern suggests that people who maintain high levels of glutathione for whatever reason, represent survivors with extreme longevity. Recently, a number of small clinical studies show that with most of chronic and infectious diseases, including AIDS, patients glutathione levels are low, compared to healthy controls.

KH: *What did you find in your study of this elderly population with regard to glutathione?*

MJ: One of the main goals of my study in Southfield, Michigan was to replicate Dr. Lang's findings on a more representative, community based sample of elderly, outside of Louisville and with a wider range of health characteristics (from very poor to excellent). The study's results confirm his findings as to the link of high glutathione levels being associated with good health and extreme longevity. Furthermore, in terms of morbidity, it confirms findings from other clinical studies of different patient populations. We have found that study participants who were diagnosed, (by our examining physicians), with heart disease, diabetes, high blood pressure, circulation problems, stomach symptoms and urinary tract infections had low glutathione. However, it was statistically significant only for the first 3 diseases, which is probably due to a small number of cases in other disease categories. In addition in the group of very old people (age 80 to 95) we found that they all had very high levels of glutathione and were diagnosed by physician as well as in their own self-reports as super healthy. Yet another collaborative study confirming those findings is a sample of post-polio victims in Michigan. Classifying the study population by levels of polio impairment as high or low, we then tested the relationship of their health status with glutathione levels. The low impairment group was similar to the general aging population, i.e. people with no other diseases (besides polio condition) had high levels, and those with one or more conditions had low levels of glutathione. However, everybody in the severely impaired polio group had higher levels of glutathione. Our interpretation is that in order to survive old age or severe impairment, one needs to be able to maintain high glutathione levels.

KH: *How do we increase our glutathione levels?*

MJ: There are very few systematic studies with definitive answers on how to correct glutathione deficiency efficiently. Two basic approaches are being explored: (1) using precursors of glutathione such as N-acetylcysteine or (2) glutathione itself. Again, depending on the purpose of the intervention, there are 2 different approaches of testing (1) to develop a preventive health supplement pill for use in general (disease free) populations and (2) to develop curative drugs to be used in patients with life threatening diseases such as carcinomas and AIDS. Dr. J. P. Richie Jr. is now conducting an intervention trial with AIDS patients. I am not at liberty to disclose what drugs are being used. However, knowing the stage of progress of that study, we should expect published results soon. To answer your questions more directly, we do not have sufficient data to categorically state which is the most effective way of enhancing glutathione in the body. However, indicators are that there will be strategies in producing effective drugs from both precursors as well as from glutathione itself.

KH: *How do we increase glutathione levels from the diet?*

MJ: Another approach in correcting glutathione deficiency, or maintaining healthy levels of glutathione, is by utilizing natural foods rich in glutathione. There are a number of research teams at different institutions analyzing food groups for glutathione content. Our colleague Dr. B.J. Mills at the University of Louisville is finishing up such an analysis. Cruciferous vegetables are rich in glutathione. However, all food groups have glutathione, but cruciferous vegetables have the highest content with a number of other nutrients (e.g. iberin, sulforaphane, preformed glutathione) that boost the utilization of exogenous as well as the production of the endogenous glutathione in the body. The cruciferous family includes cauliflower, broccoli, cabbage, kale, brussels sprouts and then some.

KH: *Until better glutathione stimulating substances are made available and discovered, the take home message would be to eat a lot of cruciferous vegetables and also supplement products already on the market which enhance the body's production of glutathione.*

MJ: We know there are very healthy ingredients in those vegetables besides glutathione. While we wait for our biochemists to discover the pathways and how to use them more efficiently, we can eat those vegetables and be healthy without completely understanding the reasons. I am currently taking glutathione, two pills per day at 500 mg, produced by Health Maintenance Programs, Inc., in Elmsford, NY 10523, (800)362-8673. I have noticed a significant improvement in energy level and fewer episodes of viral/bacterial infections. Even when I get an infection, it is much milder and lasts much shorter than before I started taking glutathione tablets.

KH: *Do you have any other parting comments about glutathione?*

MJ: It is interesting to note that many of the vitamins and nutritional supplements that have gained widespread public attention recently are also glutathione boosters. Pine bark extract (pycnogenol), melatonin, bilberry grape extract, turmeric, and other nutrients have been shown to elevate glutathione. I believe that our work will ultimately lead to the definition of glutathione as the body's master antioxidant and primary marker of aging. I have often remarked on how medicine and epidemiology often appear to be extremely errantly fixated on studying what causes disease, rather than focusing on what promotes health. In most of my study designs, I have emphasized looking at the distribution of positive health rather than disease and mortality. It appears that modern medicine and epidemiology might have an opportunity to utilize one marker for nearly all chronic and age-related disorders. This has profound implications, particularly for medicine. Instead of waiting for disease to occur and then treating it, physicians could use glutathione tests as a diagnostic tool and use glutathione in the form of drug or food supplements to slow down or reverse accelerated aging changes at the cellular level before they advance into predisease or frank disease states. Glutathione, discovered in 1888 and introduced into biochemistry in the 1920s, got its formula in the 1930's. In the late 1920s and 1930s, there was a burst of research activity on glutathione, particularly in ophthalmology. The first link between aging and glutathione was discovered in the aging human lens. Today, all eye diseases are linked to depleted levels of glutathione. The reason the research tapered off was the instability of glutathione assays. Being the master antioxidant, it is terribly sensitive to air, light and heat. It oxidizes so fast it is hard to assess its true value before it oxidizes. Developments of new methods since the 1970's makes research possible. Drs. C.A. Lang, B.J. Mills and J.P. Richie Jr. contributed significantly in developing HPLC-DEC methodology for measuring glutathione and other thiols and disulfides in blood and other tissue. Actually, Dr. Richie just published in 1995, his work on further improvement of that method which should lead to more wide spread measurement of glutathione. In 1984 when I approached them for collaboration they needed additional year to develop procedural steps so that I could store blood samples for a week, then mail them to Dr. Lang's laboratory, and still get valid glutathione readings. Until then, only blood analyzed immediately after being drawn, gave valid and reliable results. To my knowledge, even today, there are no commercial and only a few research laboratories, such as Drs. Lang and Richie that measure blood glutathione routinely. I am convinced, that in part, the relative obscurity of glutathione's role and importance for health, longevity, disease, and aging is still due to measurement problems. The other part is lack of a strong theoretical framework from which it should be studied, particularly as a marker of aging. To close our conversation on a slightly negative note, I am frustrated that when I mention glutathione, the typical reaction is "Oh it is just another antioxidant." Well it is not just another antioxidant. It is much more than that and the elements of its significance have been in the literature since 1888. ◆

Motion Sickness and P6 Acupressure

Senqi Hu, Ph.D., M.D.
Humboldt State University
Department of Psychology
Arcata, CA 95521 U.S.A.
(707) 826-5262 / (707) 826-4993 (FAX)

"P6 Acupressure Reduces the Symptoms of Vection-Induced Motion Sickness",
The Journal of Aviation, Space and Environmental Medicine, July 1995;66(7):631-634. #23069

Kirk Hamilton: Could you please share with me your educational background and current position?

Senqi Hu: I received my medical degree in China in 1977 from Shanghai Medical University. I then worked as a physician for eight years in China. I received my Ph.D. in psychology in 1990 from Penn State. Since then I have been teaching in the department of psychology at Humboldt State University. Presently, I am a tenured associate professor in this department.

KH: When did you get interested in the role of acupressure and motion sickness?

SH: I have been studying motion sickness for about 1 decade. In 1988, Dr. J.W. Dundee reported P6 acupressure reduced morning sickness. In 1989, Dr. E. Hyde confirmed that acupressure relieved symptoms of morning sickness. Since the major symptoms are nausea and vomiting for both morning sickness and motion sickness, I was inspired by these 2 reports. In 1994 I decided to test if P6 acupressure could also reduce the symptoms of motion sickness, such as nausea and vomiting.

KH: What is the theoretical mechanism by which acupressure works on motion sickness?

SH: The mechanism whereby P6 acupressure reduces nausea and other symptoms of motion sickness is still unknown. From western medical theory, my hypothesis is that P6 acupressure stimulation may increase endorphin levels in the brain, which in turn may inhibit the vomiting center in the brain. There is another explanation based on theories of Traditional Chinese Medicine. That is, various pathogenic factors (such as motion sickness) break the balance of Qi (vital energy). This imbalance occurs at the pericardium meridian (one of the 12 regular meridians in the human body), and the patient develops symptoms of nausea and vomiting. The P6 point is an important point in the pericardium meridian, so acupressure stimulation of the P6 point may restore the normal Qi's circulation of the body. Therefore the symptoms of motion sickness are reduced.

KH: Do we know what physiologic events occur along meridians?

SH: Recently Chinese medical researchers in Beijing reported that they found that meridians are organized by increased electrical resistance in each acupuncture point (such as P6) along each meridian. If the Qi circulation is unbalanced, the electrical resistance will be significantly high in the related points of the meridians. By using acupuncture treatment, the abnormally high electrical resistance can be reduced to normal levels and, at the same time, the symptoms of motion sickness will be relieved.

KH: How distinct was the difference in improvement in the P6 group versus the other controls and the sham acupressure treatment?

SH: In our study we divided 64 human volunteers into 4 groups: P6 acupressure group, dummy-point acupressure group, sham P6 acupressure group, and no acupressure control group. We found that 3 of 16 subjects in the group of acupressure developed major symptoms of motion sickness such as cold sweating and nausea while viewing an optokinetic rotating striped drum for 12 minutes. However, the cold sweating and nausea occurrence was 9 of 16 subjects in the group of dummy-point acupressure group, 11 of 16 subjects in the sham acupressure group, and 10 of 16 subjects in the control group.

KH: What type of motion sickness is this (acupressure) good for?

SH: According to my personal experience, many of my friends have told me that P6 acupressure relieves symptoms of car sickness, sea sickness, boat sickness and airplane sickness.

KH: Could this be extrapolated to have benefits with nausea and vomiting such as in hyperemesis gravidarum (morning sickness)?

SH: Yes.

KH: Were there any side effects to the acupressure therapy?

SH: The only precaution for acupressure is to use pulsed acupressure with 1 pulse for every second to protect the local skin and tissue from not being overstimulated. The local skin will be red and painful if acupressure stimulation lasts too long. Therapists should stop acupressure if local skin and tissue becomes inflamed.

KH: Could you please share how you locate the P6 acupressure point and, from your answer to the last question, what do you mean by "pulsed acupressure with 1 pulse for every second"?

SH: The P6 (The Neiguan point on the pericardial meridian) acupressure point is located about 3 cm from the distant palmer crease of the wrist, between the palmaris longus and flexor carpi radialis tendons. The pulsed acupressure means that the experimenter or therapist manually presses the local acupressure point (rhythmic intervals of applied one finger pressure) with about 1 push per second. ◆

Myocardial Infarction and Antioxidants

Ram B. Singh, M.D., DTN., H.

Heart Research Laboratory and Center of Nutrition
Medical Hospital and Research Center
Civil Lines, Moradabad-10 U.P., 244001, India
91 591 317 437 / 91 591 311 003 (FAX), 91 591 312 261 (FAX)

"Effect of Antioxidant-Rich Foods on Plasma Ascorbic Acid, Cardiac Enzyme, and Lipid Peroxide Levels in Patients Hospitalized with Acute Myocardial Infarction," Journal of the American Dietetic Association, July 1995;95(7): 775-780.   #22791

Kirk Hamilton: *Can you please share with us your educational background and current position?*

Ram B. Singh: I received my M.D. in medicine at the Institute of Medical Sciences, Benaras Hindu University, Varanasi, India in 1973. The subject of my thesis was related to digoxin, magnesium and potassium in heart disease. I am the director of the Heart Research Laboratory at Medical Hospital and Research Center and a professor of preventive cardiology and nutrition. I have contributed about 400 research papers, including 170 publications and 5 books, and I have received 5 national and international awards. During the past 25 years, I have been working on the role of fruits, vegetables, magnesium, potassium and antioxidants in the pathogenesis and treatment of cardiovascular diseases.

KH: *Why are antioxidants important during acute myocardial infarction?*

RBS: There is evidence that ischemia and reperfusion can cause the overproduction of free radicals which may be responsible for cell damage and necrosis in acute myocardial infarction. Secondly, several studies have demonstrated that in an acute myocardial infarction, there is a decrease in plasma levels of vitamins C, E and beta-carotene, selenium, zinc, magnesium and potassium which poses the possibility that these antioxidants and minerals are in increased demand during acute myocardial infarction. It is possible that treatment with antioxidants during acute myocardial infarction can provide protection against damage due to free radical stress. Antioxidants can protect myocardial cells and arterial endothelial cells, and can prevent thrombosis. Therefore, antioxidants may provide rapid protective effects.

KH: *What did you find in your study with regards to levels of vitamin C, cardiac enzymes and lipid peroxides in the heart in myocardial infarction patients?*

RBS: At entrance to this study, both groups of heart attack patients had a marked reduction in vitamin C and a rise in cardiac enzymes and lipid peroxides, which is an indicator of free radical stress. The antioxidant-rich diet group showed a smaller rise in LDH cardiac enzymes and a reduction in lipid peroxides indicating that it can provide protection against free radical damage.

KH: *Since there was an apparent benefit with consuming foods rich in antioxidants, wouldn't it be reasonable to supply antioxidants intravenously in patients having an acute myocardial infarction to help prevent myocardial necrosis and reperfusion injury?*

RBS: This is an excellent question because we have conducted a randomized trial into the role of vitamins A, C, E and beta-carotene in acute myocardial infarction. This study showed that there was a significant reduction in CPK and CPK-MB cardiac enzymes and electrocardiographic oxygen reactive species scores which suggests that treatment with antioxidants can cause a significant reduction in infarction size. After 28 days, there was a significant reduction in the cardiac event rate in the antioxidant group compared to the control group. This data was presented at the 11th Asian Pacific Conference of Cardiology in Bali, Indonesia on September 17-22, 1995 and will be published in the American Journal of Cardiology in 1996.

KH: *Magnesium has been theorized to prevent reperfusion injury if given early enough in acute myocardial infarction. Would it be reasonable to use magnesium along with an antioxidant-rich diet and antioxidant supplements?*

RBS: In one of our research papers we reported that these patients also had magnesium deficiency (Journal of the American College of Nutrition, 1994;13:139-143). In the same issue, an editorial by Dr. Seelig mentioned this article and proposed that magnesium can interact with vitamin E and can enhance its antioxidant effect, apart from providing its independent beneficial effect. Our diet included green vegetables, legumes and nuts, which are rich sources of magnesium and may have provided at least 3 times more magnesium to the antioxidant group compared to the control group.

KH: *Why weren't other antioxidants measured besides vitamin C such as beta-carotene and vitamin E?*

RBS: We were not measuring other antioxidants in our laboratory when this study was conducted. Our more recent study shows that plasma levels of vitamins A, C, E and beta-carotene are inversely related to acute myocardial infarction. A few other studies also have reported similar results.

KH: *What types of essential fatty acids are rich in walnuts and almonds?*

RBS: Walnuts contain alpha-linolenic acid which is known to prevent thrombosis and also may have an antioxidant effect. The diet also contained mustard and soybean oil, which are rich in alpha-linolenic acid and may have provided some benefit. Our new findings indicate that both fish oil and mustard oil can decrease myocardial infarction size.

KH: *Do you see a day when not only an antioxidant-rich diet will* *be given in hospitals to myocardial infarction patients but also intravenous antioxidants?*

RBS: We used intravenous vitamins A and C, and oral vitamin E and beta-carotene for the treatment of acute myocardial infarction as mentioned in the previous question. I believe this treatment may be used routinely in the near future. In another trial which is under publication in "Cardiovascular Drug Therapy" (Kluwer), it was shown that prior treatment with antioxidant vitamins E, C and beta-carotene can retard experimental atherosclerosis in rabbits. ◆

Myocardial Infarction and L-Carnitine

Ram B. Singh, M.D., DTN., H.

Heart Research Laboratory and Center for Nutrition
Medical Hospital and Research Center
Civil Lines, Moradabad-10 U.P., 244001, India
91 591 317 437/ 91 591 311 003 or 91 591 312 261 (FAX)

"A Randomized, Double-Blind, Placebo-Controlled Trial of L-Carnitine in Suspected Acute Myocardial Infarction", <u>Postgraduate Medical Journal</u>, 1995;71. #23771

Kirk Hamilton: Could you please share with me your educational background and current position?

Ram B. Singh: I received my M.D. in medicine at the Institute of Medical Sciences, Benaras, Hindu University Varanasi, India in 1973. The subject of my thesis was related to digoxin, magnesium and potassium in the heart. I am the director of the Heart Research Laboratory at Medical Hospital and Research Center and a Professor of Preventive Cardiology in Nutrition. I have contributed about 400 research papers, including 170 publications and 5 books, and I received 5 national and international awards. During the past 25 years, I have been working on the role of fruits, vegetables, magnesium, potassium and antioxidants in the pathogenesis and treatment of cardiovascular disease.

KH: When did you get interested in the role of L-carnitine in acute myocardial infarction?

RS: I became interested in carnitine in the 1980s when I read that it is a constituent of the cell and is important in cell metabolism. It was interesting to note that serum carnitine levels decrease in acute myocardial infarction similar to magnesium and antioxidants. Our experiments in the 1990s showed that pretreatment of cells with L-carnitine provides protection against damage from oxidants and preserves the cell.

KH: What was the thought behind the potential benefit of L-carnitine in acute myocardial infarction?

RS: It appeared to us that the requirement of L-carnitine increases during acute myocardial stress to maintain the cell metabolism, which is disturbed due to myocardial ischemia. It is possible that addition of L-carnitine might improve the cell metabolism and preserve the cardiac cells and enhance molecular adaptations which develop due to acute myocardial stress. L-carnitine might also preserve G-proteins or stress proteins which may prevent ventricular remodeling.

KH: Can you describe your studies and the effects of L-carnitine in a group of myocardial infarction patients?

RS: In a randomized, double-blind placebo-controlled trial, the effects of oral L-carnitine (2gm/day) for 28 days were compared in the management of 101 patients with suspected acute myocardial infarction (AMI). After 28 days, mean infarct size and lipid peroxides, as well as angina pectoris (17.6 vs. 36.0%), heart failure (23.4 vs. 36.0%), arrhythmias (13.7 vs. 28.0%) and cardiac events (15.6 vs. 26.0%) were less in the carnitine group compared to the control group (<u>Postgraduate Med. Journal</u>, 1995, *in press*).

KH: How did you pick the 2 gm dose of oral carnitine for this study?

RS: We reviewed the literature and noted that the dose of L-carnitine in AMI and angina pectoris varies between 1-6 gm/day. We wanted to test the effect of an optimal dose in view of its higher cost.

KH: Would intravenous L-carnitine have been better initially followed by oral L-carnitine throughout the days that were nonhospitalized?

RS: Yes. We are planning a study with intravenous L-carnitine because it is now available in India by Elder Pharmaceuticals Ltd., Bombay as of January 1996. We would be using it before thrombolytic therapy to prevent reperfusion ischemia.

KH: Do you see L-carnitine being used more routinely in coronary care centers?

RS: No, it is not used routinely mainly because there are no large scale trials to provide evidence that it can decrease mortality in AMI.

KH: Do you see L-carnitine and antioxidants being used together in the treatment of acute myocardial infarction?

RS: We have demonstrated that L-carnitine also possesses antioxidant effects apart from its beneficial effect on ATP and energy metabolism. More studies would be necessary to demonstrate that antioxidants plus L-carnitine can have a synergistic effect.

KH: Do you have any experience with coenzyme Q10 in the treatment of acute myocardial infarction or cardiovascular disease in general?

RS: No, it is not available in India.

KH: Would you also consider adding magnesium to this nutritional therapy in early, acute, myocardial infarction?

RS: Yes, it seems it would be interesting to test the combined effect of all the micronutrients that are deficient during AMI. ♦

Myocardial Infarction and Magnesium

Mildred Seelig, M.D.
Adjunct Professor, Nutrition,
University of North Carolina, Chapel Hill
Adjunct Professor, Family & Preventive Medicine
Emory University Medical School, Atlanta
1075 N. Jamestown Road, Apt. F
Decatur, GA 30033 U.S.A.
(404) 329-1916 (FAX/PHONE)

Ronald J. Elin, M.D., Ph.D.,
Chief, Clinical Pathology Department
Clinical Center, National Institutes of Health
Building 10, Room 2C-306
10 Center Drive, MSC 1508
Bethesda, MD 20892-1508 U.S.A.
(301) 496-5668 / (301) 402-1612 (FAX)

"Re-examination of Magnesium Infusions in Myocardial Infarction",
<u>American Journal of Cardiology</u>, July 15, 1995;76:172-174. #22865

Kirk Hamilton: Could you please share with me your educational background and current position?

Ronald Elin: I received my B.S., B.A., M.D. and Ph.D. degrees from the University of Minnesota. My internship was at the University Hospital of San Diego and I did 3 years as a research associate at the National Institutes of Allergy and Infectious Disease. I am board certified by the American Board of Pathology in anatomic and clinical pathology, chemical pathology and diagnostic microbiology.   I am currently chief of the Clinical Pathology Department and, within that department chief of Clinical Chemistry Service at the National Institutes of Health.

Mildred Seelig: I received my A.B. degree from Hunter College in New York City where I did my premedical training. I received my M.D. degree from the New York Medical College. My medical internship was at Orange County Hospital in California. I received my Masters of Public Health at Columbia University School of Public Health. I am currently an adjunct professor of nutrition at the University of North Carolina, Chapel Hill and an adjunct professor of family and preventive medicine at Emory University Medical School in Atlanta, Georgia.

KH: When did you get interested in the role of magnesium in acute myocardial infarction?

RE: From my Ph.D. thesis in 1969, I studied the biochemical and pathological changes in magnesium deficiency in experimental animals. I was the first chairman of the Gordon Research Conference on magnesium in 1978. I have followed the developing story of magnesium and myocardial infarction since the early 1980s.

MS: Since 1969 when I addressed the question of magnesium deficiency-related dangers in electrocardiography (<u>Annals of The New York Academy of Sciences</u>, 1969;162:906-917), I have published articles alone, and with others, on structural and functional cardiovascular changes caused by magnesium deficiency. An article published five years later with A. Heggtveit, reviews magnesium interrelationships in ischemic heart disease (<u>Am. J. Clin. Nutr.</u>, 1974;27:59-79). About a third of my 1980 book, <u>Magnesium Deficiency in the Pathogenesis of Disease,</u> was devoted to cardiovascular disease.

KH: What physiological effects occur with magnesium therapy that help prevent against the extension of the myocardial damage that occurs during an acute myocardial infarction?

RE: Magnesium would have 4 significant positive physiologic effects on the myocardium at the time of an acute myocardial infarction. Magnesium is nature's own calcium channel blocker. An increase in ionized magnesium concentration in interstitial fluid should diminish calcium influx into damaged tissue and limit necrosis. Secondly, magnesium is an effective vasodilator that should improve the blood supply to damaged areas of the myocardium. Thirdly, magnesium has been shown to have an antiarrhythmic effect on the myocardium. Lastly, an increase in the magnesium concentration would limit platelet aggregation and thus the extension of a thromboembolic episode.

MS: I concur with Dr. Elin's comments and would only add that magnesium stabilizes cell membranes, and functions to protect against free radicals released under stress, associated with catecholamine secretion and auto-oxidation. Recent research has shown that some of the favorable effects of magnesium are mediated by protection against endothelial damage and dysfunction, with a result that the increased magnesium favors release of endothelial-derived relaxing factors and prostacyclin, both of which increase vasodilation and inhibit platelet clumping. Low magnesium favors production of thromboxane that, with endothelial-derived constricting factor, has the opposite effects.

KH: *Could you briefly share the results of the smaller Limit-2 (Second Leicester Intravenous Magnesium Intervention Trial) study and the large ISIS-4 (4th International Study of Infarct Survival)?*

RE & MS: We believe there are the following 4 important differences in the study design between these 2 trials: 1) In the small studies (Meta-Analysis of Seven Studies, British Medical Journal, 1991;303:1499-1503) and the Limit-2 Study, the magnesium infusion was begun as soon as possible after the onset of symptoms, and before or without subsequent fibrinolysis. On the other hand, the ISIS-4 study indicates that magnesium was begun within 2 hours of the fibrinolytic therapy for about half of all randomized patients; about ¼ received magnesium between 2 to 6 hours after the onset of symptoms and subsequent fibrinolysis, and the remaining patients may have started treatment up to 24 hours after symptom onset. Because reperfusion injury begins immediately on re-establishing blood flow, and magnesium is protective, *we believe it is preferable to administer magnesium prior to fibrinolytic therapy.* 2) The amount of magnesium infused over the first 24-hour period differed between the 2 studies. In the Limit-2 Study, 73 mM of magnesium was administered during the first 24 hours. However, in the ISIS-4 and a much smaller study by Feldsted, et al, (European Heart Journal, 1991;12:1215-8) 80 mM of magnesium were administered during the first 24 hours of magnesium therapy. In both of these studies, the short term mortality was greater in the magnesium-treated group than in the control group. On the other hand, the Limit-2 Study found a 24% reduction in 28-day mortality and 5 of 7 studies in the meta-analysis, administering between 32 and 65 mM of magnesium within 24 hours after myocardial infarction, showed a mean improvement of 66% in short-term mortality. It may be that a 80 mM dosage of magnesium within 24 hours exceeds the therapeutic window for magnesium therapy and that a lower concentration is needed for a positive effect. 3) The ISIS-4 and the Limit-2 studies did not continue the magnesium infusions beyond 24 hours. However, many of the smaller studies in the meta-analysis continued magnesium beyond the first 24 hours and noted a reduction in arrhythmias. It may be that a longer duration of magnesium infusion is required to prevent tachyarrhythmias in myocardial infarction. 4) The treatment and mortality rates of control groups affect rates of improvement in the test group. The higher control mortality rate in the Limit-2 than in the ISIS-4 may reflect the fact that fewer Limit-2 controls underwent thrombolysis or received antiplatelet therapy than did the ISIS-4 controls: 30% versus 70%, and 66% versus 94% respectively.

KH: *What are the valid reasons for these differences?*

RE: We can only speculate about what factors led to the differences in the experimental design between the 2 studies. The Limit-2 study only evaluated the effect of intravenous magnesium on the outcome of acute myocardial infarction in a limited geographic area. On the other hand, the ISIS-4 study evaluated the effects of nitrates and calcium channel blockers, in addition to magnesium therapy, at the time of an acute myocardial infarction and was performed in many hospitals throughout the world. Thus, the ISIS-4 was more complicated in the experimental design, and was subject to greater variability since many patient care teams throughout the world contributed to the results.

MS: Magnesium may not have benefit when provided hours after reperfusion - especially when induced by fibrinolytic therapy. If given at the time of infarction, even the 80 mM 24-hour dose might lower mortality, although associated with a greater risk of adverse effects. Direct evidence that benefit can be accrued, can be inferred from the favorable report of the ISIS-4 study run in Poland and England, without adverse effects (European Heart Journal, 1994;15:608-619). In addition, I suggest referring to Elliott Antman's editorial: "Randomized Trials of Magnesium in Acute Myocardial Infarction: Big Numbers Do Not Tell the Whole Story", American Journal of Cardiology, 1993;75:391-393, regarding the different protocols (fixed trial pooling analysis does not account for intertrial differences, which leads to misleading conclusions) and to another article just recently published: "Magnesium in Acute MI: Timing is Critical," Circulation, November, 1995;92:2367-2372.

KH: *What is the optimum timing for intravenous magnesium in acute myocardial infarction?*

RE: We believe that intravenous magnesium should be started immediately upon hospitalization with a diagnosis of acute myocardial infarction.

MS: The earlier magnesium infusion is started, the better the chances for recovery. It may be advantageous to start a slow infusion in the ambulance.

KH: *I concur strongly with the above suggestion of magnesium's use in the ambulance. When I did paramedic work in the late 70's and early 80's all we could use for arrhythmias was lidocaine, epinephrine, atropine and cardioversion. Magnesium would have been so simple and safe to administer since you had an I.V. going at the scene, or in the ambulance, for all cardiac patients.*

What is the optimal dosage and duration of therapy for magnesium in acute myocardial infarction?

RE & MS: We would recommend administering 50 to 60 mM of magnesium during the first 24 hours of therapy followed by 10 to 20 mM of magnesium per day for the next 4 to 5 days.

KH: *What are the recommendations for the use of magnesium in acute myocardial infarction when both studies are taken in totality?*

RE & MS: This is a very controversial area. We believe that the ISIS-4 study establishes the dose of 80 mM of magnesium in 24 hours as toxic and having no benefit at the time of acute myocardial infarction. Thus, as indicated above, a reduced dose of magnesium should be given during the first 24 hours and extended for several days. Further, the magnesium therapy must be started immediately when the diagnosis of an acute myocardial infarction is made. We believe additional studies are needed to better define the optimum therapy of magnesium at the time of acute myocardial infarction. ◆

Myocardial Infarction and Magnesium

Geir Falck, M.D.
Per Jynge, M.D., Ph.D.
University of Trondheim
Faculty of Medicine
Department of Pharmacology and Toxicology
Medisinsk Teknisk Senter
N-7005 Trondheim, Norway
47 73 598851 / 47 73 59 8655 (FAX)

"High Magnesium Improves the Post Ischemic Recovery of Cardiac Function,"
Cardiovascular Research, 1995;29:439. #22164

Kirk Hamilton: *Drs. Falck and Jynge can you please share with me your educational backgrounds and current positions?*

Geir Falck: I received my doctorate of medicine degree in Trondheim in 1991 and completed an internship in Sweden in 1993. I did 6 months of service at the Department of Forensic Medicine at the Karolinska Institute in Stockholm, Sweden. Presently I am a research fellow in professor Jynge's group at the Department of Pharmacology and Toxicology, University of Trondheim with the project "Coronary Angiography; Contrast Media Pharmacology and Heart Function."

Per Jynge: I received my doctorate of medicine in Oslo in 1963. I have worked for several years as a general surgeon with special interest in experimental cardiac surgery, pathophysiology and pharmacology. I received my Ph.D. in 1980 doing research on myocardial protection in cardiac surgery and cardioplegic solutions. I became an associate professor in 1981 and a full professor in 1989 in the Department of Pharmacology and Toxicology, University of Trondheim. My recent interests are in cardiac pathophysiology including the role of Ca^{2+} and Mg^{2+} in ischemia and reperfusion.

KH: *What reasons are there to doubt magnesium's benefit in myocardial infarction?*

GF & PJ: With the publication of the 4th International Study of Infarct Survival (ISIS-4), we seriously question the role of magnesium in myocardial infarction. Previous studies were small and did not include more than a total of 1,000 patients. The Second Leicester Intravenous Magnesium Intervention Trial studies (LIMIT-2) with more than 2,000 patients, showed a beneficial effect of magnesium infusion on mortality in myocardial infarction. However, the results were only marginally significant with a mortality reduction after 28 days of 24% (95% confidence limits 1-43%). The ISIS-4 study evaluated 58,000 patients randomized into 3 main groups and a total of 8 subgroups and provided enough statistical power to detect even small differences in favor of magnesium. No such favorable effects were detected in terms of mortality reduction. At present it is fair to say that there are no grounds for the routine use of magnesium in the treatment of myocardial infarction.

KH: *Was there a harmful effect of magnesium therapy in the ISIS-4 study?*

GF & PJ: This is a difficult question. In terms of mortality in the ISIS-4 study, there were overall more deaths among those who received magnesium than those who did not (7.64% vs. 7.24%, not significant). The ISIS-4 study showed an increased incidence of heart failure and cardiogenic shock in the group receiving magnesium which was in contradiction to the LIMIT-2 study. One explanation may have been the subjective nature of diagnosing heart failure and cardiogenic shock in the 2 studies. Another explanation is that in the LIMIT-2 study, a relatively small group of doctors examined the patients whereas in the ISIS-4 study several thousand doctors were engaged. A further explanation may be the lack of placebo infusion in the ISIS-4 study. The placebo was dropped because flushing and other cutaneous signs would likely "unblind" the active treatment. The lack of placebo would probably have no importance on mortality but could bias the judgment of "soft" variables like heart failure and cardiogenic shock. The hemodynamic load produced during the magnesium infusion (50 ml/24 hours) was probably too low to explain the increased incidence of heart failure and cardiogenic shock. We see no real harmful effects of magnesium in the doses given in these studies provided that contraindications such as severe hypotension and renal failure are taken into account.

KH: *How does one explain the differences in results between these 2 studies?*

GF & PJ: The differences in the results between the ISIS-4 and the LIMIT-2 studies are not easy to explain. Even though patients with a low serum magnesium were excluded in the LIMIT-2 study, we know that magnesium deficiency might exist even with normal serum magnesium levels. Magnesium loading tests which examine the percent loss of magnesium in the urine after an intravenous dose give a far more precise estimation of the magnesium state of the patient. No such measurements were performed in any of the studies. Therefore, the patients might have been significantly different with regard to their magnesium state. In the LIMIT-2 study the patients were included from a relatively restricted area and it could be speculated that people in this area could have been magnesium deficient due to a low water magnesium. More likely reasons for a pre-existing magnesium deficiency might be the presence of magnesium depleting factors such as diuretic use, digoxin therapy, dietary deficiency or alcohol intake. In the ISIS-4 study, patients were included from more than 1,000 hospitals on 4 continents and any such regional differences would be clearly diluted. The regional characteristics might have influenced the outcome of the studies. It may be hypothesized that in the LIMIT-2 study, magnesium acted as a nutrient that raised a low serum magnesium level while in the ISIS-4 study magnesium acted as a drug which raised a normal serum level. This distinction might explain the differences in mortality rates. Another explanation is the timing of the magnesium infusion. In the ISIS-4 study half of the patients were given magnesium more than 2 hours after thrombolytic therapy, which was started with a medium time from the chest discomfort to magnesium infusion of 8 hours. In contrast, the magnesium infusion was started at a median of 3 hours after the onset of the chest discomfort in the LIMIT-2 study. Therefore, at the time of potential reperfusion by thrombolysis, the patients in the LIMIT-2 study had on the average a higher serum magnesium than the patients in the ISIS-4 study. The delay of introducing magnesium in the ISIS-4 study might partly explain the differences, although there were no favorable effects in the subgroup who were given magnesium at 0-3 hours after the onset of chest pain.

KH: In your opinion is magnesium therapy warranted in acute myocardial infarction?

GF & PJ: The routine use of magnesium in myocardial infarction does not seem to be justified. However, there might be subgroups of patients, where magnesium depleting factors are prevalent, who may benefit from early magnesium infusion. A comparison between normo- and hypomagnesemic patients utilizing the magnesium load test with regard to myocardial infarction has, to the best of our knowledge, not been performed. Such a study would indicate if magnesium acted as a nutrient, a drug, or both (or neither) in myocardial infarction. One could thus, more precisely, select patients in whom magnesium would be favorable and avoid potential side effects in patients where such therapy would have little or no effect. If there were regional differences in the magnesium state as well as regional differences in the beneficial effect of magnesium in the treatment of myocardial infarction, these differences would vanish in a large multicenter trial. If we were to treat a patient with myocardial infarction in the Leicester area we would probably give magnesium. The role of magnesium in other areas awaits further clarification.

KH: What can you conclude from the results of the LIMIT-2 and ISIS-4 studies as far as recommendations?

GF & PJ: The clinical evidence (LIMIT-2 vs ISIS-4) in favor of early magnesium infusion is controversial. Thus, no definite clinical conclusion can be reached at the present time. From the standpoint of basic researchers it would seem logical to state that the earlier the magnesium is given the better. ◆

Napping and Melatonin

Peretz Lavie, Ph.D.
Technion-Israel Institute of Technology
Sleep Laboratory, Faculty of Medicine
Gutwirth Building
Haifa 32000, Israel
972 04 226730 / 972 04 323045 (FAX)

"Melatonin Improves Evening Napping",
<u>European Journal of Pharmacology</u>, 1995; 275:213-216. #22042

Kirk Hamilton: *What is your educational background and present position?*

Peretz Lavie: I hold a B.A. in statistics and psychology from Tel-Aviv University and a Ph.D. in physiological psychology from the University of Florida in Gainesville. I completed my post-graduate training in the Department of Psychiatry at the University of California San Diego. In 1974, I joined the faculty of medicine at the Technion-Israel Institute of Technology where I established a sleep research laboratory and a clinical sleep research facility. In 1989 I became a full professor. Currently, I am the dean of the faculty of medicine.

KH: *How did you get interested in the role of melatonin and sleep?*

PL: Some years ago I was contacted by a principal of a boarding school for blind children who requested consultation concerning sleep difficulties of some of his pupils. We decided to investigate sleep in these children concomitantly with cycles of melatonin secretion. This put us on the trail of melatonin's role in sleep regulation. In that study (Tzischinsky, Skene, Epstein and Lavie, "Circadian Rhythms in Six-Sulphatoxymelatonin and Nocturnal Sleep in Blind Children," <u>Chronobiology International</u>, 1991;8:11-14), we found that blind children who had abnormally phased cycles of melatonin secretion also suffered from sleep disturbances. That is, children who showed peaks of secretion during the day had difficulties falling asleep during the night. Later (Tzischinsky, Pal, Epstein, Dagan and Lavie, "The Importance of Timing Melatonin Administration in a Blind Man," <u>Journal of Pineal Research</u>, 1992;12:105-108) we showed that exogenous treatment with melatonin can ameliorate sleep disturbances in blind children. These findings have directed us to examine the role of melatonin in elderly insomniacs (Haimov, et al, "Melatonin Replacement Therapy of Elderly Insomniacs," <u>Sleep</u>, in press) and in normal sleep regulation (Tzischinsky, Shlitner and Lavie, "The Association Between Nocturnal Sleep Gates and Nocturnal Onset of Urinary aMT6s," <u>Journal of Biological Rhythms</u>, 1993;8:199-209.)

KH: *How does melatonin work in inducing sleep?*

PL: There are several speculations concerning the effects of melatonin on sleep induction. First, it was hypothesized that melatonin does not affect sleep directly but affects the oscillator regulating the sleep-wake cycle. Second, it was hypothesized that melatonin induces sleep by reducing body temperature. And thirdly, it is also possible that melatonin affects sleep directly by influencing the brain's sleep structure directly.

KH: *Can melatonin help with sleep in different times of the day?*

PL: Yes indeed. We believe that melatonin efficacy as a hypnotic is maximal when circulating levels of endogenous melatonin are low. Thus, we showed that melatonin exerted hypnotic effects when it was administered at 12 noon, 5:00 p.m. and 7:00 p.m., but less so when it was administered at 9:00 p.m. (Tzischinsky and Lavie, "Melatonin Possesses Time-Dependent Hypnotic Effects," <u>Sleep</u>, 1994;17:638-645.); and it ameliorated insomnia in melatonin deficient elderly people (Haimov, et al, "Sleep Disorders and Melatonin Rhythms in Elderly People," <u>British Medical Journal</u>, 1994;309:167).

KH: *How specifically can melatonin can be used clinically?*

PL: Since we believe that melatonin exerts hypnotic effects primarily when its circulating endogenous levels are low, it should be used either to help with day sleep (shift workers, napping behavior) or in patients with deficient levels of melatonin (aged individuals) or abnormally phased melatonin rhythms (patients with sleep phase delay syndrome). Travelers crossing multiple time zones in the westward direction go to sleep at their new destination very late relative to their normal bedtime or very early if they fly eastward. At these times, endogenous levels of melatonin are low, and therefore exogenous melatonin may be beneficial. In such cases, melatonin also may be helpful in entraining the sleep-wake oscillator to the new time zones.

KH: *How important are levels of melatonin for the success of melatonin supplementation?*

PL: We found that either 5 mg, 3 mg, 2 mg or 1 mg administered as slow release preparations exerted hypnotic effects. We don't believe that there is a need for higher doses.

KH: *Do you think melatonin will be utilized in the future more frequently for sleep disorders?*

PL: More information on the long term effects of melatonin should be obtained before melatonin is recommended for routine treatment of sleep disorders. This is important because of the possible effects of melatonin on reproductive organs. Once its safety is demonstrated, melatonin will widely be used to treat insomnia in a variety of conditions associated with low levels of melatonin.

KH: *I have been told that melatonin is an excellent antioxidant. In fact, it is the most effective that is currently available. Do you have any knowledge of melatonin's antioxidant capability?*

PL: Indeed there is evidence that melatonin possesses antioxidant effects. However, it is still uncertain whether it is better than other types of antioxidants. As I mentioned before, we have yet to establish its long-term effects. ◆

Natural Family Planning in The 1990's

Robert Ryder, M.D.
Department of Endocrinology
City Hospital, NHS Trust
Dudley Road
Birmingham B18 7QH, United Kingdom
441 121 554 3801 / 441 121 507 4595 (FAX)

"Natural Family Planning in the 1990s", The Lancet, 1995;343:233-234. #22901

Kirk Hamilton: *Can you please share with me your educational background and current position?*

Robert Ryder: I was born and brought up in Birmingham and studied medicine at the University of Wales College of Medicine where I graduated in 1977. I pursued hospital medicine in South Wales until 1986 when I moved to Sheffield and then to the City Hospital, Dudley Road, Birmingham, as a consultant physician with an interest in endocrinology in 1991. I have held this position until the present time.

KH: *When did you get interested in natural family planning?*

RR: I am the eldest of 9 children born to Roman Catholic parents who used the old rhythm and temperature methods of natural family planning (NFP) and was therefore interested in the subject from a young age. I heard about the discovery of the cervical mucus symptoms of ovulation in the mid 1970's and immediately recognized their importance and was staggered at the complete ignorance about them in the medical and lay communities and especially in the Catholic Church. In 1976 I visited Calcutta as a medical student and found Mother Teresa's sisters teaching NFP to huge numbers of Calcutta slum dwellers with remarkable success - a pregnancy rate approaching zero. I collected and publicized this information locally on my return to the United Kingdom and the facts were later formerly studied and published in the Journal of Obstetrics and Gynecology of India in 1982 by the Professor of Obstetrics and Gynecology in Calcutta, Professor A.K. Ghosh. In 1979 I married, and my wife and I have used modern natural family planning (NFP) throughout our married life. We have 2 planned children contrasting starkly with my parent's experience using the older methods of NFP. In the mid 1980's ultrasonography became readily available as a means of identifying the exact time of ovulation and I led studies to compare the identification of ovulation using the symptoms with actual ovulation as shown on ultrasound. The study was published in the British Medical Journal in 1986 and it showed that cervical mucus symptoms identified ovulation very precisely. I have always kept track of the developments in NFP and at the time of the Earth Summit in Rio de Janeiro was particularly aware from the media coverage that the world, both medical and lay, still remained ignorant of the effectiveness of modern natural family planning or NFP. In view of this I published an article in the British Medical Journal in September of 1993 which chronicled the success of the story of modern NFP. It was followed by the biggest mail bag that the journal has ever had on a single subject with letters published in October and November and a statement by the editor of the BMJ in the November issue, stating he had changed what may have been a prejudice on his part against NFP. An article by myself and Professor Hubert Campbell in the Lancet of this year brought the data up to date in the mid-1990's.

KH: *Define the term natural family planning and differentiate, please, from the rhythm or abstinence method?*

RR: It is currently thought that the ovum is only capable of being fertilized for less than 10 hours after ovulation. Sperm can be nurtured in fertile mucus for about 5 days. So there are only a few days in each cycle during which conception can occur. Natural family planning attempts to identify the natural infertile and fertile times of the cycle so that these can be used for avoiding or achieving pregnancy according to need. The rhythm method was the earliest form of natural family planning and it used calendar calculations to identify these times. It was not a reliable way of avoiding pregnancy for many women and led to many prejudices against NFP which still exist today. The rhythm method is, however, about 30 years out of date.

KH: *Explain the changes in cervical mucus from the infertile phase to the fertile phase?*

RR: After menstruation there are a variable number of "dry days" during which there is little or no cervical mucus secretion. As the level of estrogen in the blood rises prior to ovulation a cervical mucus secretion appears and increases, changing in character, until at the time of ovulation there is an abundant discharge of the mucus which appears like "raw egg white". This is fertile mucus. With the rise in the hormone progesterone, immediately after ovulation, this fertile-type mucus disappears and there is little or no cervical mucus. The mucus at this time is usually cloudy, thick and non-stretchy. The last day of stretchy mucus with the characteristics of "raw egg white" is termed the day of peak symptoms which is a very precise marker of the time of ovulation. In the Billings method of NFP, the disappearance of dryness and onset of the fertile mucus symptoms prior to ovulation marks the end of the preovulatory infertile phase and the postovulatory infertile phase commences on the 4th day after the peak symptom.

KH: *What is the role of basal temperature in natural family planning?*

RR: In my opinion, the cervical mucus symptoms are by far the most important indicators of fertility and for most people are all that would actually be required for a highly effective form of birth control for achieving and avoiding pregnancy. There are millions of couples around the world using the Billings method or ovulation method which is the natural family planning method that uses cervical mucus symptoms only. However, there are also many users of natural family planning who feel more secure using other indicators of fertility in combination with the mucus symptoms. This has lead to the "symptothermal" method of natural family planning in which other indicators of fertility are taken into account including basal temperature. In a normal cycle, the basal temperature rises a day or two after ovulation reflecting the rise in progesterone that follows ovulation.

KH: Are there other changes which can be noted during fertility such as changes in the actual cervix?

RR: Some women experience a particular type of pelvic pain and pressure at the time of ovulation which they use as an additional indicator. During the infertile parts of the cycle the cervix is low in the vagina and closed whereas at ovulation it is high and open. Many feel that observation of this sign is unnecessary for effective NFP but some women do use it and find it a helpful adjunct to other signs of fertility. Followers of the Billings method feel that the cervical palpation is not only unnecessary but are concerned that the cervix, with its essential functions, should not be disturbed in this way.

KH: Can natural family planning be taught in under developed countries?

RR: Many studies have shown that natural family planning is as effective in the developing world as the developed. The World Health Organization undertook a major investigation in the 1970s to see to what extent women worldwide could identify their fertile and infertile times by cervical mucus observation. They found that regardless of culture and education 93% of the women could identify their ovulation symptoms in the first cycle of observation and indeed nearly half of the El Salvador Study were illiterate and yet able to recognize the mucus symptoms. It is now felt that virtually 100% of fertile women can recognize their fertility through mucus symptom observation. The potential effectiveness of natural family planning in the developing world has been highlighted by the study I have already mentioned of nearly 20,000 slum dwellers in Calcutta, 52% Hindu, 27% Moslem and 21% Christian. These extremely poor women were nevertheless highly motivated to avoid pregnancy and were taught by a considerable number of well trained and highly dedicated teachers of natural family planning. The pregnancy rate was .2 pregnancies per 100 women users yearly which is similar to that ascribed to the combined oral contraceptive pill taken by motivated users.

KH: In those who practice natural family planning fully is the period of abstinence something that is detrimental to the relationship or an enhancement?

RR: It is usually assumed that periods of abstinence associated with NFP will have, if anything, a detrimental effect on the marital relationship and the family. Some have even suggested that the abstinence is unnatural. By contrast, after its advent, many expected that the widespread availability of the oral contraceptive pill would be a step forward, improving the situation for marriages, families, couples and their children. In fact, the increasing use of the pill has been contemporaneous with a massive increase in marital and family breakdown. While this temporal association does not prove a link, it is certainly noteworthy that the advent of the contraceptive pill has not produced the expected improvement for marriages and families. In this context, Billings himself comments that the demand associated with artificial contraception for "uninterrupted availability of sexual intercourse . . . is an unrealistic expectation of any marriage and sets the course for the breakdown of the marriage".

Understanding and cooperation are necessary for natural family planning to work but also for relationships to work. Many experienced in the field report that NFP fosters marital harmony and that the mutual discipline enhances the relationship. Women in

particular, report that the times of avoidance of sexual intercourse can lead to the expression of non-genital physical love which is longed for and helps their sexual responsiveness. It has been suggested that the monthly "honeymoon" at the time of resumption after the fertile phase, provides benefits in the sexual relationship.

KH: Could natural family planning improve the capabilities of individuals to achieve pregnancy?

RR: As I have already mentioned, studies using ultrasound technology to identify ovulation have demonstrated that the peak of mucus symptom identifies ovulation with considerable precision. The time leading up to the peak symptoms is characterized by a variable number of days in which the highly fertile "egg white" mucus is seen. The chemical structure of this mucus and the nutrients contained within it are highly favorable to sperm survival. The mucus has several components, some of which it is thought, weed out poor quality sperm, allowing the highest quality sperm to be transported to the upper part of the cervix where they are stored ready to be released at the time of ovulation. Other factors in the mucus appearing at the time of ovulation release the sperm and facilitate their rapid passage towards the ovum so that conception can occur. Thus, fertile type mucus not only indicates ovulation but is also an essential component of fertility. Thus, for sub-fertile couples having difficulty with conception, the observation of cervical mucus can be used to identify the most fertile times so that intercourse can be timed to maximize the chances of conception.

KH: What kind of pregnancy rates, per 100 women years, have been achieved with committed individuals using natural family planning?

RR: In the article in the Lancet in July of 1995 on the subject, we gave the figures for the 11 studies of natural family planning so far published in the 1990s. The figures were:

United Kingdom 2.7
Indonesia 2.5
Indonesia 10.3
India 2
Germany 2.3
Liberia 4.3
Zambia 8.9
Europe 2.4
Europe 10.6
China 4.4
Belgium 1.7

These figures reflect studies from around the world, in both developed and developing countries, and Moslem, Hindu, Chinese and Christian cultures. They can be compared with pregnancy rates for artificial contraceptive methods in well-motivated couples which are said to be from .18 to 3.6. It should be remembered, however, that studies of artificial contraceptive methods in less well-motivated couples readily give much higher numbers and there are studies with pregnancy rates greater than 20. It is also worth pointing out that of the figures that I have given, the 3 studies with pregnancy rates greater than 5 were all of atypical methods of natural family planning and all the studies of standard Billings or symptothermal methods of natural family planning gave pregnancy rates less than 5. Thus, the pregnancy rates for the natural family planning so far reported in the 1990's are similar to those ascribed to artificial contraceptive methods in well-motivated couples.

KH: What in your mind would be the benefits of natural family planning if practiced on a large scale in both the developed and underdeveloped world for society as a whole?

RR: In view of the points already made, there is potential for improvement in marital relationships and perhaps less marital breakdown. The side effects of artificial contraceptives would be avoided and I believe there would be less post-pill infertility.

KH: Do you think all women should know the fundamentals of natural family planning regardless of whether they choose artificial methods or not?

RR: In view of the fact that the signs of fertility are so easily recognized by all fertile women, I never cease to be amazed by the fact that it seems only a minority of the women are provided the simple fundamental information that would give them such a power over their fertility both for achieving and avoiding conception. To me it is self-evident that the basic information about their fertility and the signs of it should be brought to the attention of all women. They would also receive the knowledge that observations of the signs of their own fertility can lead to a highly effective form of birth control and then, if they choose not to use natural family planning, they will at least have made an informed choice, rather than choosing artificial contraceptives in complete ignorance. I find that there is a considerable bias against natural family planning based on misinformation and prejudice that developed at the time when natural family planning was the "rhythm method". A major misconception that developed at the time was that natural family planning could not be used by women with irregular cycles. As the cervical mucus symptoms only occur at the time of ovulation, modern natural family planning using cervical and symptothermal observation is as effective in women with irregular cycles as in women with regular cycles. If a cycle is long and the ovulation occurs late, the mucus symptom appears late. If the cycle is short and the ovulation occurs early, the mucus symptoms appear early.

KH: Is natural family planning on the rise?

RR: It seems that the prejudices and mis-information that developed in the days of the "rhythm method" or "Roman roulette" are very deeply entrenched in society. Nevertheless, the truth about modern natural family planning is gradually percolating and there is no doubt that it is on the rise worldwide. Recent scares about the safety of the contraceptive pills have certainly increased the attractiveness of natural methods. ◆

Neural Tube Defects, Homocysteine, Folic acid and Vitamin B12

James L. Mills, M.D.
National Institutes of Health
Pediatric Epidemiology Section
Epidemiology Branch, DESPR, NICHD
6100 Executive Blvd., Room 7B03
Bethesda, MD 20892 U.S.A.
(301) 496-5064 / (301) 402-2084 (FAX)

"Homocysteine Metabolism in Pregnancies Complicated by Neural-Tube Defects,"
The Lancet, January 21, 1995;345:149-51. #21660

Kirk Hamilton: *Thank you very much for being here and your interest. Could you please share with me your educational background since college and your present position?*

James Mills: I have a master's degree in epidemiology and I am board certified in pediatrics and pediatric endocrinology.

KH: *And what is your present position?*

JM: I am the chief of the Pediatric Epidemiology section at The National Institute of Child Health and Human Development at The National Institutes of Health.

KH: *When did you get interested in homocysteine and then, subsequently, the thought of homocysteine as a risk factor for neural tube defects?*

JM: I became interested in neural tube defects at least 10 years ago when the first evidence started to appear that vitamins might be protective against neural tube defects. After doing some initial work which did not support the vitamin hypothesis, I became even more interested. Then eventually as the evidence accumulated that folate was important in preventing neural tube defects, I decided to look into the mechanism by which folate could work. It was then that we set up a study with The Health Research Board in Ireland and Trinity College in Dublin to look at specific metabolic pathways. We were very fortunate because they had just done a major study in Dublin where they collected blood on pregnant women. After the pregnancy outcomes were known, they went back and pulled out the specimens from the women who had neural tube defects and started measuring vitamin levels. The reason we were fortunate is that they found that not only was folate associated with neural tube defects, but it looked as if B12 was independently a risk factor for neural tube defects.

KH: *Was the B12 measurement just from blood levels?*

JM: That's right. In other words, they took the blood samples during the pregnancies, and then they measured the B12 and the folate after the pregnancies were over and found that B12 levels were significantly lower in the women who had offspring with neural tube defects.

KH: *And homocysteine might even be that much more prognostic or sensitive for assessing vitamin B12 levels...*

JM: That's right. But the importance, at that stage, was that up until that point nobody had any clues as to why folate worked or why folate was related to neural tube defects. Some people thought that women who had children with neural tube defects were folate deficient. Other people thought that they didn't absorb folate very well. Other people thought that there might be some metabolic abnormality. So the B12 story was an important clue that suggested that maybe it was the interaction between folate and B12 that was the critical factor. *There was only one place in the human where folate and B12 interacted and that was in the enzyme methionine synthase, which as you know, is the enzyme that converts homocysteine to methionine.* So, that gave us a very strong indication as to where to look. On top of that, we knew that these women were not folate deficient nor were they B12 deficient. So we knew it wasn't simply a case of women who were generally undernourished or generally had poor nutrition who have the neural tube defects. Most of the women in this study had perfectly normal levels of B12 and perfectly normal levels of folate. They were just in the lower range of normal.

KH: *What study was this?*

JM: This is the study that they did in Ireland before we became involved. The study told us that (a) this is not just a nutritional deficiency, and (b) it seems to be something that relates to both folate and B12. That probably means the methionine synthase enzyme and homocysteine evaluation. That is when we got involved and decided to focus on that one pathway. The results of the study, as you know, were first of all to rule out that it was just a generalized B12 problem. Because when we looked at the other major indicator of B12 activity, which is methylmalonic acid levels, they were normal and they were essentially the same in the women who had NTD offspring as they were in the women who had unaffected offspring. So we were able to exclude a B12 problem as a generalized B12 deficiency or B12 metabolic problem by showing that the methylmalonic acid (MMA) levels were normal. But we did find that the homocysteine levels were significantly higher in the women who had the NTD offspring.

KH: *Could you just backtrack a little bit and describe the amount of people in your study and exactly what you measured for?*

JM: We had 81 mothers who had infants with neural tube defects. After we supplemented the control group, for reasons I can go into later, we had 323 normal control women. As I mentioned, in this part of the study that was published recently in the Lancet, we measured MMA, controlling for B12, because if you have a low B12, you have a high MMA regardless of whether the enzymes are functioning normally. So after we matched for B12, we found that the MMA levels were no different between the mothers whose offspring had the NTDs and the controls. Then we measured homocysteine. Again, we matched for B12 levels because if you have a low B12, you can have a high homocysteine level regardless of the status of the enzyme. So the basic finding was that after you adjust for the B12 differences between the cases and controls, you still see significantly higher homocysteine levels in the cases.

KH: *Why wouldn't you just say that it is a folic acid problem strictly?*

JM: Well, it may be in the sense that folic acid is one of the critical factors in the metabolism of homocysteine. One of the major pathways for getting rid of homocysteine is using 5-methyltetrahydrofolate to methylate homocysteine, and then homocysteine becomes methionine. So folic acid is very, very important in that reaction. However, we also think that the B12 is important because of the fact that these women had significantly lower B12.

KH: *Lower normal levels?*

JM: That's right. Lower normal. Now that would be unusual in a typical population because once you have an adequate level of B12 in the average person it doesn't make very much difference if you add more B12. You basically need a certain amount to make that reaction go. But when we're looking at our women who had neural tube defects, it appeared that as B12 levels went up, the risk for having a neural tube defect went down well beyond the deficiency range. So that suggested that there may be a population out there that is at risk for neural tube defects because they need more B12.

KH: *They have a "sluggish" enzyme or something?*

JM: That's right. That is one of the things that is very intriguing about our study. There may be a group that can stimulate methionine synthase either with folic acid or B12. Of course the importance of that would be that if the B12 can help, then it may cut down the amount of folic acid that is needed.

KH: *Exactly! Tell me, you didn't happen to measure cystathionine synthase activity or B6 at all in this study?*

JM: No, we haven't. We may do that. We're discussing that now. We were very focused on the methionine synthase finding because of the B12 findings, and B12 of course is not involved in cystathionine synthase. But we are considering measuring B6 and possibly cystathionine synthase activity in some way also.

KH: *You know, it seems like a possibility that maybe lower doses of all 3 or some of the other synergistic nutrients might take the place of a very high dose of folate.*

JM: Right. And of course that would depend on what the real mechanism is. You know, we haven't really discussed that. But one possibility is that homocysteine is toxic and homocysteine's build up is causing damage to the embryo. In which case, as you say, having a more efficient cystathionine synthase might also be a way of preventing the problem. The other possibility is that it is a lack of the end product of the homocysteine-methionine reaction that is causing the problem.

KH: *So lack of methionine?*

JM: That's right. Because that is an extremely important reaction for producing methyl groups. There are a large number of

reactions that require the methyl groups. It is quite possible that it is not an excess of homocysteine but a deficiency of methionine that is really the culprit.

KH: *So is there another trial pending with methionine supplementation?*

JM: Actually there are people who would like very much to do methionine supplementation trials, but I don't think that is very cost effective or practical.

KH: *It would be so much more simple to just bump up the B vitamins a little bit.*

JM: You know what is interesting about this and different from what's going on in cardiovascular disease and cancer is those specialists think that homocysteine is important, but they don't know if homocysteine lowering therapy is going to reduce the incidence of those diseases. However, we know there is a therapy that works. We're trying to find out why it works and whether homocysteine is the critical factor.

KH: *I have seen homocysteine levels elevated in my searches in a variety of female health problems such as recurrent aborters (miscarriages), abruptio placenta, neural tube defects and also even with cancer possibly. Folic acid levels have been lower in cervical tissue and thereby may increase the susceptibility to the human papilloma virus. So I can see a day, if in fact lowering homocysteine has this clinical benefit, of homocysteine being a screen in a gynecologic and obstetric practices.*

JM: That's right. It could also be good for a lot of different conditions (cardiovascular disease, neuropsychiatric disorders, etc.).

KH: *Well, it might explain in part why many of these B12 injections or B12/folate combination injections had clinical benefit even though blood levels were low normal.*

JM: It is interesting that homocysteine levels tend to rise in older people, particularly in really elderly people. There again, it remains to be shown whether that is a result of general nutritional problems, or whether there is something specifically toxic about homocysteine or abnormal homocysteine chemistry, that is causing some kind of pathology.

KH: *As you get older, atrophic gastritis and the malabsorption of B12 becomes more of a problem. Are there any other conditions that you can see in either gynecology or pediatric medicine where a screen for homocysteine may be of benefit?*

JM: This is very, very speculative, but there is a suggestion that there may be other birth defects that are related to vitamins and possibly to folate in particular. This is very preliminary, and I don't even know that statistically you could make a good case for it at this stage at all. But in Hungary where Czeizel conducted the vitamin trial in the normal population (this is the trial that did not take women who had already had a child with a neural tube defect), he reported a lower rate of other birth defects, as well as neural tube defects, in the women who received the vitamin supplements. So there is a suggestion, but I think it is a very, very preliminary finding, that there may be some other defect(s) out there, particularly heart defects, that could benefit from folate supplementation.

KH: *Both B12 and folate are important in DNA synthesis. Could that be how it is involved in so many of those . . .*

JM: There are a tremendous number of reactions for which folate is key, and in fact in neural tube defects, generating myelin is one of them. So it is easy to find things where folate is important. The question is trying to figure out which of the many, many reactions is the important reaction.

KH: *If it was shown that when you lowered homocysteine with either B12 or folate that prenatals have enough folate, 400 - 800 mcg, might not you want to bump up the B12 a little bit, let's say in the average basic multiple? Would that seem reasonable?*

JM: I don't know. I think we're a long away from that kind of a decision yet. I haven't seen the literature on how much B12 you need to raise red cell folate to the upper range of normal which is about the only connection we can make so far between ingested vitamins and the biochemical effects in the body.

KH: *Well, Ubbink, et al, showed this in the American Journal of Clinical Nutrition, 1993:57;47-53. They took people who had subtle elevations of homocysteine and gave them 10 mg of vitamin B6, .4 mg of B12 and 1 mg of folic acid which lowered homocysteine levels.*

JM: I don't know about B6, but that is pretty high for the other two. In the Public Health Service Working Group that has been looking at strategies for actually getting folic acid to the women at risk, we have been concerned about levels of folic acid over 1 mg. So that would be a pretty high dose for the average person.

KH: *Why would you be concerned?*

JM: Because there is really no information available on the safety of that dose.

KH: *You mean chronic, long term supplementation?*

JM: Particularly chronic, long term therapy. But there is always the question of masking B12 deficiency and since that was never studied systematically for obvious ethical reasons, no one knows quite what the dose is that starts to mask B12 deficiency anemia. So 1 mg of folate was considered by most of the people in the Public Health Service Group to be about as much as one would want to feel comfortable receiving. And that is controversial because it is based on guessing rather than on any good studies. There aren't any good studies. One of the things that we were talking about in the Public Health Service was food fortification. When you fortify food, that means everybody gets it and they get it every day. We just don't have the kind of information to say, for example, that it is absolutely safe for a child to get 500 mcg of B12 every day for the next 50 years or 1 mg of folate every day. So that was more the level of concern. I don't think there are any studies that say if you take a milligram of folate for the next month you're going to drop dead. You know, that is hardly likely to happen and hardly the kind of toxicity that we would be concerned about. It is really the lack of good long term exposure data on high doses.

KH: *You bring out the age old question if you have got to do a 20-year study to be absolutely definitive in recommending a nutritional substance, more than likely a lot of people are going to suffer . . .*

JM: Actually, we have looked at that very carefully and I have even written some things about that. If you estimate how many people are going to have neural tube defects who would not have them, even if they got optimal doses of folic acid, you can come up with a pretty good estimate and that is about 2,000 people in the U.S. per year. If you gave high doses of folic acid in food and reached the absolute optimum level in all the women who might get pregnant, you would be exposing at least 1 or 2 million people to high doses of folic acid every year. So the risk of any toxicity of folic acid could be far greater than the number of neural tube defects you would be preventing. We have considered that pretty carefully. I think you have to be cautious because you're talking about a starting population of 250 million people taking folic acid if you do food fortification.

KH: *It sounds a lot easier to eat a lot of fruits and vegetables.*

JM: That's exactly it. I have been in Europe and talked to experts there about this and in several countries. They said, "We wouldn't even consider fortifying food because most pregnancies are planned. If we tell them to start taking folic acid tablets before they get pregnant, we think there is a good chance they'll do it." In the U.S., as you probably know, most pregnancies are not planned, and I suspect that most women are not going to get the message to take the folic acid tablets. It is unfortunate because that would clearly be the best solution.

KH: *Is there any generalized public recommendation that you can make from your experience looking at folic acid, vitamin B12 and homocysteine metabolism?*

JM: Right now, because we think methionine synthase and clearly homocysteine is important, the current recommendation made by the Public Health Service is an excellent one. That is that any woman at risk of getting pregnant should take 400 mcg of folic acid a day. We think that should cover people adequately to reduce the risk and still be safe. If women take a good level of vitamin B12 in their diet or take a standard supplement that contains B12, then that might even be improving their chances. But I think that their outcome should be very, very good with the current recommendation for folic acid. ◆

Neuropsychological Functioning, Elderly and Walking

Tsunehisa Satoh, M.D.
Associate Professor
Second Department of Physiology
St. Marianna University School of Medicine
2-16-1 Sugao
Miyamae-Ku, Kawasaki 216, Japan

"Walking Exercise and Improved Neuropsychological Functioning in Elderly Patients With Cardiac Disease," Journal of Internal Medicine, 1995;238:423-428. #23627

Kirk Hamilton: Could you please share with me your educational background and current position?

Tsunehisa Satoh: I studied as a cardiologist at the First Department of Internal Medicine, St. Marianna University School of Medicine. I am presently a professor at St. Marianna University.

KH: When did you get interested in the role of exercise and neuropsychological functioning?

TS: For about 20 years I have treated a significant amount of patients who complained of cardiac diseases. Many of them, especially elderly patients with acute myocardial infarction, often had experienced a gradual decline in their central nervous system function. But some of them improved with exercise through walking.

KH: What parameters can exercise improve in the neuropsychological performance of the elderly?

TS: By walking the elderly can improve their memory scale published by Hasegawa's dementia score (a modification of the Wechsler memory scale) and the areas of morphological brain atrophy by CT scanning.

KH: Do patients have to be demented to show improvement in those areas or can any elderly subject show improvement in memory and mental activity?

TS: We can estimate not only demented individuals but normal individuals about mental activities by means of the Hasegawa's dementia score.

KH: How much does a person have to exercise to improve their mental function?

TS: To improve the mental activity it is necessary to walk over 1,000 steps a day.

KH: How does exercise improve mental function? What physiologic things occur?

TS: I suspect that walking exercise promoted cerebral metabolic activity in those senile patients who walked over 1000 steps per day. This results in an increase in various neurotransmitters and high energy phosphate compounds.

KH: Is there ever an age where it is too late to start exercising to improve cognitive function?

TS: No there is not. If a individual can walk, they can participate in exercising to improve their cognitive function.

KH: Are there other types of aerobic exercise or other types of techniques such as Tai Chi that can improve the neuropsychological functioning in the elderly?

TS: Tai Chi is definitely good for improving the neuropsychological functioning in the elderly. ♦

Oral Cancer and Beta-Carotene

Harinder S. Garewal, M.D., Ph.D.

Arizona Cancer Center/College of Medicine
Assistant Director of Cancer Prevention and Control Program
1515 N. Campbell Avenue
Tucson, AZ 85724 U.S.A.
(520) 792-1450 ext. 6410 / (520) 629-1861 (FAX)

"Emerging Role of Beta-Carotene and Antioxidant Nutrients in the Prevention of Oral Cancer",
Archives of Otolaryngology--Head and Neck Surgery, February 1995;121:141-144. #22181

Kirk Hamilton: *Can you please share with us your educational background and current position?*

Harinder Garewal: I received my B.S. at St. Xavier's College in India, my Ph.D. in biochemistry from McGill University in Montreal, Canada and my M.D. from Harvard Medical School. I completed my residency at the University of Oregon Health Sciences Center and did a hematology/oncology fellowship at the University of Arizona Health Science Center. Currently, I am a professor of medicine in the sections of Hematology/Oncology & Gastroenterology at the Tucson VA Medical Center and the University of Arizona. I am also the assistant director of Cancer Prevention and Control at the Tucson VA Medical Center and the Arizona Cancer Center. I am board certified in hematology, oncology and internal medicine.

KH: *How did you get interested in the role of antioxidants and cancer and specifically the oral cavity?*

HG: I trained as an internal medicine specialist with further training in medical oncology and cancer treatment. My interest in cancer prevention developed over the years as part of an overall approach to cancer. Clearly, as is with any chronic disease, final control of this problem will depend on prevention. My interest in cancer prevention is wide, covering organs such as the colon and lung, as well as oral cavity cancer. Oral cavity cancer is an important health problem as described below and is a fascinating model for disease caused by known etiologies such as tobacco use and diet. My interest in nutritional agents is derived from initial work with vitamin A-related compounds, known as retinoids. The best known of these is Accutane or 13-*cis*-retinoic acid. These compounds can inhibit oral cancer but are simply too toxic to use for preventive purposes. Compounds such as vitamin E and beta-carotene, which exist in nature, had similar activity against oral cavity cancer in many model systems. Being non-toxic, these appeared ideal to test for prevention and therefore my interest in this subject.

KH: *What are the major risk factors for oral cancer?*

HG: The major lifestyle factors for oral cancer relate to tobacco use. In some countries tobacco, usually mixed with other products, is chewed. This is the main cause of this disease, especially in countries where oral cavity cancer is one of the most frequent cancers. Examples would be many Asian countries. Similarly, smoking tobacco is a risk factor. Alcohol use is another risk factor, which is synergistic with tobacco use. Tobacco and alcohol account for the majority of oral cavity cancers. Approximately 10% of this disease occurs in subjects without any known risk factors.

KH: *What is the prevalence of oral cancer?*

HG: Oral cavity cancer is a very common problem on a worldwide scale. It is the sixth most frequent cancer and there are parts of the world where it is the leading cancer. In the United States, there are approximately 30,000-40,000 cases per year, which puts it in the same category as ovarian cancer, leukemias, etc. In addition to mortality, which is approximately 10,000-12,000 cases per year in the United States, this disease is very morbid in that the disease and its treatment result in severe cosmetic effects that are difficult for the patient to "cover up." Furthermore, loss of functions such as swallowing or talking, which can result from removal of the larynx or other organs by surgery, can be a very psychologically distressing situation. Thus, depression and suicide are very frequent in patients even if they are cured of the oral cancer.

KH: *How do antioxidants theoretically help in cancer prevention?*

HG: Many mechanisms have been postulated for antioxidant action including free radical scavenging, immune function stimulation, etc. At this time the precise mechanism remains unknown.

KH: *Is there evidence that antioxidants can prevent disease?*

HG: Yes, although most such data currently are with beta-carotene, vitamin E is gaining increasing attention and may turn out to be the most important antioxidant for disease prevention in general. There are several theoretical reasons for this which are difficult to go into in a brief interview. One of the primary ones, in my opinion, is the difficulty in obtaining high levels of vitamin E intake via diet manipulation alone.

KH: *What are the dose levels of antioxidants needed and how toxic are they?*

HG: We have not paid close attention to the minimum doses needed for antioxidants simply because of their known lack of toxicity. Doses of beta-carotene used in clinical trials have ranged from 15 mg (25,000 units) to 180 mg daily. All these doses lead to substantial increases in plasma levels and have proven to be safe. For vitamin E, the doses used in clinical trials have usually ranged from 50 to 800 I.U. per day. Once again, because of lack of toxicity there have been no attempts to try to identify the minimum dose needed. Information from epidemiologic studies in heart disease suggests that a vitamin E intake greater than 100 I.U. per day is necessary.

KH: *What needs to be done to clarify the role of antioxidants in oral cancer?*

HG: As I have stressed recently, the perfect, placebo-controlled, blinded, randomized trial in the right population with oral cancer as the endpoint is just not possible because of logistical and practical reasons. Thus, since such direct proof will never be obtainable, we must continue to add to the numerous other indirect lines of evidence. For example, in the clinical trials arena, one could consider doing a blinded, randomized study with vitamin E versus placebo in oral leukoplakia. As I have written before, it is difficult to do a blinded study with beta-carotene because of easy recognition of the intervention arm. It also would be important to confirm results by Stich, et al, who did studies in India where the disease is very prevalent - confirmatory studies in which populations would be of great interest. Finally, another area where clinical trials are feasible includes prevention of second malignancies in patients who are cured of an initial head and neck cancer. These occur at a rate of 3%-5% per year, representing a population at high risk. In the U.S., we can only do one such study in the country at a time because these studies require approximately 1,000 subjects. Although I had initiated such a trial through the Southwest Oncology Group (SWOG), we discontinued that study at the request of other oncology groups. The reason was that there is an ongoing trial with Accutane in this setting, which has had problems with patient accrual. Opening our study was further affecting their accrual. Consequently, in the spirit of cooperating to complete clinical trials, we made a decision to have SWOG join the Accutane study and get it completed within the next couple of years. At that time, we will go ahead with our study, most likely using antioxidants. I should say that antioxidant studies in this situation are being conducted overseas, including a multi-center trial in Canada. ◆

Osteoarthritis and Glycosaminoglycan Polysulfuric Acid

Associate Professor Karel Pavelka, M.D., Ph.D.
Director of the Institute of Rheumatology Prague
Na slupi 4
128 50 Praha 2
Czech Republic
42 2 292452 / 42 2 24914451 (FAX)

"Glycosaminoglycan Polysulfuric Acid (GAGPS) in Osteoarthritis of the Knee,"
Osteoarthritis and Cartilage, 1995;3:15-23. #22891

Kirk Hamilton: *Can you please share with me your educational background and current position?*

Kavel Pavelka: I was trained as a physician, and I graduated from the Charles University of Prague in 1980. I specialized in internal medicine and rheumatology and received my Ph.D. in rheumatology. I am currently an associate professor of medicine at Charles University.

KH: *When did you get interested in the role of glycosaminoglycan polysulfuric acid (GAGPS) in the treatment of arthritis?*

KP: GAGPS has been tested in the Research Institute of Rheumatic Disease for many years both *in vivo* and *in vitro*. Clinical experience has been very positive with an acceptable frequency of side effects. There were two major goals to the studies cited above: 1. To prove the efficacy of a lower dose (25 mg/inj.) of GAGPS compared to the normal dose of (50 mg/inj.). 2. To perform the study according to new standards and the ILAR guidelines.

KH: *What is the presumed mechanism of action of GAGPS?*

KP: GAGPS has an inhibitory effect on different hydrolases, glycosidases and proteases (e.g. cathepsin Bl and elastase) which are involved in degradation of matrix. Similar inhibitory effects were demonstrated on metalloproteinases and serine proteinases. GAGPS also has shown anabolic action on chondrocytes through the stimulation of proteoglycan synthesis and collagen synthesis. GAGPS increases synovial fluid viscosity by increasing the amount of hyaluronic acid. GAGPS appears to preserve the anatomy of the cartilage in animal models of osteoarthritis both by microscopic examination and histology.

KH: *What was the protocol of your study?*

KP: The study was a 1 year double-blind, randomized, placebo-controlled parallel group study of 80 patients with osteoarthritis of the knee. The patients received 2 series of 5 intra-articular injections at 1 week intervals of 25 mg (.5 ml) of GAGPS into the knee or a placebo. The physician was blinded. Eighty patients with osteoarthritis of the knee (according to ACR criteria) with Kellgren stage II-III disease with symptoms were included. Those excluded were all with secondary osteoarthritis, inflammatory osteoarthritis, and severe disease such as those on steroids in the last 3 months. Concomitant therapy included ibuprofen 400 mg tablets. The primary parameter evaluated was the index of severity of knee osteoarthritis (ISK), and the secondary parameters were pain score, VAS, functional testing, physical examination, global assessment by the physician and patient, and ibuprofen consumption.

KH: *What were the results of your study?*

KP: The index of severity of knee osteoarthritis decreased after the end of the injection period by 34% from baseline, and this effect persisted to 26 weeks. The statistical significance compared to placebo was borderline at $P = 0.06$. The pain on the VAS decreased by 43% from baseline at week 6 and again was not statistically significant at $P = .16$. The same results were shown by other assessment criteria. The positive effects of GAGPS on pain and function were shown by all measured parameters even though the significance was only minor or not even significant. This can be explained by several reasons: 1. Not having an adequate number of patients. 2. Not finishing the second series of medications.

KH: *Can you take GAGPS orally?*

KP: GAGPS has never been tested orally in patients with chronic osteoarthritis. Some similar type drugs for the treatment of osteoarthritis are available in Europe. ◆

Osteoarthritis, Folate and Vitamin B12

Margaret A. Flynn, Ph.D., RD
University of Missouri-Columbia School of Medicine
M221 Department of Family & Community Medicine
1 Hospital Drive
Columbia, MO 65212 U.S.A.
(314) 882-2922 / (314) 882-9096 (FAX)

"The Effect of Folate and Cobalamin on Osteoarthritic Hands",
Journal of the American College of Nutrition 1994;13(4):351-356. #21184

Kirk Hamilton:　*What is your educational background?*

Margaret Flynn:　I received my bachelor's degree in clinical nutrition at the College of St. Catherine at St. Paul. Then I got a master's at the University of Iowa, Iowa City in which I also did a year residency in medical nutrition. Then, I was married and was perfectly happy with just the master's degree. I could teach in small nursing schools, etc. and we raised a family. After my husband died in 1960 I was raising a 4-year-old son and decided that if he was going to be able to get to college I better get moving and get an advanced degree which I did at the University of Missouri. I got the doctoral degree in 1966 and I have been busy clinically, teaching and doing research ever since. That's my life story.

KH:　*And your present position is?*

MF:　I am a professor at the University of Missouri Medical School and I am in the department of Family and Community Medicine. My role is teaching medical students, doing research and seeing patients.

KH:　*How did you get involved with the thought of folic acid, vitamin B12 and osteoarthritis?*

MF:　I was reading an article Carmel had written in which he had some people who were diagnosed as having pernicious anemia that were not doing well with their disease and he gave them a vitamin B12 injection. He found that in their blood, the osteocalcin, which is involved in building bone, suddenly increased in the blood after the injection. Pernicious anemia tends to occur mostly in older people and for years many family doctors have known that if the patient receives a vitamin B12 injection, the patient felt better all around. Now we're finding out that the combination of folic acid and vitamin B12 is increasingly involved in many things we were not even aware of, one of them, of course, being the red blood cell because the two vitamins work together in inducing the production of new red blood cells. Dr. Carmel also said one of his patients who was low in serum folate was being given the vitamin B12 injection and also had very good results. Vitamin B12 is necessary to induce the transformation of folic acid so that it can now become a single carbon carrier.

KH:　*With regards to osteoarthritis, how would these particular agents theoretically work?*

MF:　We don't know. This is the first time somebody has actually done a controlled study of osteoarthritis with the combinations of the 2 vitamins together or independently. We found that you need the 2 together in order to give the osteoarthritic people these changes that are very favorable to them.

KH:　*How did you choose the great disparity in dosage between folic acid and vitamin B12? You have 20 mcg of cobalamin and you have 6400 mcg of folic acid.*

MF:　The Recommended Dietary Allowance is 2 mcg of vitamin B12 and 400 mcg of folate. So already, we have that disparity.

KH:　*A 200-fold difference. Can you describe your study? What you did and what you found?*

MF:　When we decided to do this study, we had to get some money in order to be able to, first of all, buy the vitamins and secondly, to have the blood values done. The Wallace Genetic Foundation funded us because they have always looked to something that has to do with human genetics.   Then we had to find a rheumatologist who treats these kind of people and we have one here at the medical school. We asked some of his patients to volunteer and he decided that we had to restrict it to only one organ and that was the hand. If you start bringing in the osteoarthritis of the hip, knee, etc., then you get referred pain from all over and you wouldn't be able to really decide what is going on. It took us a while to acquire the 30 people that we started out with because some of them didn't want to give up their prescribed pain medicines. Some of the patients, because the therapy was prescribed by a rheumatologist who knew his business, were not reluctant to go on this 6-month study. We decided to use acetaminophen Tylenol for the pain medication. For the study to be well done, we had to give the vitamins independently, or together, or have a placebo. It was important that the pills they took looked the same and be the same size so that nobody would know what they were taking. We had a special person in the university pharmacy make up these different pills and only they knew what A, B or C pills were. They were the same color, and they were the same size. So it was only when we had finished the whole study (in which we finished with about 26 because some of them became ill during the winter and we had to take them off the study) that the pharmacist gave us the code and that is how we got our results. It was a double blind study.

KH:　*How long did it take to see benefit?*

MF:　They were on their pills 2 months each time. Every participant took each pill for 2 months during the 6 month study, going directly to the next treatment in that span of time.

KH:　*So it only took 2 months to see some benefit? And the benefits were?... A reduction in pain or were there other findings?*

MF: The one that was important to us was the grip. There is an actual instrument that measures the amount of grip these people have and if they are hurting, they are not going to be able to squeeze that bulb. So under these grip values, we knew then that they were improving. The same nurse measured the grip values, thus she was using the same degree of reading. She also then did all of the tender joint measurements so we could come up with the number of tender joints. She would look at the hand, look at the wrist and then each one of the knuckles. Then we asked them when they began feeling better and when they noticed worsening. Arthritis is very subjective. We had other measurements including blood values, food intake records and questionnaires. How did we know that they were taking the pills? Because they were doing this for the rheumatologist. This was their doctor. They wanted him to really know. So they would bring back the empty vial or whatever they did not take in the Tylenol or the treatment pills at end of each treatment. When they switched to a new treatment, we gave them a new bunch of everything. From what they brought back, we could count and we would know how much they were taking.

KH: So, in short, the folic acid alone didn't do anything. The placebo didn't do anything and the folic acid at 6400 mcg and 20 mcg of cobalamin had those positive effects? Was there a reduction in the Tylenol use in the treatment group?

MF: Yes, when they were taking the combined folic acid and B12 capsule.

KH: Was there a response within a week or could you ever delineate that?

MF: No, one week is not representative because osteoarthritics are subject to changes such as stress, weather, hand activity in work, etc. In the report, we state that we wanted to know if people were having better effects during the summer months when they were taking treatment as compared to the winter months. It really did not seem to make that much difference. We also had data as to whether in the 6 months there were any family problems that would arouse stress in these people. In osteoarthritis, patients feel worse when under stress whether it is personal stress, a disease, or your family. We also looked at whether the people with arthritis could tell you if there was a "storm coming". We did not see much of that. But who knows?

KH: So vitamin B12 and folate together were as good as . . .

MF: Were just as good as the NSAIDS.

KH: Were vitamin B12 and folate minus the Tylenol ever as good as the NSAIDS?

MF: No. We couldn't do that to them because when you have people that are in pain, you can't remove medication because then they are going to hurt and the total person is not going to give you the subjective thing that you're looking for (improved grip pain, etc.).

KH: But the people in the treatment group, which had both, reduced their Tylenol intake?

MF: Yes.

KH: So theoretically they got to a point where they had more vitamin B12 and folic acid with the same benefit as with the NSAIDS?

MF: Yes, and Tylenol is much cheaper than NSAIDS and doesn't really have any side effects if you're taking a reasonable amount. NSAIDS have frightfully bad side effects.

KH: So here we have a fairly expensive model for a chronic disease (osteoarthritis treated with NSAIDs) in the United States and if this pans out, you have created a model where we could treat osteoarthritis a lot cheaper?

MF: Yes. Most definitely.

KH: And that is the bottom line with health care reform.

MF: Absolutely.

KH: If you've read Drs. Carmel's and Lindenbaum's work, you know they look at methylmalonic acid and homocysteine as functional ways to assess vitamin B12 and folic acid. Is there a way to correlate people that have a tendency towards a better response if they had subtly elevated homocysteine and methylmalonic acid?

MF: As a matter of fact, we are right in the middle of doing a homocysteine, folate, vitamin B12 and vitamin B6 study on a different group of people. That group is my aging study in people who do have the higher homocysteine. ◆

Osteopenia and Premature Graying Hair

Clifford J. Rosen, M.D.
Maine Center For Osteoporosis Research & Education
360 Broadway
Bangor, Maine 04401 U.S.A.
(207) 942 2608 / (207) 942 4101 (FAX)

"Premature Graying of Hair is a Risk Factor for Osteopenia",
Journal of Clinical Endocrinology and Metabolism, 1994;79(3):854-857. #21006

Kirk Hamilton: *Dr. Rosen could you start off by telling me a little bit about your educational background and what your present position is?*

Clifford Rosen: I received my undergraduate degree from the University of Maine in biochemistry. I went to SUNY at Syracuse Medical School for my undergraduate medical training and then did 4 years of internal medicine residency and chief residency at the University of Massachusetts. I did a 2 year endocrine fellowship at Dartmouth Hitchcock Medical Center. For the last 10 years I have been a clinical and basic investigator in metabolic bone diseases at St. Joseph's Hospital in Bangor, Maine?

KH: *Can you define for me the difference between osteopenia and osteoporosis and make it clear?*

CR: Good question. I think this is a major issue. Osteopenia has, in the past, referred to low bone density or low bone mass detected by x-ray without any evidence of fracture. Osteoporosis is truly a syndrome composed of back pain, fractures and low bone mass. Now, because osteoporosis is a continuum, one could imagine that a person would start off with low bone mass without fracture. Prior to fracturing many people could be considered osteopenic but not osteoporotic, just the first part of that continuum. Therefore I think there is controversy about just defining everybody with low bone mass as having osteoporosis. Now, occasionally, we see patients that have low bone density but never fracture. But the relative risk of fracturing for every standard deviation below the mean, age-adjusted for bone density, is quite high. So it is very much expected that one would fracture with low bone mass.

KH: *Where I get a little confused from your abstract is when it says, "Bone density and other characteristics were not different..."*

CR: What we were trying to do was figure out if those that had premature graying of the hair had lower bone density than those that didn't. They all had osteopenia. There wasn't any difference. But we were just looking at low bone masses. A lot of these people were relatively young in their 30s and 40s. So we wouldn't have expected them to have fractures. Yet, you would expect that over time, especially in women as they enter menopause with low bone mass, that they would eventually lose more bone and fracture.

KH: *What is the definition of premature graying?*

CR: Well, there is none. And you can go as early as the 20s with more than 50% of your hair being gray or more than 50% of your hair gray before the age of 50. We chose before the age of 40 as some sort of compromise because it is published in a number of different texts. We chose people who were graying in their 20s.

Everybody gets a little gray hair in their 30s. But we wanted to see more than 50% graying before the age of 40.

KH: *How did you ever even think about this study.*

CR: Well this is very interesting and actually one of my teachers and mentors at Dartmouth, Bob Adler, who is now chief of endocrinology at the Medical College of Virginia VA Hospital, told me to always ask about graying of the hair when I was taking an endocrine history because he said there is some data that premature graying goes along with thyroid disease. So if you had somebody who had premature graying you should think about thyroid disease and conversely if you have somebody you think has thyroid disease - ask them if they have graying early. It sort of struck home in the early 80s because Barbara Bush had thyroid disease and her hair was white early. This evolved as a public image that came back to me in the early and mid 80s. We then began tracking people with premature graying and we found 2 things. One is that it was a very strong inherited trait, usually in the mother but sometimes the father. Graying would occur at just about the same age in the patient, as it did in the parent. Number two is that we found a tremendous number of subjects who had thyroid disease, premature menopause or other endocrinopathies associated with premature graying. So I went back into the library to look at this and surprisingly there was very little written on it. There is some anecdotal, non-cited references in thyroid textbooks saying premature graying may be associated with thyroid disease. My colleague, Dr. Holick, had done a lot of work on hair growth, vitamin D and skin diseases such as psoriasis. It makes sense that hair and skin may be related to bone disease or at least the physiology of bone turnover.

KH: *So what is the hormonal or biochemical link, if there is one?*

CR: We don't know why hair turns gray. We know that there is melanocyte dropout or there is depigmentation of melanocytes. But we don't know exactly why. It could be related to vitamin D because we know that in certain vitamin D resistant syndromes they don't grow any hair or if they grow hair it is thin and it is often gray. So that one link could be that vitamin D alterations occur in the hair follicle that also occur in bone. There is some recent data that alleles to the vitamin D receptor may play a role in determining peak bone density or rates of bone loss. Another thought is that skin pigmentation has some role in bone mass determination. In other words we know that blacks have considerably higher bone density than whites and this skin pigmentation tendency runs across from blacks having the highest bone density to Southeast Asian people having the lowest bone density. We wondered if maybe hair pigmentation was related to skin pigmentation which was related to either vitamin D or other proteins which regulated bone remodeling.

KH: *Tell us about your study and the results?*

CR: We looked at about 1000 patients who had bone densities and tried to sort out those that had premature graying from those that didn't. Then we looked at the rate of premature graying and the difference between those that had premature graying and those that did not. As it turned out, the ones that had premature graying, who were referred to our osteoporosis metabolic bone clinic, were primarily women concerned about their bone health. In that situation it turned out that if they had premature graying they were 4½ times more likely to have osteoporosis. We came up with 63 people who had no other secondary causes for bone loss, that is steroids, heavy smoking, alcoholism or drugs that could have caused their osteoporosis and it appeared as if those that had premature graying were much more likely to have osteoporosis or osteopenia. We subsequently expanded this study and the data seems to follow that those who become prematurely gray are much more likely to have thinner bones.

KH: *Well let's take it a step further. So let's assume that this correlation is correct. Is there a theoretic intervention?*

CR: There is probably no theoretic intervention except that those people that have that history seem to be the ones that are going to be prone to develop bone loss or inherit a low peak bone density. Those are the people that should be paying attention to their bone health by assuring they get adequate calcium, eliminating some of the risk factors and talk about this with their physician. Because those are the people who need intervention.

KH: *Can you share with us your preventive strategy - kind of 1, 2, 3 for bone health?*

CR: Let's take a 43 year old female with low bone density who may or may not have premature graying and the question is what do we do? We look, first of all, at some of her potential risk factors. Well you can't do anything about the genetics. So if she has a family history we try to optimize her calcium intake by making sure in the 40-50 year old age group that she be taking 1500 mg a day of calcium. Usually for us that means 1000 mg of supplemental calcium plus at least 500 in their diet which most people can tolerate.

KH: *And the type of calcium?*

CR: Calcium carbonate from a number of different generic products. As long as it is calcium carbonate it is reasonable with meals or calcium citrate which can be taken at any time. Citrate is a little more expensive but it is just as bioavailable. These are the two preparations that we use the most. Calcium carbonate can be consumed from TUMS or Oscal. Citracal provides calcium citrate. There are a number of different preparations. The key thing is that calcium carbonate/calcium citrate tends to be more bioavailable than calcium gluconate or calcium lactate. It is important that they get adequate vitamin D with their calcium as well.

KH: *At what dosage?*

CR: At least 2 glasses of milk a day.

KH: *Let's say I don't consume milk and what is your vitamin D dosage?*

CR: We recommend at least 1 multivitamin which has 400 units a day of vitamin D from any of the brand names, Theragram, Centrum, etc.. Vitamin D is absolutely essential for bone health.

KH: *Any other trace elements or nutrients to use?*

CR: There is a lot of debate about magnesium and it hasn't really been decided whether that is absolutely critically. Generally if they are following a pretty good diet and they are taking a multivitamin, that should give them enough magnesium. So we optimize their calcium and vitamin D intake, especially during the winter months because in the northern latitudes you can't produce enough vitamin D in the skin from solar exposure alone. You need to have that vitamin D intake, especially during the winter months, by mouth, whether it be a supplement or a milk product. Exercise is very important. Usually physical activity composed of walking 2 to 3 times a week for 15 to 30 minutes would normally make you healthy anyway and is what you should be doing for your bones. Underwater walking or exercising in a pool seems to be very helpful as well. But any activity that puts gravitation forces on the bones are going to be important. Then it is essential to avoid some of the major compounds that we know can accelerate bone loss - smoking and heavy alcohol intake.

KH: *How about salt intake? Doesn't that increase calcium spill?*

CR: Yes. If you take too much salt you can increase your calcium excretion. We tend to make sure that our patients aren't using too much. Whether or not salt consumption causes a problem in terms of bone loss has never really been established.

KH: *What about caffeine?*

CR: The coffee issue remains somewhat questionable. There is no doubt that coffee, caffeine and theophylline can increase calcium excretion in the urine. It has never been shown that this will cause significant bone loss. So it is theoretically possible but interestingly enough, if they are taking cafe ole or coffee with milk they are also getting some of the calcium they need. So those are the key elements that we work on, particularly patient education. We try very hard to have them come back in a year or two and remeasure their bone density to give us an indication of how fast they are losing bone and whether these therapeutic efforts are helpful.

Now within this preventive strategy take this 43-year-old woman, for example. Paying close attention to her menstrual status is very important. If she slows down or goes through the change of life early we would want to initiate hormone replacement therapy as a preventive strategy in order to prevent her from losing more bone than she can afford to.

KH: *In this era of health care reform and trying to reduce costs how do we screen for those at high risk? With bone density studies or risk factor assessment?*

CR: The key point is we can't screen every single perimenopausal woman for osteoporosis. Only 10 or 15% of all women are going to develop vertebral osteoporosis. Now, when you're 80 or 90 you probably will develop age-related osteoporosis and be suspect to hip fractures. But it has not been clear what percentage of the population does. Not everybody suffers a hip fracture. But certainly as preventive strategies, we're trying to identify those people who, even 40 years down the road, are going to suffer a hip fracture as well as possibly developing a spine fracture within ten years. So obviously we can't screen 115 million women, or want to at any time, so we try to identify those who are the people at risk. Even if it is genetic at least we know that those are the people that we're going to have to focus on. So I say this, "If you have got premature graying pay attention because even if it is not associated with osteoporosis it is associated with other risk factors prominent for causing osteoporosis such as hyperthyroidism, premature menopause or hyperparathyroidism. These are the kind of things which we think are important anyway as secondary causes. So I think it gives the practitioner an opportunity to screen those people and focus on whether they are at risk or not. ♦

Osteoporosis and Calcium

Felix Bronner, Ph.D.
Department of BioStructure and Function
University of Connecticut Health Center
Farmington, CT 06030-3705 U.S.A.
(203) 679-2136 / (203) 679-2910 (FAX)

"Calcium and Osteoporosis,"
American Journal of Clinical Nutrition, 1994;60:831-6. #21448

Kirk Hamilton: *What is your educational background and present position?*

Felix Bronner: I am a professor emeritus in the Department of BioStructure and Function, a department in the School of Dental Medicine of the University of Connecticut. I received my Ph.D. in nutritional biochemistry at MIT in 1952. I did postdoctoral work at Rockefeller Institute of Medical Research, now known as Rockefeller University, and I had faculty positions at Cornell University Medical College, at the University of Louisville School of Medicine, and, since 1969, here at the University of Connecticut.

KH: *How long have you been studying the role of calcium and osteoporosis?*

FB: I have studied the role of calcium all of my professional life. I did my doctoral thesis on studying what happens to calcium in human beings and did one of the first studies using radioactive calcium in human beings. I studied calcium turnover in humans, including osteoporosis, then studied calcium metabolism in rats, and then went on to study the three systems involved in handling calcium in the body, (i.e. the intestine, the kidney and the bone). What I wrote is a review article based on the literature as well as on my own work.

KH: *How important is calcium versus estrogens or gonadal hormones in the prevention of bone loss?*

FB: Calcium is part of the bone mineral that constitutes a major building block of the skeleton. If you have no calcium in the body, you obviously are not going to build up the skeleton. If you eat an adequate amount of calcium and, what that is, is still somewhat under discussion, you will develop a skeleton that represents the genetically programmed maximum. The gonadal hormones in both men and women are very important in the genetic program that defines one's size, turnover and mass of the skeleton. If you don't have gonadal hormones, you will either not reach the size of the skeleton that you would reach with gonadal hormones or, if your gonadal hormone levels decrease, you will begin losing skeletal mass; initially mostly trabecular bone, but ultimately also cortical bone. Both calcium and gonadal hormones are essential to achieving the maximum or optimum size of the skeleton.

KH: *When you say gonadal hormones, could you please define which ones you're talking about? Are you talking about estrogen, testosterone or progesterone?*

FB: The major hormone in the female is estrogen. The major hormone in males is testosterone. I don't know of any detailed studies where progesterone alone has been used. In replacement therapy for women who are menopausal or postmenopausal or who have had an oophorectomy, you take estrogens for a period of 20 to 22 days and then provide progesterone.

KH: *How important is testosterone in males in the regulation of bone, the maintaining of bone or the slowing of bone loss?*

FB: Of similar importance to estrogen in women. In women, as you know, there is an abrupt cessation in estrogen levels as a result of the menopause. In that period, there is a substantial decrease in trabecular bone, along with a modest decrease in cortical bone. In men, the drop in testosterone and the drop in bone mass are more gradual, as shown in my article.

KH: *So why don't we give testosterone to males when they have their drop?*

FB: I am not saying that you should or shouldn't. There are two aspects. First of all, there is a much more gradual drop in both testosterone and bone in men. The indication for giving replacement therapy to males may, therefore, be less evident or be later in life than women. At present, we don't have enough studies to justify treating men with testosterone. In women, estrogen replacement has really been shown to be beneficial. The number one effect is on bone. The number two effect is on cardiovascular health. Data now indicate that women who have replacement therapy will have a significantly lower incidence of myocardial infarcts. And data are now accumulating to suggest that the incidence of Alzheimer's disease is moderately diminished in women who take replacement therapy. There are no comparable studies in men. In women, there is also the obvious benefit of tissue firmness, particularly in target tissues such as the vulva and vagina. Again, there are no comparable long term studies in men. The possibility of hormone replacement in older males went into disrepute 40 or 50 years ago because people thought it would bring about dramatic results - like taking one testosterone pill and then becoming the equivalent of a 20-year-old male. But there is now talk about replacement therapy in older men, and studies are being done to see what the effect is in terms of overall bone health.

KH: *So without estrogen replacement therapy, what's the effect of calcium supplementation by itself in preventing the rapid loss of bone?*

FB: The data are not very clear. On the whole, the data suggest that calcium is of maximum help before the menopause. The problem in getting an answer to that is the following: The recommended dietary allowance for women is probably not quite sufficient. But even if it is, a large portion of women don't take as much calcium as recommended. The typical American woman may not consume more than 500-600 mg of calcium a day. The recommended dietary allowance is at least 800 to 1,000. So if you now take a woman who has a lower level of calcium in the first place and give her the higher level, you may see some benefit. But the overall data, I think, are not convincing that calcium supplementation by itself, without gonadal hormone replacement, is sufficient to slow bone loss significantly in postmenopausal women.

KH: *When is peak bone mass achieved?*

FB: Probably somewhere around the age of 30.

KH: *And therefore calcium intake or bone status in adolescence is very important I take it?*

FB: I think calcium intake in the first three decades of life is quite essential and we are now accumulating data that indicate that overall intake, especially of girls and women, is insufficient. Probably the least expensive and most nutritious source of calcium is milk. It could even be skim milk or milk that contains 1% or 2% fat. It doesn't have to be whole milk. A quart of milk a day will provide more than 1 gm of calcium. In addition, it is an excellent source of protein. Girls in their teens are very concerned about their figure and may not drink milk. It is very popular now to take calcium pills. People talk about eating crushed oyster shells, but most of that is highly insoluble calcium in the form of calcium carbonate and calcium metaphosphate, both of which have very low bioavailability. A soluble calcium salt - calcium malate citrate for example - - seems to be a very good preparation. I would like to emphasize that if you drink milk it would be cheaper, and you will be better off than if you are taking pills. Some people are lactase deficient and consequently cannot handle milk, but there are special lactase-treated milks available. I am not giving individual advice, that's the physician's responsibility. But on a population basis, there is no doubt that calcium intake is important throughout life, but especially in the first three decades.

KH: *If you took a supplement, you're saying one of the most absorbable forms is calcium citrate malate?*

FB: Right.

KH: *Are we talking about a 10% improvement in absorption or are we talking about 1%? My understanding is that most calcium pills are not absorbed very well at all, less than probably 30% to 40% maximum.*

FB: Calcium absorption involves two processes: a saturable, vitamin D-dependent transcellular step that is down regulated when calcium intake is high, and a concentration-dependent nonvitamin regulated, essentially passive movement that is paracellular. Passive absorption is somewhere in the neighborhood of 15% or 16% per hour, so in adults the typical percentage absorption is somewhere in the neighborhood of 25%. How much improvement do you get by consuming more soluble calcium? The data suggests you get enough to make it worthwhile.

KH: *Are there any other minerals that you know of that are beneficial in the maintenance of bone, such as magnesium, copper or manganese?*

FB: We're always coming back to that. Our country is dedicated to taking all kinds of vitamin and mineral pills. If you eat a reasonably balanced meal you don't really need most supplements. The data on low intake of certain minerals are variable and not convincing. Manganese, magnesium, copper, even zinc

supplementation . . . there is still a fair amount of controversy as to whether such supplementation is beneficial in any real sense to the ordinary population. And as far as trace elements for the skeleton, it comes right back to the question as to how important it is to supplement. Your ordinary intake of trace elements is generally adequate. I suppose if you tried to survive on french fries and coke alone without eating anything else - - if you tried to survive on highly purified specialized foods - - you would obviously end up with nutritional deficiencies. Most of us don't do that. Personally, I don't believe it is necessary to add these trace elements to the ordinary diet.

KH: *What about the role of increased protein intake and bone loss or urinary calcium spill?*

FB: The suggestion that high protein intake is responsible for thinner bones or osteoporosis is not well supported by available data. There are data in the literature to suggest that there is an increase in urinary calcium output if you have a high protein diet. There are no good data to indicate that this continues and leads to osteoporosis. People jump to conclusions on it. There are also data that suggest you can get increased urinary calcium losses with lots of protein intake. Other data have been published that show there is no real effect. So, I would not think this is a major factor.

KH: *How about vitamin D deficiency in elderly as being a risk factor to bone loss?*

FB: There are data to suggest that elderly people who don't have an opportunity to get out into the sunlight have marginal levels of vitamin D or 1,25 dihydroxyvitamin D_3. The elderly population that is institutionalized or has inadequate vitamin D intake may have low vitamin D levels. Whether you can ensure adequate vitamin D levels by providing pasteurized, vitamin D supplemented milk or by some additional vitamin D supplement depends on the individual's situation and the food intake. It is certainly a factor that the dietitian needs to think about. The fact that an elderly population may not be able to chew very well or taste things very well needs to be thought about when providing sources of calcium and vitamin D. You've got to make the food attractive, interesting and variable in order to meet the dietary needs of the institutionalized elderly.

KH: *What about lifestyle factors and the prevention of bone loss such as exercise, smoking, etc. What do you recommend?*

FB: There is reasonable evidence that exercise will help build bone. Increased muscle activity will lead to greater bone mass. People who don't exercise are not as well off as people who exercise moderately and frequently. On the other hand, there are no good data to support the notion that if you take a postmenopausal woman and make her exercise, that will significantly arrest the bone loss if you don't at the same time provide her with hormones and an adequate amount of calcium. In the presence of both, exercise is beneficial. And it is also beneficial, of course, for cardiovascular and other reasons.

KH: *If I could paraphrase in a nutshell your bone loss prevention program, the consumption of dairy products to get an adequate calcium intake during the first three decades of life is probably the most cost-effective strategy. If for some reason you need to take a supplement, a more soluble form might be better such as the calcium citrate malate. And, estrogen replacement therapy is definitely something that you would recommend for the prevention of bone loss.*

FB: Adequate calcium intake throughout life is highly recommended. Gonadal hormone replacement, certainly in women, is now the consensus approach. You know, it is very important and I would like to emphasize one thing: I am talking in terms of population statistics. If you are the examining physician, you have to know what the patient is about. Not every woman will adequately tolerate gonadal hormone replacement. You need to figure out how or what to do; it isn't an automatic kind of thing. These are very powerful drugs, and you need to know what you are doing. But on a population basis, there is very little doubt in my mind that postmenopausal women should be supported with gonadal hormone replacement as well as adequate nutritional measures. ◆

Osteoporosis, Calcium Citrate and Trace Elements

Paul Saltman, Ph.D
Department of Biology 0322
University of California at San Diego
La Jolla, CA 92093-0322 U.S.A.
(619) 534-3824 / (619) 534-0936 (FAX)

"Spinal Bone Loss and Postmenopausal Women Supplemented With Calcium and Trace Minerals," Journal of Nutrition, 1994;124:1060-1064. #22291. "The Role of Minerals in Osteoporosis," The Journal of the American College of Nutrition, 1993;12(4):383-389. #18815.

Kirk Hamilton: Can you please share with me your educational background and current position?

Paul Saltman: I received my Bachelor of Science in Chemistry from the California Institute of Technology in 1949. I received my Ph.D. in Biochemistry from the California Institute of Technology in 1953. I was on the faculty for 14 years at the University of Southern California in the Department of Biochemistry. Since 1967 I have been a Professor in the Department of Biology at the University of California at San Diego.

KH: When did you get interested in the role of trace elements and bone loss?

PS: When I learned about the problems of Bill Walton's basketball injuries, I realized that his dietary regimen was not ideal.

KH: Could you share your experience with the chronic foot fractures of the professional basketball player, Bill Walton and the role of the trace elements (manganese) in resolving this problem?

PS: Bill Walton was an excellent basketball player who was crippled by various bone and joint injuries. At the time he was very much involved in a dietary regimen that was fundamentally vegetarian and lacked foods that were good sources of both calcium and trace elements, particular iron, copper, zinc and manganese. We tested his serum and found that he was low indeed in manganese, copper and zinc and was excreting large amounts of calcium. We supplemented him and he appeared to recover. He did not continue to participate in our study so we went on to study the problem initially in rats and then in a clinical study involving postmenopausal women.

KH: How might the trace elements zinc, copper and manganese physiologically help with bone loss?

PS: Zinc is a trace element which is required by over 300 different enzymes, particularly those involved in nucleic acid protein metabolism. But more specifically, there is an alkaline phosphatase involved in bone metabolism for which zinc is a cofactor. Copper is involved as an oxidase metallic cofactor which is involved in the cross-linking and synthesis of collagen needed in the organic matrix of bone. Manganese is involved in the transglycosylation reactions in the synthesis of proteoglycans of the organic matrix of bone.

KH: What did your study show of postmenopausal women who took either calcium citrate malate alone; the trace elements zinc, copper and manganese alone; or in combination?

PS: Our studies showed that calcium citramalate (*please note it is not calcium citrate but a citramalate complex that we tested*) reduced the rate of bone loss, while the combination of the trace elements and citramalate actually increased bone density. Trace elements alone had no effect on bone metabolism in the women that we tested.

KH: What were the doses of zinc, copper and manganese that were used?

PS: The doses of zinc, copper and manganese that were used were the U.S. RDAs and were approximately 15 mg of zinc, 2.5 mg of copper and 5.0 mg of manganese per day.

KH: Is calcium citrate malate a better form of calcium to use in general or just for specific subgroups of high risk patients? Is there any concern about excess aluminum absorption from calcium citrate ingestion?

PS: Extensive studies showed that calcium citramalate has an increased absorption when compared with calcium carbonate in general human studies. It is a function of the enhanced solubility of calcium and its ability to be transported more effectively. There is no fundamental concern about aluminum absorption as a serious health problem with calcium citrate.

KH: Where do you advocate getting your calcium in foods from?

PS: The primary source of calcium in food is from dairy products. There is no question about that. Whether the milk is homogenized or skimmed makes no difference. Cheese and ice cream and other dairy products are excellent providers of calcium. It should be noted that some forms of tofu, involve calcium precipitation of the soybean protein. Corn products made in Mexican style where calcium hydroxide is used to prepare the corn, are also rich in calcium. These latter foods can be consumed by individuals who don't care to consume dairy products.

KH: Do you encourage red meat consumption since it is a good source of trace minerals?

PS: Yes.

KH: Does a high protein diet cause excess spill of calcium from the urine?

PS: There is some evidence, but it is weak, that high protein diets cause chelation and loss of calcium in the urine. It is certainly not a major problem for most people in our society. The major problem is calcium and trace element insufficiency.

KH: *Is there any evidence that the higher protein intake from milk or red meat might offset the benefit of calcium and trace elements due to excess calcium spill?*

PS: No.

KH: *Do you have any experience with magnesium or boron in the prevention of bone loss?*

PS: I have not done any experiments with magnesium or boron. There are experiments in the literature that would indicate that both of these play some role in bone loss. It is unlikely that boron deficiency is a major problem in osteoporosis. Magnesium also seems unlikely to play a definitive role.

KH: *What are your bottom line recommendations for the prevention and building of new bone in postmenopausal women?*

PS: My bottom line is to get enough calcium either from food or supplements as the case may be. It does not matter where you get the calcium, only that you get the calcium. Beware of using sources of calcium that may contain heavy metal toxicity such as dolomite. Trace elements are absolutely necessary and they should be obtained from food, primarily from meats, fish and chicken but also available in trace element supplements. Under *no* circumstances should macro doses or mega-mineral therapy be utilized. ◆

Pancreatitis (Acute) and Sodium Selenite

Bodo Kuklinski, M.D.
Klinikum Sudstadt
Head of Clinic for Internale Medicine
Suedring 81, D-18053 Rostock, Germany
49 0381 4 40 12 03 / 49 0381 4 40 16 33 (FAX)

"Reducing the Lethality in Acute Pancreatitis With Sodium Selenite,"
Med. Klin., 1995;90:Suppl. I:36-41. #22503

Kirk Hamilton: Could you please share with us your educational background and current position?

Bodo Kuklinski: I received my medical education at the University of Leipzig Medical School in Germany. After 16 years as a specialist in internal medicine with a focus on trace elements and vitamins, respectively, I finished my appointment as University Lecturer with the topic "Infusions with HDL-Cholesterol in Diseases with Arteriosclerotic Origin." By having a chance to work in all areas of internal medicine, I remained a generalist. Since 1988, I have been head of the Hospital of Internal Medicine in Rostock, Germany. We have been measuring the concentrations of metabolic products of lipid peroxidation (thiobarbituric acid reactive substance-TBARS) in healthy volunteers, premorbids and morbids routinely for more than 15 years. We also have been monitoring the redox potential of the plasma, as well as the plasma concentrations of the trace elements like selenium, zinc, etc.. After critical intensive investigations, we realized that the molecular or atomic basis for all acute and chronic diseases is "free radical" based. No other disturbances behind that are possible. At the level of the proton/electron homeostasis, diseases have no "faces." After having investigated about 1,000 various foods and toxic pollution substances, we found that the need for antioxidant nutrients has increased dramatically by negative interaction between the environment, food chain and disease.

KH: When did you begin to think that selenium played a role in acute pancreatitis?

BK: We knew from our investigations that acute pancreatitis is positively correlated with the degree of lipid peroxidation. We looked for a radical scavenger with rapid solubility and good permeability and discovered selenite. This substance has a redox potential of -740 mV during acidotic metabolism. Thus, selenite is a unique and highly effective powerful acceptor of electrons. In the beginning we thought this was due to an increase in glutathione peroxidase activity. We found that maximal selenium supplementation does not maximize glutathione peroxidase activity before the end of 3 days. At this time selenite has already established its protective effects. Its efficacy shows immediately. In 1984, we showed the suppression of late potentials and life threatening arrhythmias by selenite in 43 pigs with myocardial infarction which occurred immediately after ligation of the coronary artery. While all the animals in the control group (n=21) died after 13 minutes due to myocardial infarction (fibrillation), the trial had to be stopped after 60 minutes in the animals who received the selenite treatment (n=22). We could not see any arrhythmias. Therefore, it seemed to us that there must be an immediate membrane stabilizing effect of selenite which cannot be explained by the glutathione peroxidase synthesis or its activity.

KH: What is the mechanism of the damage to the pancreas in acute pancreatitis?

BK: In acute pancreatitis, either of alcoholic, biliary or idiopathic origin, the source is from free radical damage. We found low concentrations of glutathione, selenium, vitamins C and E and methionine, and high concentrations of TBARS in all forms of pancreatitis independent of the inducing substance. During the course of the disease, a latent, chronic oxidative stress suddenly changes into an acute event. Massive injury occurs from the uncontrolled activation of phospholipase A2, the arachidonic acid cascade and the production of lysolecithin.

KH: What were the findings of your study on the use of selenium in acute pancreatitis?

BK: Development of necrosis was blocked during the toxic phase. During therapy with selenite, which was started immediately after the beginning of symptoms, total necrosis could not be observed. Besides the detrimental septic phase, development of abscesses in multi-organ failure was blocked, and invasive operation in intensive care was not necessary. Since the surgeons in the hospital have taken over the responsibility for therapy, no patients have died. We have treated 342 patients with selenium since that time, with results remaining successful. The protocol for the therapy includes sodium selenite on the first day, which provides 1,000 mcg of selenium. On the second day, 500 mcg is consumed. This is provided in intravenous fluids with carbohydrates and electrolytes (no calcium!). The total fluid is approximately 3 to 6 liters. Analgesics are given by enemas 3 times per day. In spite of this treatment, the patients developed exudation in the abdomen and pleura, and an atonic bowel during the first 3 to 5 days. Very early the efficacy of treatment can be seen by the rapid lowering of malondialdehyde in the blood and the normalization of calcium values.

KH: Might other antioxidants have benefit in conjunction with selenium such as vitamin E, C, glutathione and beta-carotene?

BK: Yes. After the occurrence of motility of the colon, we gave orally 400 I.U. of vitamin E, beta-carotene 15 mg, vitamin C 500 mg two times a day, methionine 400 mg, zinc 50 mg, magnesium 600 mg, vitamin B6 20 mg, selenium as selenomethionine 200 mcg, acetylcysteine as three 200 mg tablets and folic acid at 500 mcg.

KH: Were you surprised at the dramatic results of the selenium therapy given early in the disease with regards to lethality?

BK: Yes. Absolutely! That a simple substance could work so dramatically was remarkable. There is a high affinity of the pancreas to selenium. The scintigraphic investigation of the pancreas has been done with selenocysteine marked with radioactivity some years ago. Besides, the redox potential is unique. Yes, we were indeed surprised with the results since the lethality of the acute pancreatitis was 34.4%, and in alcoholic forms it was even 80%.

KH: Has this therapy with selenium been accepted as a treatment of choice in hospital settings or are further trials ongoing?

BK: The method is still in discussion. The reaction to our results which we presented at the "Deutscher Pancreas Club" was refusal, despite that J. Braganza (Manchester) found similar results to ours. Up to now, there have been 2 studies with selenite in 2 surgeon hospitals. They found a decrease in oxidative stress and an improvement in the antioxidative status. No difference in lethality could be seen because all patients had undergone surgery. But every surgery is an enhancer of oxidative stress. The advantage of therapy with selenium becomes negated. Under early treatment with selenium, there is no need for surgery. It seems to us that the surgeons do not have the courage to wait.

KH: Can you see selenium being of benefit in other free radical-initiated diseases or acute illness such as multi-system organ failure and sepsis?

BK: We did studies about the treatment with selenite in other diseases. In a 1 year double-blind, controlled trial after myocardial infarction, no patient died under antioxidative treatment, but 20% in the control group did. The treatment was done with selenite, coenzyme Q10, selenocysteine, beta-carotene, vitamin C, vitamin E, zinc and B6. The renal excretion of albumin was reduced by vitamin E, thioctic acid and selenite in diabetic late syndrome patients. Diabetic late syndrome refers to late complications in long-term diabetic patients with retinopathy, nephropathy and neuropathy. Peripheral diabetic neuropathy improved in 60% of the patients. In patients with intensive alcoholic liver damage, lethality was reduced to 6% under treatment with antioxidants, and in the control group the lethality was 40%. The redox potentials of the different antioxidants are as follows: +0.100 ubiquinone, +.080 ascorbate, -0.120 riboflavin, -0.220 cysteine, -0.230 glutathione, -0.290 thioctic acid, -0.320 NADH and -0.740 of selenite.

In septic patients, chronic renal insufficiency, dialysis, allergies, epileptic patients, Alzheimer's disease, multiple sclerosis, Parkinsonism, psoriasis, myopathies, chronic fatigue syndrome and multiple chemical sensitivity disorders caused by exposure to halogenated xenobiotics, we have had positive results with antioxidant therapy.

Further, patients with leukemia, cervical dysplasia, a stage III pap smear, cystic fibrosis, chronic ischemic heart disease, cardiomyopathy, arrhythmia, cutaneous and pulmonary sarcoidosis, chronic pancreatitis, chronic arthrosis, non-HIV immune suppression and HIV infection (n=200) have received benefit from antioxidant therapy. We investigated 6,000 patients with cancer in whom an extreme high oxidative stress level could be measured. More of the results have not been published yet. In general, all elderly people from 65 years on should receive antioxidants since nearly all of them show a chronic oxidative stress.

The antioxidants which are used by us are as follows: selenite, selenium, vitamins B1, B2, B6, pantothenic acid, folic acid, vitamin E, vitamin C, choline, coenzyme Q10, L-carnitine, dimethylsulfoxide, bioflavonoids, methionine, cysteine and alpha-lipoic acid. In patients who show very low levels of malondialdehyde as in neurodermatitis, we treat them with n-3 fatty acids, magnesium, zinc, manganese, copper, titanium, molybdenum, glutamine and anthocyanines in most cases. It is our own experience in experimental work which convinced us to follow this way. In the meantime, a lot of severely ill patients living in a country where they are confronted with enormous environmental pollution every day could be stabilized with therapeutics that basically are free of side effects. As long as enrichment of food is not common here and people eat with a low concentration of essential nutrients, we have to support at least basic essentials to assist the body in the healing process. ◆

Pemphigus, Nicotinamide and Tetracycline

David P. Fivenson, M.D.
Department of Dermatology Henry Ford Hospital
2799 W. Grand Blvd.
Detroit, MI 48202 U.S.A.
(313) 876-2600 / (313) 876-2093 (FAX)

"Nicotinamide and Tetracycline Therapy For Bullous Pemphigoid",
Archives of Dermatology, June 1994;130:753-758. #20381

Kirk Hamilton: *Dr. Fivenson could you share with us your educational background and what your present position is.*

David Fivenson: I received my undergraduate and medical school training at the University of Michigan in Ann Arbor. I interned at St. Joseph Mercy Hospital in Ann Arbor. I did a immunodermatology fellowship at University of California at San Diego and my dermatology residency training at the University of Cincinnati. I completed my postdoctoral training in 1989. I joined the dermatology staff at Henry Ford Hospital in Detroit Michigan in July of 1989.

KH: *How long have you been treating pemphigus with the tetracycline and nicotinamide combination.*

DF: For approximately 7 years.

KH: *What are bullous pemphigoid and pemphigus vulgaris and the differences between the two?*

DF: Bullous pemphigoid is an autoimmune blistering disease that is characterized by tense blisters or blebs that come on suddenly and can be widespread across the skin. It normally lasts 2 to 3 years and is treated with steroids or other immune suppressive drugs.

Pemphigus vulgaris is also an autoimmune blistering disease but it is characterized by flaccid blisters which easily break and often times patients only have skin erosions. This can start earlier in life whereas bullous pemphigoid usually starts in the patient's 60s or 70s. Pemphigus vulgaris can start in the 30s and 40s - the prime years of life. Pemphigus vulgaris is harder to treat and often requires higher doses of immune suppressive drugs and is a life long condition. Pemphigus vulgaris is also more associated with genetic tendencies than bullous pemphigoid in that patients with pemphigus vulgaris typically are of Mediterranean descent and there is an increased incidence in people from that area who are Jewish.

KH: *Why did you consider an alternative approach to pemphigus such as nicotinamide and tetracycline?*

DF: Any alternative to immunosuppressive drugs, especially in bullous pemphigoid patients who are older, would be advantageous as it would help avoid some of the side effects of steroids and other immunosuppressive drugs. My particular interest in this combination was sparked by a preliminary report from the University of Chicago citing that 4 patients had been treated with tetracycline and nicotinamide in the early to mid 1980s in an uncontrolled trial. There had been isolated case reports throughout the 70s and 80s of patients with bullous pemphigoid or pemphigus responding to various antibiotics but these were all anecdotal or serendipitous studies with no organized trials being performed.

KH: *What were the doses of nicotinamide and tetracycline?*

DF: In our studies we have been using, as a starting dose, tetracycline 500 mg 4 times daily and nicotinamide or niacinamide administered 500 mg 3 times daily.

KH: *Why did you choose nicotinamide or niacinamide versus niacin?*

DF: Studies have shown that nicotinamide is a moderately effective immunosuppressive agent through a number of pathways, whereas studies using niacin have not shown the same efficacy in suppressing the immune response. Also, this high dose of niacin would be almost universally associated with severe flushing sensations, whereas nicotinamide is generally not associated with any symptoms when taken at this dose.

KH: *You mention in your article reasons why nicotinamide might work - electron scavenging, phosphodiesterase inhibition, increased conversion of tryptophan to serotonin, an antihistamine effect, inhibition of neutrophil and eosinophil chemotaxis and secretion, and gene regulation. In your opinion, can you hone in on which one is the most significant?*

DF: My most educated guess would probably be the effect on neutrophils and eosinophils because those are the two most active cell types in these autoimmune blistering diseases. Histologically these diseases are characterized by extensive infiltrates of eosinophils and/or neutrophils.

KH: *In comparing nicotinamide and tetracycline treatment to prednisone, the thought that obviously comes up in this era of health care reform is the comparison of the cost of this treatment versus immunosuppressive drugs and their side effects.*

DF: Prednisone is pretty cheap as is nicotinamide and tetracycline. A month's supply of nicotinamide is about $5.00 at the health food vitamin counter and tetracycline is probably not a whole lot more than that as it has been available in generic form for many years. Prednisone, likewise, is very inexpensive. *However, the main motivation for the alternative therapy is to avoid some of the side effects associated with chronic steroid administration and that is where the real difference in health care costs will add up. We expect to see, and our initial studies have shown, that the two therapies are equal as far as their effect on the disease and that patients who take the tetracycline-nicotinamide combination have less side effects and, therefore, there is less health care costs associated with long term administration.* ◆

Preeclampsia and Lipid Peroxides

Scott W. Walsh, Ph.D.
Medical College of Virginia
Department of Obstetrics and Gynecology
P.O. Box 980034
Richmond, VA 23298-0034 U.S.A.
(804) 828-8468 / (804) 828-0573 (FAX)

"Lipid Peroxidation in Pregnancy",
Hypertension In Pregnancy, 1994;13(1):1-32 #20802

Kirk Hamilton: *Thank you very much for being here. Could you please start off by giving me your educational background from college up to your current position.*

Scott Walsh: I received my Ph.D. degree from the University of Wisconsin in Madison in 1975. I then taught or did research at the Oregon Regional Primate Research Center, Michigan State University and the University of Texas Medical School at Houston. Currently I am a professor in the Division of Maternal - Fetal Medicine in the Department of Obstetrics and Gynecology and I hold a joint appointment in the Department of Physiology at the Medical College of Virginia, Virginia Commonwealth University, Richmond, Virginia.

KH: *Could you please explain the differences between preeclampsia, eclampsia and pregnancy-induced hypertension? I get them kind of mixed up.*

SW: There is a lot of confusion with those terms and they are often times misused. There is a clear distinction between preeclampsia and eclampsia. Eclampsia is a very severe form of preeclampsia in which convulsions occur. When the disease progresses to the point where the mother starts to convulse, it can become life threatening. Preeclampsia is hypertension that occurs during pregnancy with proteinuria. Pregnancy-induced hypertension is often times used synonymously with preeclampsia but most people now recommend the term preeclampsia rather than pregnancy-induced hypertension because there can be a hypertension that occurs during pregnancy that is not associated with proteinuria which is referred to as gestational hypertension. This does not seem to be as serious a problem as preeclampsia where there is proteinuria.

KH: *I've got to thank you for that. You don't know how long I have struggled with those definitions. I always get confused.*

SW: Another term you see a lot is toxemia of pregnancy which is the same as preeclampsia.

KH: *How did you get interested in lipid peroxides in relationship to pregnancy, preeclampsia and eclampsia?*

SW: My interest actually stems from work that we did in the early to mid 80s in which we were studying placentas obtained from women with preeclampsia and found that there was increased thromboxane and decreased prostacyclin production. Now thromboxane is a very potent vasoconstrictor and stimulator of platelet aggregation whereas prostacyclin opposes those actions. It is a potent vasodilator and an inhibitor of platelet aggregation. So when we found this imbalance of increased thromboxane and decreased prostacyclin, it could explain a number of the clinical signs of preeclampsia. The increase in thromboxane production by the placenta to me indicated that there was an increase in the activity of the cyclooxygenase enzyme which is responsible for converting arachidonic acid into thromboxane and other prostaglandins. After moving to the Medical College of Virginia, I learned that when the cyclooxygenase enzyme is activated it generates oxygen radicals. Since the placenta is a very rich source of polyunsaturated fatty acids, it seemed to me that if there was increased activity of the enzyme with generation of oxygen radicals, there would be an increase in lipid peroxide production by the placenta, and that is indeed what we found.

KH: *Isn't thromboxane A2 more vasoconstrictive than thromboxane B2?*

SW: No, thromboxane B2 is the stable breakdown metabolite of thromboxane A2 and that is the one that everyone measures. Thromboxane A2 is too short lived to be measurable. So we look at the stable breakdown metabolite.

KH: *But thromboxane B2 doesn't have the same activity.*

SW: No, it does not have the activity of vasoconstriction or stimulating platelet aggregation.

KH: *What have you found with regards to lipid peroxides . . . and when you measure lipid peroxides what are you talking about? Malondialdehyde, thiobarbituric acid substances (TBA). . .*

SW: In our first report of blood levels of lipid peroxides in women with preeclampsia, we used the malondialdehyde or TBA assay, but we are now using a different assay. We use an assay that is more specific for peroxides. We actually utilize enzymes that naturally occur in the body, glutathione peroxidase and glutathione reductase. Glutathione peroxidase is an antioxidant enzyme that is specific for inactivating peroxides - hydrogen peroxide and lipid peroxides - and we have incorporated it into an assay which was described by other workers. So the assay we use actually measures specifically peroxides, and mainly lipid peroxides, not an indirect product such as malondialdehyde.

KH: *So you have found those elevated in preeclamptic women?*

SW: Yes, we found elevated placental production of lipid peroxides in women with preeclampsia. We also found them elevated in the blood of the mother and we found that the placenta secretes lipid peroxides primarily towards the maternal circulation. So if you have an abnormal increase in placental lipid peroxides that are secreted into the maternal circulation, that would explain at least one of the sources for increased lipid peroxides in the mother with preeclampsia.

KH: *Is there actual tissue destruction? How does the hypertension, proteinuria and all these things resulting from lipid peroxides being released affect the mother or fetus?*

SW: Well one of the ways for hypertension to occur by the cyclooxygenase enzyme is shown by taking human placentas and perfusing them with an exogenous peroxide. We can stimulate the activity of the cyclooxygenase enzyme with peroxide to increase production of thromboxane, and then the thromboxane brings about the vasoconstriction in the placenta. But the peroxides can also enhance vasoconstriction by directly stimulating an increase in intracellular calcium which then enhances the overall vasoconstrictive response. As far as the proteinuria and edema, lipid peroxides and oxygen free radicals have been shown to increase the permeability of membranes to ions and also to proteins. So if you increase the permeability, for example of the endothelial cells in the glomerulus of the kidney, that could directly result in proteinuria. And if you increase the permeability of the endothelial cells in the systemic vasculature, that could directly result in edema. You can also get damage of the cell membranes by circulating lipid peroxides.

KH: *You have just given me a hint on how magnesium may possibly benefit in preeclampsia when you said that the lipid peroxides cause increases in intracellular calcium. Magnesium can act as a kind of a natural calcium channel blocker. I assume, in part, that is why advanced eclampsia is treated with magnesium.*

SW: We have actually just been looking at that. We have just completed some studies where we have perfused placentas with a hydroperoxide to induce vasoconstriction and then perfuse it with magnesium sulfate. We found that magnesium sulfate does in fact inhibit the peroxide-induced vasoconstriction and we think it is primarily by blocking the calcium channels because we can reverse the effect by increasing the amount of calcium in the perfusion media. We are preparing that study right now for submission to a meeting next spring.

KH: *It is interesting that there is a hot debate right now in whether to use magnesium versus classic anticonvulsants in eclampsia which has frequently been present in the literature the last year or so. I don't normally see this explanation when they talk about magnesium.*

SW: Yes. I haven't seen the explanation either. Certainly the reason magnesium sulfate is mainly given is to prevent convulsions and it seems logical that it would do that by blocking calcium effects. It has also been shown to stimulate prostacyclin production. Prostacyclin is a vasodilator, so that may be another mechanism of action of magnesium sulfate.

KH: *Well you know you're drawing a beautiful model for an anti-inflammatory approach to preeclampsia using antioxidants or also maybe a low arachidonic acid based diet. A diet including more fish and less preformed arachidonic acid from dairy products or meat fat, and more antioxidants might be a way to reduce the risk in a high risk population.*

SW: Certainly diet is one of the things people have considered, and interestingly, vegetarians have a very low incidence of preeclampsia. Also studies of Eskimo's in Greenland and people of the Faroe Islands, where they eat diets high in fish, have shown these populations have very low incidences of preeclampsia and heart disease. So there is some interest in the N-3 fatty acids having a protective effect against preeclampsia.

KH: *They can actually displace arachidonic acid and here you're drawing the model for not just prevention of preeclampsia but for all the inflammatory conditions. There are a lot of them. You know, the general antiinflammatory type of diet and regime. I just got finished reviewing the article "Preeclampsia and Antioxidant Nutrients: Decreased Plasma Levels of Reduced Ascorbic Acid α-Tocopherol, and Beta-Carotene in Women With Preeclampsia", Mikhail, Magdy S., M.D., et al, American Journal of Obstetrics and Gynecology, July 1994;171(1):150-157 which notes reduced levels of antioxidants in preeclampsia.*

SW: They found a decrease in vitamin C, beta-carotene and also vitamin E. We had originally published back in 1991, not only an increase in lipid peroxides in women with preeclampsia, but also a significant decrease in vitamin E. Now more people are interested in the antioxidants and finding more deficiencies in antioxidants. I should point out that the first report on increased lipid peroxides in preeclampsia was actually published by a Japanese worker back in 1978 and then there were a couple of other papers in 1981, but it has only been recently that there has been more interest in this area as we started to recognize the importance of oxygen free radicals and antioxidants.

KH: *Obviously once these things happen at the end stage of pregnancy it is very expensive to deal with the complications. If you could prevent this with a basic multiple vitamin/mineral supplement rich in antioxidants and magnesium this would be a great study.*

SW: We have found some other deficiencies too. In studying the placenta we found a deficiency in superoxide dismutase, which inactivates the superoxide anion, and we also found a deficiency of glutathione peroxidase, which is probably one of the most important antioxidants in the tissue for inactivating lipid peroxides.

KH: *We'll you're setting the stage for selenium supplementation since it is the cofactor for glutathione peroxidase and for SOD there are 2 forms, the zinc:copper and manganese forms.*

SW: We found the zinc:copper form is the one that is deficient and apparently no difference for the manganese form which is the inducible form of the enzyme.

KH: *You're setting the perfect stage here. Is there somewhere a trial that is going on that is going to test some of these basic antiinflammatory, antioxidant type of nutrients. Or where are we going with this?*

SW: Most of the attention recently has been with low dose aspirin, but I think there is more attention now being given to the lipid peroxides and antioxidant side. I currently don't know of any trial that is started with the antioxidants. There was one report back in, I believe, 1988 from Italy that combined low dose aspirin with vitamin E and reported a beneficial effect. But they didn't give very many details. Certainly I would think that the stage is set for doing some clinical trials with low dose aspirin plus maybe a combination of antioxidants. A number of studies have been published (smaller studies) using low dose aspirin, and here we're talking anywhere from 60 to 150 mg of aspirin a day, or what many people use is 1 baby aspirin a day. The earlier, smaller trials, found a significant decrease in the incidence of preeclampsia, as much as 94%. Some of these earlier trials showed a really significant decrease in the incidence of preeclampsia, but a couple of later larger trials are not showing quite as much of a decrease in the incidence and there may be some reasons for that. One reason is that we may need to combine aspirin with antioxidants.

KH: If I recall vitamin E happens to modulate cyclooxygenase...

SW: There is some data on vitamin E that it can increase prostacyclin production. It may modulate cyclooxygenase activity in that it inhibits lipid peroxidation. By decreasing the level of lipid peroxides, it would decrease the activity of cyclooxygenase. This would decrease thromboxane. But since lipid peroxides also inhibit prostacyclin synthase, by inhibiting lipid peroxides you have an additional beneficial effect of increasing prostacyclin. ◆

Pregnancy, Homocysteine and Vitamin B12

Jack Metz, M.D.
The Royal Women's Hospital
Division of Pathology
720 Swanston St.
Carlton VIC 3053, Australia
61 613 9347-6346 (FAX)

"Biochemical Indices of Vitamin B12 Nutrition in Pregnant Patients With Subnormal Serum Vitamin B12 Levels", <u>American Journal of Hematology</u>, 1995;48:251-255. #22217

Kirk Hamilton: *What is your educational background and present position?*

Jack Metz: I received my undergraduate medical school training at the University of Witwatersrand, Johannesburg, South Africa. I subsequently trained in hematology and pathology at the South African Institute For Medical Research (SAIMR). I was director of the SAIMR and chairman of pathology at the university until 1990 when I moved to Australia, where I am currently the director of hematology at the Royal Women's Hospital and principal consultant hematologist at the Royal Melbourne Hospital.

KH: *When did you get interested in the role of homocysteine as a marker of vitamin B12 deficiency in pregnancy?*

JM: Following the publications of Robert Allen and his group at Denver, in which they showed that serum homocysteine was a marker for vitamin B12 deficiency, I became interested in the possibility that serum homocysteine could be used to evaluate the significance of the commonly observed fall in serum vitamin B12 levels in pregnancy.

KH: *In your opinion, is serum vitamin B12 an accurate indicator of vitamin B12 deficiency in pregnant females?*

JM: Serum vitamin B12 is not an accurate an indicator of vitamin B12 deficiency in pregnant females, as the vast majority of pregnant women with low serum vitamin B12 levels show no clinical hematological or biochemical evidence of deficiency, and a low serum level returns to normal after pregnancy.

KH: *Do you see the day where homocysteine and methylmalonic acid may be routinely used in pregnant females as a screen for folic acid and vitamin B12 deficiencies?*

JM: As our study suggests, serum methylmalonic acid levels may be elevated in pregnancy in the absence of vitamin B12 deficiency. I do not believe that it will be used as a screen for deficiency in pregnant females. Homocysteine could well be applied to routine screening in pregnant women, but this would depend on the development of an assay that is simpler and cheaper than the current HPLC method. As raised homocysteine levels may occur with either folate or vitamin B12 deficiency, a positive homocysteine screening result would need to be followed by serum vitamin B12 and folate assays.

KH: *How do you document folate status if homocysteine is elevated to determine whether it is a B12 deficiency or not?*

JM: The best way to document folate status is to measure red cell folate concentration.

KH: *If homocysteine is elevated, are there other things that can elevate homocysteine such as vitamin B6, betaine and choline deficiency along with deficiencies of folic acid and vitamin B12?*

JM: Causes of elevated homocysteine other than folate or vitamin B12 deficiency include impaired renal function, deficiencies of vitamin B6, betaine or choline, and inborn errors of metabolism. Impaired renal function is readily excluded by suitable tests. Homocysteinemia, due to vitamin B6, betaine or choline deficiency, is probably quite rare in humans. However, inborn errors of metabolism leading to elevated homocysteine may be more common, particularly due to a genetic defect of the enzyme methylene tetrahydrofolate reductase. Thus, in any patient with raised homocysteine, serum vitamin B12, folate levels and renal function should be checked. If these are normal, methylene tetrahydrofolate reductase abnormality would be likely. Unfortunately, a therapeutic trial of folic acid may not differentiate between homocysteine due to folate deficiency from other causes. This is due to the fact that folic acid appears to lower homocysteine levels irrespective of the cause of the homocysteinemia.

KH: *How do you see homocysteine being used in either gynecologic or obstetric practices?*

JM: I do not see measurements of homocysteine being clinically used in gynecologic practice. However, in obstetrics it could replace vitamin B12 and folate serum assays as a screening test for deficiencies of these vitamins in pregnancy. ◆

Pregnancy-Induced Hypertension and Calcium

Patricio Lopez-Jaramillo, M.D., Ph.D.
Director, Mineral Metabolism Unit
Medical School, Central University
P.O. Box 17211060
Quito, Ecuador
593 2 439168 / 593 2 544597 / 593 2 461115 (FAX)

"Calcium Supplementation Prevents Pregnancy-Induced Hypertension By Increasing the Production of Vascular Nitric Oxide," Medical Hypothesis, 1995; 45:68-72. #23717

Kirk Hamilton: *Can you please share with me your educational background and current position?*

Patricio Lopez-Jaramillo: I received my undergraduate medical school training at the Central University of Quito, Ecuador. I subsequently trained in endocrinology and pharmacology at the Medical School of Ribeirao Preto, Sao Paulo University, Brazil, where I received my Ph.D. degree. I also was in a postdoctoral position in Wellcome Research Laboratories, Pharmacology Department, Beckenham, Kent, United Kingdom. I am presently professor and director at the Mineral Metabolism Unit, Medical School, Central University and a nutrition national consultant for the Pan American Health Organization.

KH: *What got you interested in the potential role of calcium supplements to prevent pregnancy-induced hypertension?*

PLJ: In 1980, following the publication of Jose Belizan and Jose Villar at Guatemala (American Journal of Clinical Nutrition, 33:2202-2210) in which they proposed a causal inverse relationship between calcium intake and pregnancy-induced hypertension (PIH), I became interested in the possibility that calcium supplementation to poor Andean pregnant women, a population with very low calcium intake (mean 400 mg/day) and a high incidence of PIH (18%), could be useful in the prevention of PIH. The results of two clinical trials (British Journal of Obstetrics and Gynaecology, 1989; 96:648-655; Lancet, 1990;335:293) demonstrated that in these populations, calcium supplementation is an effective and safe intervention to decrease the risk and prevent PIH.

KH: *Do we know the mechanism which triggers pregnancy-induced hypertension?*

PLJ: There are several hypotheses to explain the pathophysiology of PIH. However, we do not know yet the exact triggers for PIH. Recently, an important body of evidence suggests a crucial role of the vascular endothelium in the normal hemodynamic adjustments during pregnancy, especially mediated by the production of vasoactive substances such as prostacyclin and nitric oxide. In PIH there is an alteration of the production of the vasodilators which could explain the clinical manifestations of the disease (hypertension, edema, proteinuria, platelet activation, etc.)

KH: *How does calcium play a role in preventing PIH?*

PLJ: In 1987, (American Journal of Obstetrics and Gynecology, 156;216-262) we proposed that calcium supplementation increased the vascular production of prostacyclin because its synthesis is partially dependent on the levels of extracellular calcium, which are maintained between the narrow physiological range by calcium supplementation. However, later on we demonstrated that supplementation with 2 gm per day of elemental calcium in the second half of pregnancy does not increase production of prostacyclin by maternal-fetal tissues (Journal of Obstetrics and Gynaecology, 1991; 11:93-96. Recently we have demonstrated (British Journal of Pharmacology, 1990; 101:489-493) that serum ionized calcium levels are crucial for the production of endothelial nitric oxide (NO). Nitric oxide plays a fundamental role in the control of blood pressure, blood flow and platelet function. In my view, dietary calcium supplementation reduces the frequency of PIH by maintaining the serum ionized calcium.

KH: *What is the role of vascular nitric oxide (NO) in pregnancy-induced hypertension and its relationship to calcium?*

PLJ: In animals it has been demonstrated that calcium-dependent nitric oxide synthase activity in maternal tissues rises and is associated with an increase in cyclic GMP, the second messenger of NO. Furthermore, it was reported that inhibition of NO synthesis in rats during pregnancy produces signs similar to those of PIH. Recently, we have shown that in human pregnancy (British Journal of Obstetrics and Gynaecology, 1996;10:33-38) the synthesis of nitric oxide is increased and that in preeclampsia there is a reduction in plasma concentration and urinary excretion of cyclic GMP. Interestingly, hydralazine, a vasodilator compound used as an antihypertensive drug in patients with PIH, produces an important increase in plasma levels and in the urinary excretion of cyclic GMP. The release of nitric oxide is dependent on transmembrane ionized calcium flux. So, it is likely that any significant decrease in levels of calcium necessary for this process of adaptation will favor the generation of PIH.

KH: *What dosages are we talking about with regards to calcium supplementation and its preventive role?*

PLJ: In most clinical trials, the supplement was either 1.5 or 2 gm of calcium. Supplementation was by tablet rather than by dietary modification. However, this is an intake which can be achieved by changes in the diet or by adding calcium to certain common foods.

KH: *Is calcium something that could be taken either orally or intravenously for an acute episode of pregnancy-induced hypertension or is it something that we should get in a preventive type of approach?*

PLJ: Calcium supplementation during pregnancy appears to reduce the risk of PIH. It cannot be recommended for the treatment of PIH.

KH: *Are there any adverse consequences to calcium supplementation?*

PLJ: There is a theoretical concern that increasing calcium intake during pregnancy could increase the risk of urinary calculi which occurs in approximately 1 in 1500 pregnancies. However, a recent report (New England Journal of Medicine, 1993; 328:833-838) suggests that dietary calcium intake is inversely related to the risk of symptomatic kidney stones. At the moment, calcium supplementation during pregnancy appears to be safe, efficacious and a cost-effective preventive measure which can significantly reduce the risk of PIH.

KH: *What further studies need to be done to confirm calcium's role in this condition?*

PLJ: Despite the promise from the results of calcium supplementation trials, these are too small to provide reliable information about the effects on substantial measures of outcome, such as mortality. Additional large trials are required. ◆

Premature Rupture of Fetal Membranes and Antioxidants

Bridgett Barrett, Ph.D., RD
Ross Products Division
Abbott Laboratories
Dept. 105200 - DN3
625 Cleveland Avenue
Columbus, OH 43215-1724 U.S.A.
(614) 624-3571 / (614) 624-3453 (FAX)

"Potential Role of Ascorbic Acid and β-Carotene in the Prevention of Preterm Rupture of Fetal Membranes," International Journal of Vitamin Nutrition Research, 1994;64:192-197.   #21209

KH: Please describe your educational background since college.

BB: I received a bachelor's degree in dietetics from the University of Dayton in Dietetics and a Master's of Medical Science from Emory University in Atlanta, Georgia. I also did a dietetic internship at Emory University and became a registered dietitian. I did my Ph.D. work on nutrition and pregnancy at the University of Georgia in conjunction with the Center For Disease Control in Atlanta.

KH: What is your current position?

BB: My current position is a clinical research associate with Ross Product Division, Abbott Laboratories.

KH: How did you get interested in the particular topic of antioxidants in the prevention of preterm rupture of fetal membranes (PROM)?

BB: Actually, I became interested in vitamin C and its relationship to premature rupture of membranes because of the important role vitamin C has in collagen synthesis. There had been some actual *in vitro* work done on tissue cultures evaluating the role of vitamin C in the synthesis of collagen in the chorioamnion. This experimental work is what led me to conduct some observational research on pregnant women. I also had an interest in other antioxidant vitamins because they may be important in the overall picture, especially in women who smoke during pregnancy. In my first study (Biology of the Neonate, 1991;60:333-335), I found a relationship between smokers and vitamin C in the amniotic fluid. Women who smoked had a vitamin C level 50% lower in the amniotic fluid than women who didn't smoke. Perhaps smoking increased fetal utilization of vitamin C.

KH: Your first explanation was vitamin C is important in collagen synthesis. But the theoretic mechanism that antioxidants work by is preventing free radical damage to tissue. So you have two mechanisms?

BB: The mechanisms are really not known, however, speculation would suggest two mechanisms. Vitamin C is important in both free radical formation and, as we know, collagen synthesis. My most recent research indicates that concentrations are significantly lower in amniotic fluid of women with premature rupture of fetal membranes (PROM). However, lower serum vitamin C levels were not detected in women with PROM. Perhaps the placental transfer of the vitamin is impaired or the requirement is increased for pregnant women with PROM. Another interesting finding was smokers who did not have PROM had a significantly higher serum beta-carotene level. Beta-carotene in maternal serum may play a role in protecting the fetoplacental unit from free radical damage caused by cigarette smoking. Whether high concentrations of beta-carotene in maternal serum alter antioxidant capacity in the fetoplacental unit remains to be elucidated.

KH: In other words, vitamin C is the first line of oxidant defense. If these females were low in other antioxidants, maybe you might get a lower amount of ascorbate?

BB: This is not known. To understand the role of antioxidant vitamins in the prevention of PROM, more studies directed towards the exploration of the effects of ascorbic acid and beta-carotene in the fetal membrane are needed.

KH: Is beta-carotene an essential nutrient during pregnancy and what dose would you look for in a prenatal vitamin?

BB: There is no evidence that beta-carotene is an essential nutrient (no RDA) during pregnancy. However, it's probably important during pregnancy, especially for those women who smoke. I can't really say what the dose would be.

KH: How about a dose range?

BB: I would say 20% to 30% of the actual amount of vitamin A should be as beta-carotene. Beta-carotene not only is an antioxidant, but is a nontoxic form of vitamin A. When pregnant women select a prenatal vitamin, they should select one that has beta-carotene.

KH: I recently interviewed Dr. Scott Walsh from the Medical College of Virginia who evaluated lipid peroxidation products during pregnancy. There seems to be a trend of lower antioxidants and increased lipid peroxidation products in preeclampsia.

BB: I have reviewed some research in this area.

KH: Is there a trial in the future of antioxidants?

BB: Not that I am aware of. Based on our results, a prospective randomized study is warranted to expand and support the present findings. Fifteen to 40% of all preterm births can be attributed to PROM. Strategies to help pregnant women receive adequate nutritional intervention as well as cease smoking should be pursued.

KH: How did you get these samples of fluid? Before delivery or after delivery?

BB: Amniotic fluid was obtained from each patient by either sterile speculum exam or amniocentesis during the third trimester prior to delivery. A simultaneous venous blood specimen was collected. Both amniotic fluid and serum specimens were analyzed for ascorbic acid, beta-carotene, retinol and vitamin E. Beta-caroten/e was not found in amniotic fluid.

KH: If you had to pick out a vitamin C dose that was reasonable in a multiple or prenatal, what would you suggest?

BB: For a smoker?

KH: A smoking pregnant female.

BB: I would say 100 mg, which is the new RDA for smokers. For somebody who wasn't smoking but pregnant, I would say the RDA, which is 70 mg for pregnancy. The other very interesting finding of this study is that vitamin C levels in the amniotic fluid did significantly correlate with dietary intake. This was an unexpected finding, and whether or not dietary vitamin C is adequately transferred to the amniotic fluid/fetus in all pregnancies is unknown. Many factors (i.e., blood volume expansion) can influence the placental transfer of vitamins/minerals during pregnancy.

KH: Were concentrations of vitamin C better correlated with amniotic levels than serum levels?

BB: Yes. Serum didn't correlate at all.

KH: So you just found a new assessment technique for vitamin C values.

BB: Yes. However, this would not be practical in the clinical setting.

KH: How would you know how to select a good prenatal vitamin? What would you look for?

BB: I would look for a prenatal vitamin that is based on the 1989 RDAs and contains beta-carotene as part of the vitamin A requirement. ◆

Psychiatry and Inositol

Jonathan Benjamin, M.D.

The Soroka Medical Center
P.O. Box 151
Beer-sheba, Israel 84101
972 7 400783 or 400351 / 972 7 274696 (FAX)

"Inositol Treatment in Psychiatry,"
Psychopharmacology Bulletin, 1995;31:167-175. #23703

Kirk Hamilton: *Can you please share with me your educational background and current position?*

Jonathan Benjamin: I trained as a physician and psychiatrist at Ben Gurion University, Beer-sheba, Israel. In 1993-1995 I was a visiting associate and visiting scientist at the National Institutes of Health in Bethesda, Maryland.

KH: *When did you become interested in the role of inositol in psychiatric disorders?*

JB: Actually, it was my mentor R.H. Belmaker, a life-long student of lithium, who built on the suggestion that lithium might be working by lowering inositol levels. He showed that exogenous inositol could reverse lithium effects in animals and lithium side-effects in man. Then he found a report of low CSF inositol levels in the depressed patients and he and J. Levine showed that inositol could treat clinical depression.

KH: *What are the psychiatric disorders that inositol may have the most benefit in?*

JB: We have thus far found inositol helpful in double-blind studies of depression, panic disorder and obsessive-compulsive disorder.

KH: *What are the theoretic mechanisms by which inositol might work in depression and panic disorder?*

JB: Inositol is a precursor of phosphatidylinositol biphosphate, which is split into two second messengers when certain noradrenaline and serotonin receptors are activated. So pharmacological doses of inositol may be affecting noradrenaline and serotonin systems at the second-messenger level. Another possibility is effects on membrane stability; inositol is a constituent of membrane lipid structures.

KH: *At what therapeutic dose range has inositol been used in clinical trials with success in depression and panic disorder?*

JB: Six to twelve grams a day. The situation may resemble that of L-tryptophan where large doses of natural substances are required before a pharmacologic effect is apparent.

KH: *What is the upper limit with regards to side effects of inositol therapy?*

JB: We and others have given 20 gm a day without any ill effects.

KH: *What is the best form of inositol to use in therapy?*

JB: The only form we have worked with is oral powder mixed in juice.

KH: *Do you see any other psychiatric disorders where inositol may be used in clinical practice?*

JB: We have performed negative studies in autism, schizophrenia and dementia. Inositol *may* be contraindicated in mania. ◆

Rheumatoid Arthritis and Fish Oil

Dr. P. Geusens, M.D., Ph.D.
Dr. L. Willems Institute
Clinical Research Center for Bone & Joint Disease, Belgium
Universitaire Campus, Gebouwen A en C
B-3590 Diepenbeek, Belgium
32 11 26 92 11/ 32 11 26 93 12 (FAX)

"Long-Term Effect of Omega-3 Fatty Acid Supplementation in Active Rheumatoid Arthritis: A 12-Month, Double-Blind Controlled Study", <u>Arthr. and Rheu.</u>, June 1994;37(6):824-825. #21724

Kirk Hamilton: *What is your educational background and present position?*

Piet Geusens: I am currently a professor at the Doctor Willems-Institute and the Limburg University Center in Belgium. Formerly I was a consultant at the Catholic University of Leuven, where I trained in Internal Medicine and Rheumatology. Here, I also received my M.D. and Ph.D. degrees with Professor Dr. J. Dequeker. I am now head of the Clinical Research Center For Bone and Joint Diseases, doing clinical and basic research mainly on rheumatoid arthritis and osteoporosis.

KH: *What is the theoretical basis for the use of omega-3 fatty acids as antiinflammatory agents?*

PG: The theoretic rationale for the use of omega-3 fatty acid supplements is based on the finding that fatty acid metabolism is involved in inflammation. Fatty acids are incorporated into the cell wall of inflammatory cells. When these cells become activated, the metabolism of arachidonic acid is activated, resulting in the production of inflammatory active metabolites. These metabolites consist of 2 main groups, the prostaglandins and the leukotrienes. Prostaglandins are more proinflammatory than some of the leukotrienes. If more omega-3 fatty acids are present in the food then there is more incorporated in the cell wall proteins, less inflammatory active leukotrienes are released, and general inflammation is lower.

KH: *How might fish oils (omega-3 fatty acids) have benefit in rheumatoid arthritis?*

PG: From a theoretic standpoint a fish-based diet should have benefit in reducing rheumatologic symptoms as they contain more unsaturated fatty acids. However, the dose-effect of fish oil supplements we used in the study as omega-3 fatty acids would be the equivalent to a huge amount of fish, which cannot be achieved on a regular basis. It is, however, important also for the treatment of rheumatoid arthritis (RA), to reduce the intake of saturated fatty acids as found mainly in red meat and, consequently, to increase the intake of 'white meat' and/or fish.

KH: *What was the main finding in your study regarding the long term use of omega-3 fatty acids in rheumatoid arthritic patients?*

PG: The main findings in our study on the use of omega-3 fatty acids in rheumatoid arthritis is the positive effects on the evolution of the disease as perceived by the patients which resulted in even a lower consumption of other antirheumatic therapies, many of which are potentially toxic. The favorable effects of omega-3 fatty acids was already known from short term studies. But the main new insight of this research was that this effect is long-lasting. Also, this occurs possibly because patients are already treated with antirheumatic drugs.

KH: *How practically can we incorporate omega-3 fatty acids into the diet?*

PG: The practical implication for utilizing this high dose of omega-3 fatty acids in clinical practice is that normal dietary manipulation, switching from saturated to unsaturated fatty acids, is not sufficient on its own, as lower doses of omega-3 fatty acids was not able to induce improvement. The other consequence is that high doses used are quite expensive, at least in Europe. Furthermore, patients should take these supplements in plastic gelules 6 per day, but, there was excellent gastro-intestinal tolerance.

KH: *Are there any other nutrients that may help modulate inflammation?*

PG: Whether other accessory nutrients may help modulate the inflammatory cascade as fish oil is not known. Some rheumatic diseases are well treated by dietary manipulation such as purine deficiency in the treatment of hyperuricemia in gout. Gout is, however, very different from rheumatoid arthritis, as its inflammatory problems are secondary to the deposition of uric acid by a disturbed metabolism, while the pathophysiology of rheumatoid arthritis is not fully understood and of autoimmune origin. As long as no definitive treatment for rheumatoid arthritis is available, every new medication or dietary manipulation is a welcomed additive. Although there were some initial concerns that the use of omega-3 fatty acids could result in a person being predisposed to bleeding (as they also interfere with blood clotting mechanisms), no such problems were observed at either dose used. Interestingly, most patients participating in this trial were treated with several other antirheumatic drugs, combinations of which were well tolerated.

KH: *What is the role of food in rheumatoid arthritis?*

PG: Other influences of food are well known in rheumatoid arthritis. One of the most impressive is the antiinflammatory effect of fasting, a therapy which can however not be performed in the long term.

KH: *Is there any evidence of abnormal bacteria in the bowel and altered intestinal permeability in rheumatoid arthritic patients?*

PG: Since the beginning of the study of rheumatoid arthritis, many investigators have studied the possibility of infection, also in the intestines and increased permeability of the gastrointestinal tract wall. In some forms of arthritis, such as spondyloarthropathies and reactive arthritis, there is some evidence that infection - especially in the gut - could initiate or perpetuate the disease. However, again, these diseases are different from the clinical picture in rheumatoid arthritis. Although infections can aggravate the same course of the disease in rheumatoid arthritis, the relation between infection and rheumatoid arthritis lies on the possibility of molecular mimicry between the infectious agents and components of the joints. In this way, antibodies to proteins that are found in infectious agents or its byproducts could cross-react with similar proteins in the joint, initiating or perpetuating the disease in this way. ◆

Sarcoidosis and Melatonin

Matteo Cagnoni, M.D.
Department of Dermatology
University of Siena
Via Bolognes vecchia
178-50139, Florence, Italy
39 55 412 178 / 39 55 410 183 / 39 55 422 3549 (FAX)

"Melatonin For Treatment of Chronic Refractory Sarcoidosis,"
<u>The Lancet</u>, November 4, 1995;346:229-230. #23549

Kirk Hamilton: Could you please share with me your educational background and current position?

Matteo Cagnoni: I am a dermatologist at the Department of Dermatology at the University of Siena in Italy.

KH: How did you come up with the idea of using melatonin in sarcoidosis?

MC: We and other researchers shared the opinion that melatonin, besides exerting a "scavenger" activity, might modulate the immune system. For this reason we proposed melatonin's use in diseases which involved an immunologic mechanism in their pathogenesis.

KH: What is the physiological mechanism by how melatonin may work in sarcoidosis?

MC: This answer is similar to the answer above which is that melatonin acts as a modulator of the immune system.

KH: These two case reports in <u>The Lancet</u> dramatically showed resolution of symptoms. Have you utilized melatonin in other cases of sarcoidosis?

MC: We have also administered a long-term melatonin treatment to many other patients affected by sarcoidosis, always obtaining significant clinical improvements. However, we have chosen two of these treated cases for publication, because they seemed particularly significant. These cases in fact were not responsive to long-term corticosteroid therapy and were chronic evolving sarcoidosis. We believe that the results obtained are well worth mentioning because of the failure of previous long-term steroid therapy, the improvement during melatonin treatment in the second patient, the worsening which followed the precocious interruption of that treatment, as well as the rapid improvement obtained with its resumption.

KH: How did you come up with such a supraphysiolic treatment dose of 20 mg per day of melatonin?

MC: In the treatment of endocrine diseases, dosages higher than physiologic levels are currently being used. The choice of the dosage is derived from the experience acquired for the treatment of autoimmune disease (rheumatoid arthritis and scleroderma) and in particular of neoplastic disease.

KH: Is melatonin's antioxidant properties the probable reason for benefit in this condition or is it a hormonal effect?

MC: Melatonin is a substance which modulates the neuro-immuno-endocrine system. Other researchers and ourselves have the opinion that melatonin can explicate a "scavenger" activity and an immunomodulary activity (so modifying the abnormal immunologic response which characterizes these diseases).

KH: Do you know of any other uses of melatonin as a medical treatment?

MC: We have utilized melatonin also in patients affected by systemic sclerosis (scleroderma) and in patients affected by rheumatoid arthritis. In the first group of patients we obtained encouraging results, both in those affected by the diffuse form and in those affected by localized scleroderma. Patients affected by rheumatoid arthritis can be treated orally or, when it is indicated, intra-articularly. In these cases, we had the clinical impression of slight improvement. In our center a larger trial has been started to confirm the efficacy of melatonin in these diseases.

KH: What is the safety of this dose of melatonin (20 mg/d)?

MC: Many experiences in this field have permitted us to assess an absolute absence of side effects even at much higher doses than those we use (i.e. up to 5 g/day in Parkinson's disease). In the majority of cases, hormonal treatments are performed at doses which are much higher than physiologic ones. ◆

Silicone Breast Implant Syndrome

Frank V. Vasey, M.D.
University of South Florida College of Medicine
Division of Rheumatology
12901 Bruce B. Downs Blvd., Box 19
Tampa, FL 33612-4799, U.S.A.
(813) 974-2681 / (813) 974-5229 (FAX)

"Clinical Findings in Symptomatic Women With Silicone Breast Implants",
Seminars in Arthritis and Rheumatism, August 1994;24(1)/Suppl. 1:22-28. # 20882

Kirk Hamilton: *What is your educational background from college and what is your present position?*

Frank Vasey: I am currently a professor of medicine at the University of South Florida, College of Medicine. I received my undergraduate degree from Cornell College in Mt. Vernon, Iowa. I started medical school at the University of North Dakota in Grand Forks and after 2 years transferred to the University of Pennsylvania in Philadelphia where I received my M.D. degree. I did 2 years of general internal medicine at the Oakland Alameda County Hospital in Oakland, California and then 2 years in the Navy at Mare Island Naval Shipyard in Vallejo. I did 1 year of rheumatology at Queens University in Kingston, Ontario, Canada and went with my training supervisor then to McGill University in Montreal where I finished the rheumatology program. I was on the faculty for 1½ years as an assistant professor of medicine and rheumatology. Then I relocated to the University of South Florida where I have been since 1977.

KH: *When did you start to get interested in silicone breast implants and the suspected autoimmune/rheumatologic condition that everybody is speaking about?*

FV: Even though there were a couple of papers in the literature as far back as 1979, the paper that I first noted was in 1984 in Arthritis and Rheumatism. Since that time, I have worked closely with Luis Espinosa, M.D. who is now chief of Rheumatology at Louisiana State University. I saw a patient about 1986 that had aches and pains in her upper back and neck and I didn't know she had breast implants at the time. I followed her for about 2 years and then one day she stopped me out in the hall and said, "Guess what happened, my breast implants eroded through the skin. I took the implants out and now I feel so much better." I saw other patients with similar stories. Dr. Espinosa was following some scleroderma patients and a lupus-like patient all of whom were reported in the medical literature in 3 separate reports. They took out their implants and all tended to improve. So in 1990 we summarized all the patients that we had and reported them at the national American College of Rheumatology. By early 1991 we had 50 patients. I think we were somewhat fortuitously located. I think more women had implants in California, Texas and Florida. Actually Steven Weiner from Los Angeles had a similar experience to ours writing up patients in the late 80s. He described an unusual arthritis in 3 patients with breast implants. Then he also became actively involved seeing many women with breast implants and systemic symptoms. So we became convinced there was a problem based on our clinical experience and we suggested the possibility to the patients that they remove the implants. We were gratified that the majority of patients seemed to be improving after they took out the implants. It appeared unlikely

that these experiences were a coincidence.

KH: *So this experience has really been over the last 10 years. With the removal of the implants (and we're talking specifically about silicone) can you give a ballpark percentage of the females that have their symptoms improve?*

FV: In the article you reviewed in Seminars in Arthritis and Rheumatism we looked at 50 patients. Thirty-three removed their implants. Only 1 woman of the 33 continued to worsen after she took out her implants and she appeared to have natural rheumatoid arthritis. About 30% seemed to stabilize and 70% improved with an average of 2 years of follow-up.

KH: *Are there individuals who have risk factors that are more susceptible to the silicone implant problem?*

FV: There probably are genetic factors. I've have seen 3 sets of identical twins. In 2 sets there was a very similar illness at a similar pace in both sets of women. In the third set the woman here says her sister in Los Angeles insists that she is not sick but the sister here isn't quite sure. She thinks perhaps the sister in Los Angeles is in denial. There probably are genetic factors that increase the likelihood of some women's immune system reacting to the silicone material that is escaping from the implants and other women's bodies are going to tolerate the same material.

KH: *So there is not any lifestyle factors that you have been able to correlate?*

FV: Anything that encourages the escape of the material from the implant. So I think physical forces could be a factor there. I have seen deep sea diving put more pressure against the implants for example.

KH: *Let me ask you this - Is it definitely your opinion that silicone is the problem?*

FV: Well that's not totally resolved either. I think it is clear that the women who are symptomatic have an excited immune system basically. Now the question of what aspect of the implants are causing this immune activation is still unresolved. The possibilities include some component of the gel and the amorphous silica in the wall of the envelope. The problem is not just the gel. The macrophages from the immune system attack the envelope. That is what gradually weakens the implant. So we know now that after 10 years they are largely ruptured which is a recent recognition. They have been putting implants in for 30 years and now we find they are mostly ruptured after 10. That is from a paper in <u>Plastic and Reconstructive Surgery</u> in April of 1993. The reason that they rupture is that the immune system nibbles away in a sense at the envelope.

KH: *And when you say the envelope - that is the actual encasing of the...?*

FV: That is hard silicone. But it still isn't all that hard.

KH: *In a saline implant, what is the envelope made of?*

FV: It's still silicone.

KH: *So, it could be the same problem?*

FV: Our preliminary observations suggest symptomatic women who replace gel filled implants with saline filled do not do as well as those who remove them and don't replace them. Still they meet the psychological need so each woman has to balance the risk and the benefit. Certainly if your condition continues to worsen you should then consider removing the saline filled silicone envelope implant.

KH: *So, in the saline implant, the fluid is saline. When you say gel, what is that?*

FV: That's silicone gel.

KH: *So you've got a silicone envelope and you have got silicone gel.*

FV: Right.

KH: *Now I am clear. Then you have a silicone envelope again with saline.*

FV: Right. And a lot of women are confused too. The surgeons talk about saline implants and everybody assumes they don't have any silicone.

KH: *Is there any kind of antibody testing that you do that is a generic kind of screen for these individuals?*

FV: I don't, but Dr. Kissovsky, a pathologist in Los Angeles has been working on this longer than I have and has evolved an antibody test to the silicone material which would be a marker of immune activation in a sense. I think it is certainly a fascinating research tool. I don't personally have enough experience with it to know exactly how useful it might be. The approach I take depends on the clinical symptoms the patient has. In other words if they are tired and they have aches and pains and a chronic flu-like state and swollen lymph nodes then I say consider taking the implants out. *I don't treat the laboratory findings because generally in this setting they aren't very helpful. Most of the time the tests are all normal.* About 25% of the time, the people do have a positive ANA. That is an antinuclear antibody test for lupus. But again most of the time they don't have lupus. They don't have a butterfly rash, renal failure, seizures or the typical things of lupus. They just have aches and pains and a fibromyalgia-like state plus the breast implants.

KH: *Do you absolutely not recommend anybody put in silicone implants... should they be taken off the market?*

FV: I do feel that the gel filled implants should be off the market and I think the saline filled implants need to be studied. The problem is the saline implants are going to rupture at some point as well.

KH: *They all rupture at about 10 years?*

FV: They will likely all rupture at some point. Certainly at 10 years most of them are ruptured. So, I mean it would be nice to be able to tell the women, "Listen, you can put this thing in but it is going to go flat like a tire in 5 years or 2 years or 10 years or something and then you're going to have to replace it". Then the question of how many women's immune systems are going to react to the saline filled implant? Some women's bodies are not going to tolerate even the saline filled.

KH: *How long have we been doing this experiment with saline implants?*

FV: I think they were invented in the 70s even or maybe even in the late 60s but they weren't used very much because, again, it had a watery texture rather than a breast-like texture. So the women preferred the gel filled.

KH: *Is there kind of a battle line being drawn between plastic surgeons and rheumatologists?*

FV: There is to some degree. I mean at this point there is still no absolutely definitive study. So basically each physician has to make up his/her own mind based on their own experience and following their own patient. Now some plastic surgeons, for example Leroy Young in St. Louis, has written that he is basically on the same page I am. He sees the chronic fatigue, aches and pains syndrome in his women with breast implants. Yet most plastic surgeons take the position, "Well there is no epidemiological study that proves this yet so we're going to hesitate to think there is an association until it is absolutely proven beyond a shadow of a doubt."

KH: *Do the plastic surgeons have an alternative?*

FV: No they don't at this point other than tissue transfer procedures. They can take stomach muscle tissue and move it up to the chest. It is a fairly large procedure and better discussed with a plastic surgeon. But I have seen some patients who are happy with the procedure. I have also seen some who were unhappy. It turned out to be a bigger procedure than they thought. Rarely the transplant material can die because it has sort of a tenuous blood supply and that is a disaster too. So it is not an easy operation I don't think.

KH: *This has been a great interview. I have learned so much and I am sure our reading audience will appreciate it.*

FV: I have written a book. Do you know about that? It is entitled <u>The Silicone Breast Implant Controversy</u>. If you call Crossing Press they are at 1 (800) 777-1048 you can get a copy of this book. ◆

Sleep Problems, The Elderly and Caffeine

S. Lori Brown, Ph.D., M.P.H.
Epidemiology Branch, HFZ-541
Division of Postmarket Surveillance
Office of Surveillance and Biometrics
Center for Devices and Radiological Health
Food and Drug Administration
1350 Piccard Dr., Room #3060
Rockville, MD 20850 U.S.A.
(301) 594-0610 / (301) 594-0050 (FAX)

"Occult Caffeine as a Source of Sleep Problems in an Older Population",
Journal of the American Geriatric Society, 1995;43:860-864. #23013

Kirk Hamilton: *Could you please share with me your educational background and current position?*

Lori Brown: I have a Ph.D. in medical sciences (immunology) from the University of New Mexico School of Medicine and a Masters of Public Health from Johns Hopkins University School of Hygiene and Public Health. I am currently a Research Scientist Officer at the Food and Drug Administration in the Center For Devices and Radiologic Health, Epidemiology Branch.

KH: *When did you get interested in the role of caffeine and sleep disorders?*

LB: I became interested in this area while I was working at the National Institutes of Health at the Institute on Aging. Much of the work that I did there was with a study called the Established Populations for Epidemiologic Studies of the Elderly. One of our co-authors, Dr. Tamara Harris, was looking at a list of drug ingredients and was struck by the number of participants in our study who had reported using medication containing caffeine. In fact, Dr. Harris thought that these participants were taking over-the-counter products that contained caffeine to help them stay alert or awake. Closer analysis indicated that these were not what they were taking but that a majority of them were taking over-the-counter analgesic products such as aspirin or acetaminophen that contained caffeine. I wondered if those taking medications with caffeine in them were aware that the medication contained caffeine and whether those who took medication with caffeine might have sleep problems related to consumption of that medicine.

KH: *Is caffeine's use in medications and/or recreational drink consumption significantly related to sleep disorders?*

LB: In our study of 2,885 men and women in the Iowa 65 Plus Rural Health Study, those participants who reported taking medication that contained caffeine were more likely to report trouble falling asleep than those not taking a medication with caffeine. Those drinking either tea or decaffeinated coffee did not report trouble falling asleep and, oddly, those reporting drinking coffee were slightly, though not significantly, <u>less</u> likely to report having trouble falling asleep. We think that this is because those that have trouble falling asleep may intentionally avoid beverages that they know contain caffeine, such as coffee.

KH: *How does caffeine affect sleep?*

LB: Caffeine works by biochemically stimulating cortical arousal. The effect of caffeine on sleep was reported widely to delay the onset of sleep and increase the number of arousals during sleep including early waking.

KH: *How prevalent is caffeine in over-the-counter medications and what kind of medications most commonly contain caffeine?*

LB: Over-the-counter products which may contain caffeine are analgesics (pain relievers) or cold preparations for such common ailments as headaches, stomach ailments or pain. They may contain 30 mg of caffeine or the equivalent of a weak cup of coffee. The reason that caffeine is included in these medications is that it is reported to potentiate the effect of common analgesics such as aspirin or acetaminophen. Also, caffeine is reported to have a slight analgesic effect of its own. Many people do not realize these common remedies contain caffeine.

KH: *What is the message to health care workers with regards to caffeine- containing medications?*

LB: Health care workers should counsel their patients that over-the-counter products may contain caffeine. If patients are complaining of sleep difficulty, OTC medications should be considered as a possible source of the problem. Patients should be counseled to avoid such caffeine-containing products, particularly if they are reporting sleep problems such as delayed onset of sleep, repeated night time arousal or early waking. Clearly, other factors should be taken into consideration too.

KH: *How can the elderly avoid using these products?*

LB: Many people limit their consumption of caffeine-containing beverages intentionally, but they may be unaware that medications they are taking are a source of caffeine. Manufacturers are required to label OTC medications so that all of their ingredients are known. Consumers should read these labels carefully so that if they are sensitive to the effects of caffeine they can avoid these products. ◆

Stroke, Transient Ischemic Attacks, Vitamin E and Aspirin

Manfred Steiner, M.D. Ph.D.
Professor of Medicine
Hematology/Oncology Section
School of Medicine
Brody 3E-127
Greenville, NC 27858-4354 U.S.A.
(919) 816-2560 (dept), (919) 816-2558 (of), (919) 816-3418 (FAX)

"Vitamin E Plus Aspirin Compared With Aspirin Alone In Patients With Transient Ischemic Attacks", American Journal of Clinical Nutrition, 1995;62(suppl):1381S-1384S. #23791

Kirk Hamilton: Can you please share with me your educational background and current position?

Manfred Steiner: I went to medical school at the University of Vienna, Austria, and subsequently trained in internal medicine and hematology at Tufts University, New England Medical Center in Boston, and received a Ph.D. in biochemistry and nutrition from the Massachusetts Institute of Technology. Until 1994 I was head of the Hematology section, Brown University. In 1994 I moved to North Carolina and I am director of hematology research at East Carolina University School of Medicine.

KH: When did you get interested in the role of vitamin E and cerebrovascular disease, and in particular, transient ischemic attacks?

MS: I have been interested in vitamin E for many years, having studied its effect on platelet aggregation, on lipid peroxide production and platelet adhesion. I became interested in the possibility that vitamin E might offer a logical additive to a strong aggregating agent in the treatment of transient ischemic attacks when I discovered that vitamin E inhibited the shape change of platelets - the very first stage in the activation of platelets and important for the anchoring of platelets to the adhesive surface.

KH: What did you find from your study with regards to aspirin and vitamin E at 400 I.U./d versus aspirin alone?

MS: My colleagues and I detected that vitamin E offers additional protection (beyond that provided by aspirin) against the progression of transient ischemic attacks or incomplete strokes to complete strokes. We estimated an additional 25% (above the 20% reduction due to aspirin) reduction in the risk of developing ischemic strokes in patients who were taking 400 I.U. vitamin E plus one aspirin (325 mg) per day.

KH: Are there any suspected side effects to the vitamin E therapy at the dose of 400 I.U. per day?

MS: Vitamin E was tolerated well by our patients when they took it in the prescribed doses.

KH: Is there an increased risk of hemorrhagic stroke with vitamin E supplementation?

MS: Our studies have shown that there were more patients who developed hemorrhagic strokes when they took vitamin E plus aspirin versus aspirin alone. The difference between the two groups was not statistically significant, however. Nevertheless, there appears to be a trend that vitamin E-supplemented individuals under appropriate circumstances (e.g. high blood pressure, etc.) may be more prone to develop hemorrhagic strokes than those taking aspirin alone. There is also some evidence from epidemiologic studies that supplemental vitamin E intake may be associated with a higher incidence of hemorrhagic stroke. If vitamin E, in fact, will be shown to enhance the occurrence of hemorrhagic strokes, it would be an effect that is in line with its purported mechanism of action, i.e., inhibition of platelet adhesion to adhesive surfaces such as subendothelial tissue exposed to the flowing blood in areas of endothelial cell discontinuity.

KH: How do you think vitamin E helps protect against transient ischemic attacks?

MS: I believe that vitamin E is a very effective inhibitor of platelet adhesion and shape change which together with aspirin-induced inhibition of platelet clumping in the circulating blood may reduce the occurrence of platelet aggregates that can be dislodged by the flowing blood and temporarily obstruct small vessels in areas of the brain. ◆

Sudden Infant Death and Iron

Eugene D. Weinberg, Ph.D.
Indiana University
Department of Biology/Jordan Hall 142
Bloomington, Indiana 47405-6801 U.S.A.
(812) 855-4842 / (812) 855-7323 / (812) 855-6705 (FAX)

"The Role of Iron in Sudden Infant Death Syndrome",
Journal of Trace Elements and Experimental Medicine, 1994;7:47-51. #22201

Kirk Hamilton: *Can you please share with us your educational background and present position?*

Eugene D. Weinberg: I received my Ph.D. in microbiology at the University of Chicago in 1950. Since then I have been a faculty member at Indiana University in Bloomington. In 1963 I became head of the microbiology section of the University's Medical Sciences Program. I have published approximately 175 full-length papers that are concerned with the interactions of microbial and animal cell physiology in determining the outcome of infectious and neoplastic diseases. A few of these publications have been designated as bench mark papers in microbiology. During the past 30 years I focused mainly on the offensive strategies whereby pathogenic microbes and cancer cells obtain iron from their hosts and on the defensive measures by which the hosts attempt to withhold iron from the invaders. I am retired from the USPHS Commission Corps Reserve where I held the rank of scientist director. I retired from classroom teaching in 1992, and I am now occupied with full-time studies on iron.

KH: *What got you involved in iron's role in possibly causing disease?*

EW: My students and I participated in the discoveries in the 1940s and 50s concerning the need for iron for bacterial growth.

KH: *How does iron play a role in Sudden Infant Death Syndrome?*

EW: Iron enables toxigenic bacteria to seed in the infant gut.

KH: *Can you share why formula fed infants have a greater risk to SIDS?*

EW: Iron is a risk factor for salmonellosis, botulism, and SIDS because it enables the toxigenic bacteria that cause these diseases to seed in the infant gut. Infants who die of SIDS usually have a history of receiving iron supplements or iron enriched formulas; their livers have 3 times the amount of iron as do infants who died of non-infectious causes.

KH: *Do we know the mechanism of how iron might cause SIDS?*

EW: SIDS infants have more of various bacterial toxins in their gut and bloodstream. A number of microbiology labs in the United States, England and Australia are studying specific bacterial species and strains to determine precise etiologies.

KH: *How much iron in comparison to breast-fed infants is in regular formulas?*

EW: Milk formulas contain an enormous range of iron; the highest ones have 155 times more iron than is contained in maternal milk.

KH: *How does the excess iron in infant formulas effect gut ecology?*

EW: Iron is necessary for growth of all bacteria except lactobacilli. The latter grow in the infant gut when breast milk is used. Lactobacilli are nontoxigenic! When supplemental iron is given, the lactobacilli are crowded out by the harmful bacteria.

KH: *What are your recommendations for iron in infant formulas?*

EW: Excessive quantities of iron should be removed from formula. The amount to be retained needs to be more than is present in maternal milk but should be just sufficient for good nutrition of the infant.

KH: *You probably encourage, very avidly, females to breast feed?*

EW: For many reasons, including that of optimal nutrition, breast milk is best. ◆

Surgery, Critical Illness and Glutamine

Stephen M. Pastores, M.D.
Albert Einstein College of Medicine
Department of Anesthesiology
Montefiore Medical Center
111 East 210th Street
Bronx, NY 10467-2490 U.S.A.
(718) 920-2449 / (718) 652-2464 (FAX)

"Immunomodulatory Effects and Therapeutic Potential of Glutamine in the Critically Ill Surgical Patient," <u>Nutrition</u>, September/October 1994;10(5): 385-391.   #21498

Kirk Hamilton: Could you please share with me your educational background since college and your present position?

Stephen M. Pastores: I received my B.S. in biology at the University of St. Thomas in Manila in the Philippines. I earned my medical degree at Northwestern College of Medicine, also in the Philippines. In 1984 I started a surgical residency at the Cabrini Medical Center in New York.   I then did 4 years of internal medicine at the Metropolitan Hospital Center in New York - the fourth year acting as chief resident. I then went on to do a pulmonary critical care fellowship at the New York University Bellevue Hospital Center from 1990 to 1992. From there I did a surgical critical care fellowship in 1992-1993 at Mt. Sinai Medical Center in New York. Since July of 1993, I have been an assistant professor of anesthesiology and an instructor of medicine at the Montefiore Medical Center at Albert Einstein College of Medicine in the Bronx, New York.

KH: When did your interest in glutamine and critical care come about?

SP: I worked with a few investigators who had done some earlier work in the area of nutrition and metabolism, mainly work using branch chain amino acids. One of the investigators, a Ph.D. Dr. David Katz, happened to be a frequent guest editor for a nutrition journal and had wanted to do a review on glutamine. I worked primarily out of the Surgical Intensive Care Unit and had expressed an interest, since my fellowship, into looking at nutritional support in surgical, critically ill patients. We did some small trials and tried using nutritional interventions in surgically ill patients. That got me into reviewing the area of glutamine.

KH: When you say nutritional intervention, what actually are you talking about? Could you be specific?

SP: There certainly has been a lot of controversy in the areas of nutritional support in the critically ill. Much of the nutritional support of critically ill patients has essentially evolved with time. There have been a lot of changes in our recent concepts of how we should be providing nutritional support to critically ill patients. The traditional way in which we provided nutritional support was to provide essential nutrients like ordinary carbohydrates, lipids and amino acids. In the last 10 to 15 years there has been a better understanding that providing nutrition not only means trying to conserve lean body mass, but it also affects various cellular and metabolic responses which, in the critically ill, may be very important. The whole thinking behind nutritional therapy is changing more into

directing studies, to at least try to provide nutrients that have not only the provision of energy requirements, but also affect cellular and metabolic function that may be important in the critically ill patient.

KH: Could you list a few of the nutrients of interest?

SP: The major nutrients that have been of interest over the last decade or two have been branch chain amino acids, arginine, glutamine and growth hormone.

KH: Is glutamine essential?

SP: Glutamine is not considered an essential amino acid. It is better described as a conditionally essential amino acid. It has been recognized, until very recently, that glutamine actually is one of the major amino acids that happens to be preferentially used up very early in catabolic patients. It is one of the primary nutrients that has to be provided in that early phase of catabolism.

KH: What are some of the functions of glutamine?

SP: Glutamine functions as an essential nutrient for enterocytes, the cells lining the intestinal mucosa of the bowel.

KH: Now is that the small bowel or the large bowel?

SP: Mainly the small bowel. It also has a lot of functions in terms of providing the energy stores for immune cells, primarily lymphocytes and macrophages, which are the primary cellular elements that are important in trying to provide cellular immunity in patients that are sick. Glutamine also has a role in the provision of nitrogen substrates for renal ammoniagenesis. It also serves a role in protein and glycogen synthesis. It functions not only to provide amino acids required for energy, but it also has other roles, primarily immunomodulation.

KH: Is the most important effect of glutamine on the gut or is it systemic?

SP: It seems to be in the gut. This is the area that has been most intensely investigated. As you are probably aware, the role of the gut and gut barrier failure has been an area of intense research both experimentally and clinically. There has been a lot of emphasis on the thinking that the gut may actually be the primary organ system that gets deranged very early in very critically ill patients. This is what we call gut barrier dysfunction. It seems to initiate release of intestinal bacteria which trigger various cytokine responses that seem to generate what we now call "The Multiple Organ Dysfunction Syndrome." This appears to be a major pathway in which most sick patients get into and ultimately succumb.

KH: That is a term that maybe you can help clarify for me . . . bacterial translocation? When you have trauma or significant stress you have increased utilization of glutamine or not enough in the gut. Then somehow the barrier breaks down and the bacteria that are normally there...

SP: The bacteria breaks down. The endotoxin that is normally contained in an intact gut is then able to translocate through various circulations - circulatory beds like the portal and systemic circulation, where it can then trigger various cytokine responses responsible for the inflammatory response we now call "Multi-System Organ Failure."

KH: If the gut was intact and the bacteria stayed where they are supposed to stay then these effects wouldn't happen?

SP: A lot of the work on bacterial translocation has tried to assume that this hypothesis is real. To be honest with you, bacterial translocation, as far as I know, has never been proven to actually occur clinically in humans. But there is a lot of work experimentally to suggest that this is what occurs. This whole idea behind the "gut hypothesis" for multiorgan failure in humans still remains kind of controversial.

KH: There have been some trials utilizing glutamine. What are the benefits in humans, or are there any proven yet?

SP: There have been limited clinical trials but several experimental studies. But then again, glutamine is just one of those amino acids in most catabolic patients, particularly surgically ill catabolic patients, that tend to have inefficient utilization of protein. It is not only glutamine that probably is depleted but other amino acids as well. The provision of glutamine alone may be one essential need that has to be provided. You have to understand that there also is an interplay of other amino acids that may be relevant. What we do know is that at least in experimental work, the provision of glutamine, either enterally or mixed in parenteral solutions, seems to improve gut immune function and seems to prevent the development of gut barrier dysfunction. There have been a lot of studies in rats and dogs showing that the provision of glutamine seems to not only increase glutamine levels but also prevent bacterial translocation from occurring. However, in humans the studies have been few. And the ones that have been done have mainly shown reductions in morbidity but not really changes in overall outcome in sick patients.

KH: Define the term morbidity for me please.

SP: Most of the morbidity is related to either reductions in length of hospital stay or decreases in incidence of infection....

KH: But wouldn't that save a significant amount of dollars right there?

SP: Oh yes. It certainly may be very relevant in terms of decreasing costs. If you have a patient that can stay a week or two less in an intensive care unit because you have reduced infection rates and you have been able to decrease the overall length of stay, then there definitely is significant cost savings.

KH: Are there any other benefits that have occurred with glutamine supplementation?

SP: In the limited clinical studies done so far, overall nitrogen balance seems to be improved, and with that there has been an associated reduction in the patient's length of stay as well as overall reductions in morbidity from the reduction in infection. But they are very limited studies.

KH: Well, it would seem to be an area to pursue since the health care dollar is shrinking.

SP: The only difficulty with glutamine, as far as being part of our routine administration, is that glutamine for intravenous use has not been FDA approved yet.

KH: Tell me . . . I kind of hinted to this earlier. It seems to me that these are still essentially macronutrients, and it always amazes me why the micronutrients (vitamins and minerals) aren't looked at because they are actually the cofactors which make these amino acids convert from one to another.

SP: Oh yes. They are certainly very, very important.

KH: I recall one study in an intensive care setting in which patients on Lasix therapy were assessed for vitamin B1 status using the transketolase enzyme test. Many patients turned out to be functionally deficient, and vitamin B1 injections helped improve their ejection fractions. And this is just one micronutrient. I am sure a lot of these critical care patients, if they were ever assessed, (by functional means for micronutrients) would show significant multiple deficiencies.

SP: The problem is that it is a very complex interplay. I think provision of single nutrient vitamin interventions are probably hard to look at in overall terms. But I think at least as far as surgical critical illness, the only reason we were interested in patterns of amino acid release, breakdown, utilization and so forth is because we know that a lot of these patients tend to be very catabolic very early. Much of the catabolism is protein depletion and now we know that there are certain amino acids that have been traditionally considered nonessential that may be of benefit with supplementation.

KH: Is there a routine multivitamin that gets put in with this solution?

SP: Yes. Parenteral solutions generally have multivitamins incorporated in them.

KH: Just on an RDA type of level?

SP: Right. Usually just on an RDA level unless you have a suspicion or a clinical marker that suggests that you may be specifically deficient in a specific vitamin or if you pull a level....

KH: Yes. But you know the point is that the RDA's are designed for essentially all healthy people, and here you have the stressors of the critical care and surgery? These critically ill surgical aren't in the category of "essentially all healthy people" by any means!

SP: A lot of the early attempts to provide some form of nutrition tried to incorporate supplements like vitamin E, zinc and things like that. We tend to like to have those on board in most of our big surgical cases, but it is not routine to pull levels of vitamins looking for specific deficiencies. Much of the time the regular, routine, parenteral vitamin preparations are what are incorporated in regular hyperalimentation solutions.

KH: Well, I can see from my perspective, if there was a way to get a vitamin/mineral panel or functional enzyme tests at a reasonable cost and "turn-around", you could look at all the micronutrients. You would see gross functional deficiencies.

SP: Most of these are cofactors of the metabolic pathways which may be very important because those are the respondents (cytokines) that essentially mediate all of the various organ dysfunctions that we see in patients who are very ill. ◆

Surgery, Inflammatory Disease and Selenium

Klaus Winnefeld, M.D.
Surgical Clinic
Friedrich-Schiller-Universitat Jena
Institute For Clinical Chemistry and Laboratory Diagnostics
Naturwissenschaftligh-technischer Bereich
07740 Jena, Germany
49 3641 633 127 (PHONE/FAX) / 49 3641 639 212 / 49 3641 639 343 (FAX)

"Selenium and Serum and Whole Blood in Patients With Surgical Interventions,"
Biological Trace Element Research, 1995;50:149-155. #23738

Kirk Hamilton: *Dr. Winnefeld could you please share with me your educational background and current position?*

Klaus Winnefeld: I am a chemist with postgraduate study in the fields of analytical atomic spectroscopy and clinical chemistry. Since 1968 I have engaged in the determination of trace elements in medicine in the surgical clinic setting initially, and now in the Institute of Clinical Chemistry at the Friedrich Schiller-University Jona. From the work in that domain of trace elements, I realized the importance of antioxidants in many disciplines of medicine. Currently, I am vice director of the Institute of Clinical Chemistry.

KH: *Why might selenium be important to the surgical patient?*

KW: At present, more and more attention is being paid to radicals and reactive oxygen compounds in metabolic processes because an increased occurrence of such highly reactive species can be found in numerous diseases. Radicals are involved in the etiology of many diseases such as pancreatitis, renal failure, sepsis and cancer among others. Preventive measures include utilizing dietary components with antioxidant effects but also drug therapy, using antioxidants, have found their way into medicine. As a prerequisite for such treatment, the status of the antioxidant needs to be characterized with the help of suitable markers. One marker is the status of selenium in the human organism. In many countries there exists a malnutrition of selenium. Therefore, the correction of the imbalance of selenium before large surgical interventions is necessary.

KH: *What are some of the physiologic effects of selenium in relation to inflammatory conditions?*

KW: Selenium as an essential trace element plays an important role in many diseases. It is supposed to be toxic and carcinogenic, but can also have a protective function against free radicals. Over the last several years there has been accumulating evidence that reactive oxygen species, and therefore selenium status, are significant in the pathogenesis of various diseases. Glutathione-peroxidase (GSH-Px), an enzyme containing selenium, has an antioxidant effect. Glutathione peroxidase is involved in the "destruction" of reactive oxygen species (ROS). Furthermore, a number of selenium proteins have been identified whose exact functions are as yet unknown. Alongside this indirect effect of selenium, there is reason to assume that another antioxidant mechanism of action must exist as selenium has a very rapid antioxidant effect in acute pancreatitis. Inflammatory syndromes decrease over a very short period of time with selenium therapy.

KH: *How did you get interested in the role of selenium and surgical outcome?*

KW: Every operation represents a stress reaction for the patient which diseased body has to compensate for, and in this process selenium can turn out to be of vital importance. On the other hand many patients awaiting surgical treatment showed decreased selenium concentrations in the serum and whole blood which result in reduced antioxidant capacity.

KH: *What dosage of selenium did you add to the parenteral nutrition?*

KW: The dosage was fixed according to the selenium concentrations in the serum and whole blood and was 58-410 ug Se/d over a period of 10 days after the operation.

KH: *What parameters of selenium status were normalized and how long did it take to achieve this in this study?*

KW: With the number of patients examined, we only monitored the selenium concentrations in the serum and whole blood as well as selenium balance (intake and excretion in the urine) over a period of 10 days.

KH: *How was it shown that selenium supplementation improved resistance to oxidative stress in these patients?*

KW: The patients who received selenium replacement overcame the surgical stress more quickly and showed fewer complications in the postoperative phase.

KH: *How serious a problem is oxidative stress in the surgical patient?*

KW: All inflammatory processes are accompanied by a generation of free radicals/reactive oxygen species. In the case of surgical interventions carried out in the state of bloodlessness, there will be a massive generation of free radicals during reperfusion. This same release of free radicals will occur in organ grafting, interventions on the vascular system or bones, neurosurgical operations and burn injuries.

As 30% of all newly operated patients show malnutrition prior to operation, which among other things also reflects their selenium status, monitoring the selenium status is being recommended even for patients who receive postoperative parenteral nutrition over a short period of time. Numerous authors have associated the risk of sepsis in newly operated patients with a selenium deficiency. Lowered selenium levels have been documented in sepsis patients irrespective of the type of pathogen involved. Tumor patients very frequently show dysfunctions of antioxidant status.

KH: *Did these patients who received selenium have better outcomes such as reduced hospital stay or reduction of infections?*

KW: The patients were treated and monitored over 10 days after surgical intervention. During this time the group substituted with selenium showed fewer complications than those who did not received selenium substitution. The selenium balance in the treatment group versus the control group all turned out to be positive.

KH: *Dr. Winnefeld, do you think that selenium should be routinely given to all surgical patients and, if so, at what dose?*

KW: Selenium should not be given routinely without documenting a deficiency. But in those who have a deficiency, selenium should be given at a dosage of 200-1000 mcg/d. All patients undergoing a large surgical operation should have their selenium status evaluated. ◆

Vaginal Candidiasis and Beta-Carotene

Magdy S. Mikhail, M.D.
Albert Einstein College of Medicine
Department of Obstetrics and Gynecology
Jacobi Hospital Rm #709
Pellham Parkway South & East Chester Road
Bronx, NY 10461 U.S.A.
(718) 918-6311 / (718) 918-6300 / (718) 824-2894 (FAX)

"Decreased Beta-Carotene Levels in Exfoliated Vaginal Epithelial Cells in Women With Vaginal Candidiasis," American Journal of Reproductive Immunology, 1994;32:221-225. #21510

Kirk Hamilton: What is your educational background and your present position?

Magdy: I'm currently an assistant professor at Albert Einstein College of Medicine. I am the deputy directory of obstetrics and gynecology at the Bronx Municipal Hospital Center. I did my medical training and postgraduate work in Cambridge, England. I did my undergraduate work back in Egypt.

KH: How did you get interested in beta-carotene and vaginal candidiasis?

MM: Dr. Romney, who is the head of our research group and is a professor and ex-chairman here at Albert Einstein, and the rest of the group have published extensively on beta-carotene and other antioxidants such as vitamin E and vitamin C, particularly in relation to cervical cancer and cervical dysplasia.

KH: What is your impression of the role of antioxidants in cervical dysplasia or cervical cancer?

MM: We reported before that women with cervical dysplasia have decreased dietary intake of antioxidants. In separate studies we showed that these women also have decreased plasma levels of antioxidants. We later reported that they have decreased concentrations of antioxidants in the cervix itself.

KH: Is there a correlation between the dietary intake of antioxidants and the cervical and plasma levels?

MM: There is a correlation between dietary intake and plasma levels. But, there is no good correlation between dietary intake and tissue levels.

KH: So what you found is that they were essentially low in the dietary intake?

MM: They are low in dietary intake. They are low in plasma levels and they are low in tissue concentrations. If you take the risk factors for cervical cancer and cervical dysplasia, like the human papilloma virus (HPV), smoking and long term use of oral contraceptive pills, studies have shown that these conditions are associated with low antioxidant levels.

KH: Could it be that the low antioxidants in the cervical tissue set the stage for the invasion of the human papilloma virus? Or is it the other way around?

MM: It could be that the low level started first and that is why you ended up with the lesion, or it could be that the lesion started first and you ended up with the lower levels. However, because the antioxidant levels really are decreased in precancer levels, which is the cervical dysplasia, you would then tend to support the view that the antioxidant deficiency starts first as a risk factor and that may lead to the lesion later on. We think the reason it works is because antioxidants protect against free radical damage that can occur to the cell, particularly to the cell DNA.

KH: What is the basic bottom line findings from your article?

MM: This was a small study. It serves as a preliminary study for what may come later on. There was also a limitation to the study. The diagnosis of candidiasis was established on clinical grounds that the patient has symptoms of a cheesy vaginal discharge consistent with candidiasis, and also on the identification of the candida itself by doing a positive potassium hydroxide slide. That was the criteria used in this pilot study to make the diagnosis of candidiasis. The best way, however, to make a diagnosis of candidiasis is by doing a culture. So these are the two limitations of our study. Having said that, we found that women who have vaginal candidiasis as compared to women who do not, had lower concentrations of beta-carotene in the exfoliated vaginal cells. The way we collected the vaginal cells is actually a technique that the group developed in making a diagnosis of human papilloma virus infection -- we wash the cervix and the vagina with saline and then collect the lavage, centrifuge it, get a pellet and then analyze that pellet itself. In the past, we submitted it for human papilloma virus detection. We now take the same technique and apply it to measure antioxidant concentrations locally in the vagina or in the cervix.

KH: Is this a fairly simple technique that the average gynecologist could do?

MM: You just get a syringe, fill it with saline and flush it onto the cervix and vagina. You then collect it again into the syringe and spin it down.

KH: What did you find with your study?

MM: We found that women who had a diagnosis of vaginal candidiasis had a significantly lower beta-carotene concentration in the exfoliated vaginal cells. The P value was less than .001.

KH: *Do you think it is the candidiasis invasion that reduces the local antioxidant level?*

MM: In order to find that out for sure, we need a significant number of patients and follow them for a long time. We studied beta-carotene because beta-carotene has a significant immunologic enhancement function starting with its activation of cytotoxic T-lymphocytes and natural killer cells. It protects against free radical damage which has immunotoxic effects. Beta-carotene has been shown to increase T-helper cells. I wonder if somebody may look into AIDS patients and try to find out if there is any correlation there.

KH: *I believe that beta-carotene supplementation has been done in AIDS patients at 60 to 180 mg/d. The one study increased natural killer cells and the other study increased T-helper cells.*

MM: Beta-carotene also has been shown to increase the production of interferon by T-lymphocytes. Another study showed that if you incubate lymphocytes with carotenoids, you then activate natural killer cells. Another study showed that beta-carotene stimulated macrophage cytokine production. Yet another study showed that carotenoids act as enhancers of antigen presentation. Other studies have shown enhanced intracellular killing of microorganisms by human neutrophils with beta-carotene. There are a lot of case-reported immuno-enhancing functions of beta-carotene. One of the most common risk factors in women with candidiasis is when their host immune response is suppressed, for whatever reason. That is how we came up with this idea. If beta-carotene, and possibly other antioxidants, stimulate the immune response and if candida flourishes and overgrows when the immune response is suppressed, then we wanted to look at this relationship to see if women who have candidiasis could have decreased beta-carotene and other antioxidant levels. If that is true then it could be that the decrease in antioxidant levels could have suppressed the immune response, and that may be a factor in the development of vaginal candidiasis. If this is confirmed in a larger study, we could then recommend eating rich sources of beta-carotene and antioxidants such as green leafy vegetables and colored fruits, which may enhance the immune response and help to prevent vaginal candidiasis.

KH: *Is there any research that shows females with chronic candidiasis have an increased susceptibility to cervical cancer?*

MM: No. There is no direct relationship. However, women with AIDS have increased susceptibility to candidiasis and, if you depress your immune function, you are at increased risk of cancer. That's why AIDS female patients are at increased risk for cervical cancer.

KH: *For our audience, what are your recommendations for prevention of cervical cancer with insights from this study and just in general?*

MM: I will tell you something else about our work. We just recently published a study in the <u>American Journal of Obstetrics and Gynecology</u> showing women with preeclampsia, which is hypertension in pregnancy, having significantly decreased antioxidant nutrient levels. By that I mean ascorbic acid, vitamin E, and beta-carotene. We found out that if you have mild disease, you have a decreased level of ascorbic acid alone. If you have a severe disease, you have decreased levels of vitamin C, vitamin E and beta-carotene. ◆

Vitamin B12 Deficiency In The Elderly

John Lindenbaum, M.D.
Columbia-Presbyterian Medical Center
Department of Medicine
630 West 168th Street
New York, NY 10032 U.S.A.
(212) 305-9178 / (212) 305-8466 (FAX)

"Prevalence of Cobalamin Deficiency In the Framingham Elderly Population",
The American Journal of Clinical Nutrition, 1994;60:2-11. #20547

Kirk Hamilton: *Please describe your educational background and current position?*

John Lindenbaum: I went to Harvard Medical School and did my internship and residency at Columbia-Presbyterian in New York City. I then did fellowship training in hematology at Columbia. I worked at the Cholera Research Hospital in Dhaka in Bangladesh for three years and I came back to New York and have been at Columbia since. I am now associate chairman of the Department of Medicine at Columbia University College of Physicians and Surgeons.

KH: I have followed your work since 1988 when your paper entitled "Neuropsychiatric Disorders Caused By Cobalamin Deficiency in the Absence of Anemia or Macrocytosis" in the New England Journal of Medicine, June 30, 1988;318-1720-8. In my opinion, that article heralded a new era in medicine which I think could be described as the era of functional medicine, where you intervene early on by a functional test such as homocysteine or methylmalonic acid. I have eagerly followed your work because, being in clinical practice, we have observed that B12 shots work and no one really knew why. I was pleased to see maybe that was an answer for why some of these patients responded who had normal or low normal B12 levels and yet no anemia or macrocytosis. In a recent article in the American Journal of Clinical Nutrition, you survey a group of Framingham patients (548) and the general conclusion was that approximately 12% of this free-living elderly population was cobalamin deficient. I am wondering if you could define what vitamin B12 deficiency really is?

JL: There are various ways of defining deficiency and one could say that deficiency develops in stages. People don't become depleted of their body stores of a vitamin, particularly like cobalamin, overnight. For some reason, vitamin B12 is one of the vitamins that is stored very extensively in the body compared to a lot of other vitamins, such as folic acid or vitamin K where you could become deficient in weeks or months on a deficient diet, or if you had poor absorption. In a normal person, let's say a vegetarian, it takes years to deplete the body stores of vitamin B12. The depletion progresses through various stages. The early stages are biochemical. The standard way we assess this is through serum vitamin levels. But we think a more accurate and more specific way of figuring out whether somebody is in the early stage of cobalamin deficiency, as well as in a late stage, is to look at the enzymes in the body that require vitamin B12 as a coenzyme. The two things you would predict that would accumulate would be (1) methylmalonyl CoA, which is converted by another enzyme to methylmalonic acid. So we can measure methylmalonic acid because the step whereby vitamin B12 converts methylmalonyl CoA to succinyl CoA is blocked in the absence of vitamin B12. We can measure whether that reaction is running correctly in the body by measuring methylmalonic acid levels in the serum or in the urine. The other step (2) is the conversion of homocysteine to methionine which can be assessed by measuring homocysteine levels. These are the 2 reactions that require vitamin B12.

Let me say that as one becomes more and more depleted of the vitamin, you go beyond these biochemically detectable events and you begin to see clinical abnormalities. People develop anemia. People develop trouble walking - paresthesias. Some people develop dementia and so forth. So, at a further stage of depletion of the vitamin, you have a whole variety of interference with organ system function.

KH: Where do you get methylmalonic acid measured?

JL: I have been collaborating with Bob Allen at the University of Colorado since 1985. Before he developed these assays, it was felt that methylmalonic acid (MMA) could not be measured in normal serum as it was present in such small or trace amounts. But the assays he has developed will pick up, in every normal person, a certain minimum amount of MMA.

KH: Could I interject here. Would you say then that there is laboratory variation in the homocysteine or methylmalonic tests compared to Dr. Allen's?

JL: Well, I think initially, and perhaps still, some people have had difficulty with the MMA assay. There is a lot of assays for homocysteine out there that were developed previously and subsequently. Some laboratories have had trouble with the methylmalonic acid but I think they are getting better at it - the reference laboratories. I have been checking some of the reference laboratories by sending sera to them occasionally, at least the ones that are used in my area, where I know the methylmalonic acid is measured by Dr. Allen. I know at least a couple of the laboratories that have set up their own methods who are doing it accurately. I could not vouch for every laboratory. But it does not have to be done at Dr. Allen's lab I guess is the point I am making.

KH: Methylmalonic acid is specific for B12 whereas...

JL: Homocysteine goes up in folate deficiency.

KH: And B6 deficiency?

JL: That is correct. Homocysteine is not a very sensitive test for B6 deficiency. Homocysteine does not go up very early in the course of vitamin B6 deficiency in comparison to folate or cobalamin deficiency where it goes up early.

KH: In getting back to your work, it seems like there is a much larger group of people, especially the elderly, that you're recognizing as being B12 deficient that were unrecognized before. I wonder if you can share with us the clinical impact of this?

JL: It has been known for 30 years or so that elderly folks tend to have low serum B12 levels compared to younger people. People wondered whether the range of normal in the elderly was different or whether these individuals were actually deficient in vitamin B12. We first found that if a patient had tissue manifestations of deficiency, for example megaloblastic anemia, one or the other or both (MMA or homocysteine) were elevated in virtually 100% of patients with cobalamin deficiency. The evidence for that is published in the March 1994 issue of The American Journal of Medicine where we have a series of 434 patients with proven cobalamin deficiency. There was one patient of the 434 that had both MMA and homocysteine in the normal range. So, we think the combined use of the tests pick up virtually every patient with obvious or clear cut deficiency. We then looked at people with pernicious anemia who have a life long requirement for vitamin B12 who hadn't had any maintenance injections for 2 or 3 months, or sometimes as long as 6 months (American Journal of Hematology, 1990). We found that they were dependent on their B12 shots and, if you stop their shots, they gradually - over usually 2 or more years - develop anemia again. So, if you catch one of those people during the first months after a B12 shot, they are in a very early stage of vitamin B12 deficiency of recurrence. *What we found was that the metabolites were frequently elevated when the serum B12 was still normal.* In other words it looks as if the metabolites, in the average patient or person, are elevated in the serum before the serum B12 drops below the lower limit of normal.

KH: If you intervene when these metabolites are elevated versus when the serum B12 is low you can prevent neurologic damage?

JL: Yes. We found there were actually patients, maybe 5 to 10%, with clear cut deficiency with neurologic damage, without megaloblastic anemia or a high MCV. There are clearly patients with low normal serum B12 levels that are frankly deficient. The most persuasive evidence is that if you give them vitamin B12 therapy, their clinical syndrome, neurologic damage, and megaloblastic anemia improve, and their high metabolite levels come down to normal. When we realized that you could have frank deficiency and still have a normal serum B12 level and, that in early deficiency, the metabolites were elevated before the B12 level fell to levels low enough to be considered low, we then thought that these metabolites were a more sensitive test for either early or advanced B12 deficiency than the serum B12. We then applied this to the Framingham population in a consecutive group of elderly survivors and we found that a lot of people had high metabolite levels and whose serum B12 levels are at the lower end of the normal range (200-350). If you treat these elderly people that have a low normal serum B12 and elevated metabolites with vitamin B12, the metabolites come down to normal.

Now, the real key question is the one that you asked but I haven't answered yet and that is what is the clinical significance of this? Well, I think one could say the following: Some of these elderly people are going to go on to develop frank tissue manifestations of deficiency; some of them are going to develop neurologic damage; some of them are going to develop anemia. What we don't know is what percentage of them are actually going to get into trouble clinically.

KH: We haven't even asked the question about neurologic damage. We also haven't asked the question about cardiovascular damage if there is any?

JL: If you look at people who are developing cobalamin deficiency, and we looked a long time ago in a paper we wrote in 1983 in patients with pernicious anemia who had interrupted their vitamin B12 therapy, we found that it took an average of 6 years for these people to develop a clinical recurrence of their cobalamin deficiency. So one clear finding is that cobalamin deficiency develops very slowly. I think a lot of these elderly people in our study, that had high metabolites and a normal serum B12, may have to go 10 years before they get evidence of tissue deficiency. They may not live long enough to develop B12 deficiency. Others will develop B12 deficiency. So, I don't know if you take 12% of the Framingham population, whether 2% of the population is eventually going to show clinical evidence of deficiency or whether it is 1%, 3%, or 5%. I am sure it is not all of them. Some are at risk I think.

KH: So, would you in this 12% encourage them to take a B12 supplement or a vitamin B12 injection once in a while?

JL: We do not know how serious a problem this is in terms of eventually developing things like neurological damage. I think if the percentage is at least 12%, the most cost effective way to do it in the long run would be to treat everybody. That may also have some implications for vascular disease. So, before one embarks upon a program to give all the elderly people in the United States vitamin B12 for the rest of their life, I would favor doing a controlled study because I think sometimes we have our prejudices and we're surprised by the results of a controlled study.

KH: Do you have any feelings about what dosage you would use? You mentioned 500 or 1000 mcg?

JL: I would use very large oral doses of vitamin B12 because some of the elderly with metabolic evidence of deficiency can't absorb small doses of B12 because they have pernicious anemia. They have a lack of intrinsic factor.

KH: Is a large dose 500 to 1000 mcg?

JL: Exactly. And those doses have been shown to be absorbed by patients with pernicious anemia given by mouth or some other mechanism. If you present the intestinal cells with a huge concentration of cobalamin in the lumen, you can get 1% or something like that across the mucosa.

KH: I actually read an internal medicine magazine 2 or 3 years ago where, in a European country, they don't even use the injection. They use 3 to 5 mgs or something. I read an article several days ago from Japan where they were giving vitamin B12 as methylcobalamin orally at 60 mg for multiple sclerosis. Can you share with us the range of vitamin B12 in the serum?

JL: Well, we think that an elderly person, at least, and sometimes a younger person with a serum cobalamin say below 350 pg/ml, may be deficient. Now I am not saying that this should become the low limit of normal for the B12 assays because most people with a level of 300 pg/ml are not deficient. Their metabolites will be normal and they won't have any evidence of tissue deficiency. So if one started doing a big work-up on everybody with a serum B12 of 300 you would work-up thousands of people unnecessarily. What we would prefer to do is say that, for example, if a patient has dementia or a macrocytic anemia, and a serum B12 of 250 or 300, then you might realize that a low normal level does not rule out deficiency. Then you could get homocysteine and methylmalonic acid levels.

KH: *What implication does your work have on the RDA level of vitamin B12 ... which you know I have to plead ignorance because I don't even know what it is?*

JL: It is in the ball park of a few micrograms. But the RDA is set up for normal people and, when we're talking about this problem in the elderly, we have a subgroup of elderly where the prevalence of pernicious anemia is about 1%. So it is appreciable. We are talking about people that can't get B12 out of the diet and so the RDA is a dietary value level that a normal person should take - but these are people that have a defect in the absorption of B12 from food. So they have a disease that the general recommendations for the population does not account for.

KH: *Are you saying all these people here have pernicious anemia? The 12%?*

JL: No, I think most of them don't. I think most of them could be managed with 5 or 10 mcg a day in a supplement which is the level in a lot of vitamins.

KH: *That is what I was getting at. If somebody was looking for a basic multivitamin and mineral to take to keep the metabolites normal or keep the B12 level in the normal range, 5 or 10 micrograms would be sufficient?*

JL: There were a few people that were taking vitamin supplements with this kind of level of B12 in them that had high metabolites. So if the histories are correct, taking 5 to 10 micrograms will not eliminate this problem of B12 deficiency in the elderly. It will just reduce it.

KH: *Essentially B12 is pretty innocuous...correct?*

JL: That's right. That is one of the reasons why I don't have any hesitation in recommending 1000 times the daily requirement.

KH: *I have read about elevated homocysteine levels in multiple sclerosis, myocardial infarction, neural tube defects and in strokes. Homocysteine, to me, is a model for functional medicine because it is elevated in a wide variety of different chronic diseases. The hope would be that if you could even intervene with a good diet or a multivitamin and mineral supplement then you could reduce the risk to some degree to these diseases.*

JL: Now that's another thing that requires an intervention study and I think they are planning to do one in Europe within the next year - giving probably a tablet or a capsule that has a high level of B12 in the range we are talking about, as well as folic acid and pyridoxine to see whether they have an impact on the incidence of stroke, heart attack and peripheral vascular disease.

KH: *I have always felt that B12 and folate would be very beneficial in nursing home patients and I would love to evaluate homocysteine and methylmalonic acid in those patients and then give ½ of the hospital vitamin B12 and folate by injection and ½ of the hospital a placebo just to see what happens. Because I believe from the experiences in our clinic that a lot of people are going to "wake up"!*

JL: Are we looking for a needle in the haystack or are we looking at half the haystack? I think that some people are going to wake up but I am not sure whether it is 1%, 5% or 15%. And, that

is why we need controlled trials. ◆

Vitamin D Deficiency and the Elderly

F. Michael Gloth, III M.D.
The Union Memorial Hospital
Chief, Division of Geriatrics
Department of Medicine
33rd Street Professional Bldg., Suite #415
201 East University Parkway
Baltimore, MD 21218-2895 U.S.A.
(410) 554-2923 / (410) 554-6794 (FAX)

"Vitamin D Deficiency in Older People",
Journal of American Geriatric Society, 1995;43:822-828. #22863

Kirk Hamilton: *Could you please share with me your educational background and current position?*

Michael Gloth: I am a graduate with a Bachelor of Science degree in chemistry and biology from the College of William and Mary in Williamsburg, Virginia. In 1984, I received my medical degree from Wayne State University School of Medicine in Detroit, Michigan. Between 1984 and 1987, I completed an internship and residency in internal medicine at the Union Memorial Hospital in Baltimore, Maryland. In 1987, I was an assistant chief resident of internal medicine here, and between 1987 and 1990 I became a fellow in the division of geriatric medicine and gerontology at the Johns Hopkins School of Medicine in Baltimore, Maryland.

KH: *Is vitamin D deficiency prevalent in the elderly?*

MG: There is good reason to believe that vitamin D deficiency is prevalent amongst the elderly. A recent European study published in the British journal "Lancet" indicated that 36% of elderly men and 47% of elderly women in the general population had a low vitamin D status. A study by Omdahl, et al, from New Mexico showed almost a third of individuals to have a low vitamin D status. It is important to note, however, that elderly individuals who are healthy and ambulatory and get adequate amounts of sunlight are likely to have adequate vitamin D stores. However, for individuals who are sunlight deprived, depending upon their location, we can expect a third to half of those individuals to have a low vitamin D status based on data that we have collected and presented previously before the American Geriatrics Society.

KH: *Can you briefly explain how vitamin D is converted from sunlight into its active forms in the body?*

MG: The ultraviolet wavelengths from sunlight stimulate the formation of precursor molecules in the skin to vitamin D. Vitamin D is then transported through the bloodstream to the liver where it is converted into a more active form (25-hydroxyvitamin D), whereby it is then transported to the kidneys. There it is converted to the most active form which is 1,25-dihydroxyvitamin D.

KH: *What are the risk factors for vitamin D deficiency in the elderly?*

MG: The biggest risk factor for vitamin D deficiency in the elderly is total lack of sunlight, but other risk factors would include

medications (i.e. seizure medications), diseases such as malabsorption, or surgical procedures such as partial gastrectomy that affect the absorption of vitamin D in the diet.

KH: *What are the consequences of vitamin D deficiency in the elderly?*

MG: Vitamin D deficiency has been associated with bone loss and increased risk of fractures, muscle weakness, pain and impairment of immunologic function. There have been weaker associations with other diseases as well.

KH: *Aside from bone metabolism, can vitamin D deficiency result in chronic pain and muscle weakness?*

MG: As noted in the previous question, pain and muscle weakness can be associated with vitamin D deficiency. Pain can take a variety of forms including tenderness to light touch, or a deep musculoskeletal discomfort that is often associated with osteomalacia. Muscle weakness can occur with atrophy of some of the Type II muscle fibers. This can occur with prolonged periods of inadequate vitamin D stores.

KH: *Do we know the role of vitamin D in immune function and in the prevention of cancer?*

MG: There has been a link between vitamin D and diminished function of white blood cells. There also has been a link between vitamin D and cellular differentiation. Some individuals believe that vitamin D plays a role in the prevention of a variety of cancers including prostate, breast and colon cancer.

KH: *How should a physician assess for vitamin D deficiency? What tests can they use?*

MG: The simplest way to assess for vitamin D deficiency is to perform a simple serum test of 25-hydroxyvitamin D. This is the predominant storage form of vitamin D. Usually a clinician will also obtain a 1,25-dihydroxy D level, the most active metabolite. Although this may provide some contributory information, clearly the 25-hydroxyvitamin D is the more important of the two in assessing vitamin D stores.

KH: *What forms and dose regimens should be prescribed if the patient is found deficient?*

MG: There is some debate about the best form and the dose regimen for vitamin D, however, we recommend using either 100,000 I.U. of vitamin D every 3 months or 800-1600 I.U. of vitamin D daily for individuals who are sunlight deprived and cannot get into direct sunlight. This is a maintenance schedule and, if someone is found to be vitamin D deficient, it would be worthwhile giving larger doses such as 50,000 to 100,000 I.U. 2 or 3 times during the first week and then placing the patient on maintenance dosing. If an individual is not sunlight deprived and does not have one of the other risk factors for vitamin D deficiency, it would be worth repeating a level to be sure that adequate stores have been obtained.

KH: *When you say supplement with vitamin D, what form are you recommending? Is one form of vitamin D more bioavailable than another?*

MG: Vitamin D supplementation when administered, is usually administered as either vitamin D2 or vitamin D3, sometimes called ergocalciferol or cholecalciferol. This form of vitamin D is similar to the form of vitamin D that is produced in the skin. This form actually goes through some conversion until it reaches the kidney, where it is converted to the most active form of vitamin D, the 1,25-dihydroxyvitamin D metabolite. It is of interest to note that some individuals who have severe renal disease are not able to manufacture enough of the most active metabolite, the 1,25-dihydroxyvitamin D. In that circumstance, the recommendation is to administer 1,25-dihydroxyvitamin D itself. When this is done, particular attention needs to be addressed to monitoring calcium levels. Adverse events are probably more likely with this form of supplementation and, for this reason, this type of supplementation is reserved for people who have severe renal disease. Vitamin D2 (ergocalciferol) and vitamin D3 (cholecalciferol) are believed to be equal in bioavailability in humans....now if you're a chicken, that's a different story.

KH: *How readily can exposure to sunlight improve vitamin D status in the elderly?*

MG: Sunlight exposure can improve vitamin D status in the elderly. Although changes occur with age, and the skin's ability to manufacture the active forms of vitamin D, it is reasonable to expect that 30 minutes of sunlight 2 to 3 times a week should lead to adequate vitamin D stores. The further north one goes, the less effective this exposure. The further south and the higher in altitude, the more direct the needed wavelengths of ultraviolet light can be obtained. It should be noted that the wavelength necessary to convert precursor molecules to vitamin D is blocked out by glass and, therefore, sitting in a solarium provides no benefit with regards to vitamin D status. ◆

Wilson's Disease, Zinc and Molybdenum

George J. Brewer, M.D.
The University of Michigan Medical School
Professor of Medicine and Human Genetics
Department of Human Genetics
4708 Medical Science II
Ann Arbor, MI 48109-0618 U.S.A.
(313) 764-5499 / (313) 763-3784 (FAX)

"Treatment of Wilson's Disease With Ammonium Tetrathiomolybdate. I. Initial Therapy In 17 Neurologically Affected Patients", Archives of Neurology June 1994;51:545-554. #20382

Kirk Hamilton: *Thank you very much for being with me today. Can you please start off by giving me a little bit of your educational background and where you are professionally at the moment?*

George Brewer: I went to medical school and did an internal medicine residency at the University of Chicago and then did postdoctoral work in human genetics at the University of Michigan. I was accepted for a faculty appointment at the University of Michigan in 1963 and have been there ever since. Currently, I am a professor of human genetics and internal medicine at the University of Michigan Medical School.

KH: *I have followed your work with zinc in Wilson's disease for some time and zinc, if my understanding is correct, has been used more as a maintenance type of approach versus when there is an acute problem with Wilson's disease. Is that correct?*

GB: Yes.

KH: *Could you give me a brief definition of what Wilson's disease is, its frequency, and the adverse side effects if it goes on undiagnosed?*

GB: Wilson's disease is an autosomal recessive, inherited disorder of copper accumulation. It typically presents in the late teenage years or 20s. The usual presentation is the appearance of liver disease, such as hepatitis or chronic cirrhosis not unlike that of alcoholic cirrhosis, or, it can present with acute hepatic failure and in some of those patients the only way to prevent death is liver transplantation. About ½ of the patients present with neurologic disease rather than liver disease. Those patients always have some underlying liver damage, but it hasn't presented itself clinically. The neurologic disease is called a movement disorder. The parts of the brain affected are those that have to do with coordination and movement. Speech, sometimes swallowing, and the coordination of fine movements of the hands and, later, controlled movements of the arms and legs and the rest of the body can be affected.

KH: *It sounds like it almost has a silent killer effect like blood pressure. You don't recognize it until something acute happens?*

GB: That is certainly true of the liver disease. The neurologic disorder, on the other hand, is rather tangible. That is, patients and their families begin to notice they are talking different and there is a rather slowly progressive movement problem that may progress over 2, 3 or 4 years.

KH: *Are these effects permanent, or can they be reversed with not* only the zinc and the tetrathiomolybdate therapy, but with any copper lowering therapy?

GB: No, they are not permanent. It is a progressively fatal disease if not treated. The treatments developed include penicillamine, a chelator-type drug that will get rid of copper by causing excessive excretion in the urine. There is another chelator developed later called trientine, which also causes increased copper excretion in the urine. Both of those drugs are rather toxic, so we have developed zinc for maintenance therapy, which acts differently than the other drugs. It acts by affecting the intestinal tract so copper is no longer absorbed and has essentially no toxicity. Tetrathiomolybdate is used for the initial treatment of the patient who presents with acute illness of neurologic type. As far as reversal of damage is concerned, generally speaking, Wilson's Disease is quite reversible. The drugs are used to control copper and get the levels down, and then the brain and the liver, to a certain extent, repair themselves generally over about a 2-year period.

KH: *When did you start becoming interested in zinc? Where did that concept come from?*

GB: We had been using zinc as a therapeutic trial in sickle cell disease and, as a side effect, we began to induce copper deficiency. The reason we saw this and others didn't, was because we switched to zinc acetate because zinc sulfate was irritating to the stomach. The zinc sulfate had been given with meals to reduce the unpleasant gastrointestinal effects. When we switched salts and used zinc acetate, we gave it away from food and found the absorption was much greater. When we gave zinc away from food, it suddenly became an effective anticopper agent and we thought of using it in Wilson's disease. We tried it and it worked very well. We now have about 115 patients across North America on maintenance zinc therapy. You asked about the incidence of the disease. It is not a common disease. It's called an orphan disease, and affects about 1 in 40,000.

KH: *I have always been a little bit confused on how to diagnose Wilson's disease by laboratory assessment once you have suspicion. What are the tests that you do?*

GB: The best screening test is a urine copper. It has to be a 24-hour urine copper measurement. The collection is in a trace element-free container and measured accurately with atomic absorption or another sensitive technique. The gold standard for diagnosis is the quantitative copper in a liver biopsy. It is a more invasive procedure, but it is the gold standard for diagnosis.

KH: *What level of urinary copper triggers your suspicion?*

GB: The normal level is 20 to 50 mcg for 24 hours. Anything more than 100 in a well-performed test is virtually diagnostic of Wilson's disease. The one exception is obstructive liver disease - it will also cause an elevation in both hepatic and in urine copper.

KH: *Ceruloplasmin plays no role in diagnosis?*

GB: Ceruloplasmin is a guide. It affects the index of suspicion when it is low, which is about 90% of the time. About 10% of patients have a normal ceruloplasmin and about 10% of carriers of the gene have a low ceruloplasmin, even though they will never be ill. It is not diagnostic. It is measured usually and does affect your index of suspicion.

KH: *Just out of a curiosity, you were talking about chelating agents - has EDTA ever been tried?*

GB: It is not nearly as good as penicillamine, the reason probably being that penicillamine is a reductive chelator. It reduces the copper, which decreases the copper's affinity for protein, whereas EDTA just competes with the protein to which the copper is bound and isn't very affective.

KH: *Tetrathiomolybdate - where did the concept of utilizing this substance come from?*

GB: It has an interesting history. It started in New Zealand and Australia where ruminants (cattle and sheep) in certain pastures developed a disease syndrome which was later found to be copper deficiency. Then the soil was found to have a high level of molybdenum. Molybdenum given to ruminants then reproduced copper deficiency, but molybdenum given to rats had no effect. It took quite a while to figure this puzzle out. It was later realized that the rumen of ruminants has a very active sulfide metabolism, because of the sulfur in the grass, so the molybdenum was really being converted to a sulfur molybdenum compound. In other words, a thiomolybdate. Then when thiomolybdates were given to rats, they were found to be very effective. There can be 1, 2, 3 or 4 sulfhydryl groups. The tetra substituted is, by far and away, the most potent. Tetrathiomolybdate is the most potent anticopper agent that has been discovered.

KH: *Can you give the dosages you use with zinc acetate and tetrathiomolybdate?*

GB: Zinc is used at 50 mg of elemental zinc 3 times a day, separated from food by an hour. Food includes beverages other than water because there are a lot of substances in food that can complex zinc and prevent the intestinal cell from ever seeing it. The 150 mg per day is about 10 times the recommended dietary allowance. For young patients, we usually use 25 mg, 3 times a day. It is 100% effective. With zinc maintenance therapy, the only thing that needs to be followed is the urine copper and zinc. Zinc therapy is much easier to follow than the older therapies. In the case of zinc therapy, the urine copper is a very good reflector of the body load of copper. There will be a gradual reduction in urine copper with therapy and, so we usually do every 6 months, a 24-hour urine copper and zinc. We do the zinc to see if the patient is complying well or is faltering on their therapy. We expect the zinc to be at least 2 mg a day in the urine when the patient is taking their medicine. When they start going below that level, we know the patient is having a problem and the urine copper will start going up later. So those 2 things are very good monitoring tools; switching to tetrathiomolybdate (TM). The protocol we're using at the moment is a little bit complicated and is basically a research procedure. We'll probably have to simplify it somewhat for general clinical use. But at the moment, we give it 6 times a day - 3 times with meals and 3 times between meals. The way TM works is it forms a complex of protein and copper. It is a 3-way complex, a tripartite complex. If you give TM with meals, it complexes the copper of the food and of the secretions of the body (the saliva and gastric juice) and prevents its absorption. There is more copper in those 2 secretions than you eat each day. So one result is an immediate negative copper balance. No copper is being absorbed when you start giving TM with the meals. Then we gave 3 doses in between meals and it absorbed very nicely into the blood where it forms complexes with copper in the albumin. That copper is no longer toxic because it can't be taken up by cells. So rather quickly, by escalating that dose, we can titrate the potentially toxic copper of the blood. That copper is in equilibrium with the potentially toxic copper in the organs and so, in a matter of a week, we can usually nullify copper toxicity with this drug. We treat for 8 weeks with this 6 times a day dose schedule and then switch over to maintenance therapy. But because that protocol is rather early in its developmental stages and because this drug really isn't available, I don't think it is something that clinicians are going to be able to use right away. *We do accept patients here for the clinical trial of TM and everything is free except for the transportation to get here.*

KH: *Can you get zinc acetate anywhere or do you order from a particular pharmacy or company?*

GB: What you can get in drug and health food stores is usually zinc sulfate and zinc gluconate. For the most part, zinc acetate isn't available. It is being made by a company called Lemmon in Sellersville, Pennsylvania [(215)-723-5544] and they, and we, have a new drug application into the Food and Drug Administration under the Orphan Drug Act. Once that is approved by the FDA, they will be distributing zinc acetate around the country. In the meantime, people can use zinc gluconate. It is almost certainly equivalent. I wouldn't use zinc sulfate because it is so irritating.

KH: *How about the tetrathiomolybdate?*

GB: It is not really available. You can, of course, buy it chemically, but what we get is purified for human use and it has to be watched for loss of potency because the sulfur replaces the oxygen if it is exposed to air for extended periods of time. I really wouldn't recommend other people using this at the moment. They should send their patient here for that trial.

KH: *Why is TM such an important new therapy?*

GB: When the patient presents with neurologic disease, if they are treated with penicillamine, 50% of them get worse and a lot of them never recover. The reason is if the penicillamine mobilizes large stores of copper from the liver and flushes it through the brain, this makes a whole range of neurologic symptoms worse. Zinc is kind of slow acting for these acutely ill patients so that is where TM fits in. If the patient presents with neurologic disease, it is really a magic drug for that kind of patient. We have treated 25 so far and have lost no neurologic function in any of these patients and then they go on and recover later on.

KH: *So the side effects for both drugs are obviously better than penicillamine?*

GB: There are no side effects of zinc other than the gastric irritation that an occasional patient will get. With TM, we haven't discovered any side effects. It is a very toxic drug in animals if they are not protected with copper because it makes them copper deficient very quickly. If you protect with copper, there is no known toxicity.

KH: My last question is the cost of your treatment with zinc acetate and tetrathiomolybdate - is that going to be comparable, or more or less, than penicillamine in the overall picture?

GB: Zinc is dramatically cheaper. Penicillamine and trientine are rather expensive. I would imagine zinc would be 10% of the cost of chelation-type drugs. It is pretty hard to predict for TM because it will have its manufacturing costs and it won't have a very large market presumably. So it is a little hard to predict what will happen to that. ◆

Subject Index

The Experts Speak 1996